BLUEPRINTS IN OBSTETRICS AND GYNECOLOGY

Blueprints: USMLE Steps 2 & 3 Review Series

General Series Editor:

Bradley S. Marino, MD, MPP
Department of Pediatrics
Johns Hopkins Hospital
Baltimore, Maryland

CURRENT BOOKS IN THE SERIES:

Blueprints in Medicine
Blueprints in Pediatrics
Blueprints in Psychiatry
Blueprints in Surgery

BLUEPRINTS IN OBSTETRICS AND GYNECOLOGY

Tamara L. Callahan, MD, MPP
Clinical Fellow in Obstetrics,
Gynecology and Reproductive Biology
Harvard Medical School
Resident in Obstetrics and Gynecology
Brigham and Women's Hospital
Massachusetts General Hospital
Boston, Massachusetts

Aaron B. Caughey, MD, MPP
Clinical Fellow in Obstetrics,
Gynecology and Reproductive Biology
Harvard Medical School
Resident in Obstetrics and Gynecology
Brigham and Women's Hospital
Massachusetts General Hospital
Boston, Massachusetts

Faculty Advisor:
Linda J. Heffner, MD, PhD
Associate Professor of Obstetrics,
Gynecology and Reproductive Biology
Harvard Medical School
Chief, Maternal-Fetal Medicine
Department of Obstetrics and Gynecology
Brigham and Women's Hospital
Boston, Massachusetts

Contributing Editors:
Annette Chen, MD
Clinical Instructor of Obstetrics,
Gynecology and Reproductive Biology
Harvard Medical School
Clinical Fellow in Gynecological Oncology
Department of Obstetrics and Gynecology
Massachusetts General Hospital
Boston, Massachusetts

Bruce B. Feinberg, MD
Assistant Professor of Obstetrics,
Gynecology and Reproductive Biology
Harvard Medical School
Attending Physician in
Maternal-Fetal Medicine
Department of Obstetrics and Gynecology
Brigham and Women's Hospital
Boston, Massachusetts

b
Blackwell
Science

Blackwell Science
Editorial Offices:
350 Main Street, Malden, Massachusetts 02148, USA
Osney Mead, Oxford OX2 0EL, England
25 John Street, London WC1N 2BL, England
23 Ainslie Place, Edinburgh EH3 6AJ, Scotland
54 University Street, Carlton, Victoria 3053, Australia

Other Editorial Offices:
Blackwell Wissenschafts-Verlag GmbH Kurfürstendamm 57, 10707 Berlin, Germany
Blackwell Science KK, MG Kodenmacho Nihombashi
Chuo-ku Tokyo 104, Japan

Distributors:
USA
Blackwell Science, Inc.
Commerce Place
350 Main Street
Malden, Massachusetts 02148
(Telephone orders: 800-215-1000
or 781-388-8250; Fax orders: 781-388-8270)
Canada
Login Brothers Book Company
324 Saulteaux Crescent
Winnipeg, Manitoba
Canada, R3J 3T2
(Telephone orders: 204-224-4068
Australia
Blackwell Science Pty., Ltd.
54 University Street
Carlton, Victoria 3053
(Telephone orders: 03-9347-0300;
Fax orders: 03-9349-3016)
Outside North America and Australia
Blackwell Science, Ltd.
c/o Marston Book Services, Ltd.
P.O. Box 269, Abingdon
Oxon OX14 4YN
England
(Telephone orders: 44-01235-465500;
Fax orders: 44-01235-465555)

Acquisitions: Joy Ferris Denomme
Production: Karen Feeney
Manufacturing: Lisa Flanagan
Typeset by Publication Services
Printed and bound by Capital City Press

Printed in the United States of America

98 99 00 5 4 3 2

Library of Congress Cataloging-in-Publication Data

Callahan, Tamara.
Blueprints in obstetrics and gynecology / by Tamara Callahan, Aaron Caughey:
Faculty advisor, Linda Heffner.
p. cm.—(The blueprints series)
Includes bibliographical references and index.
ISBN 0-86542-505-1 (pb.)
1. Obstetrics—Outlines, syllabi, etc. 2. Gynecology—Outlines, syllabi, etc.
I. Caughey, Aaron. II. Heffner, Linda. III. Title. IV. Series.
[DNLM: 1. Pregnancy Complications. 2. Genital Diseases, Female.
WQ 240 C156b 1997]
RG112.C35 1997
618—dc21
DNLM/DLC
for Library of Congress 97-9851
CIP

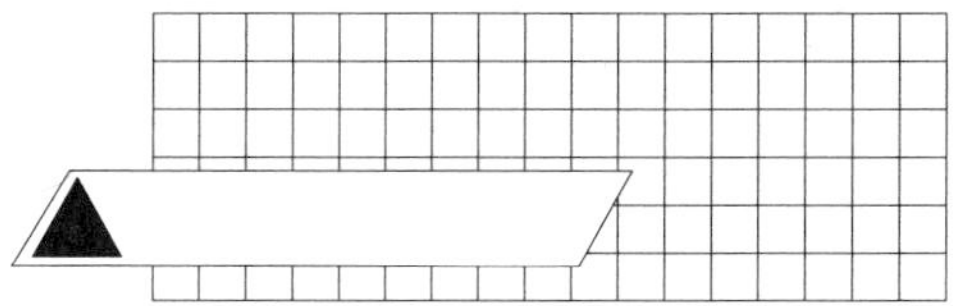

Contents

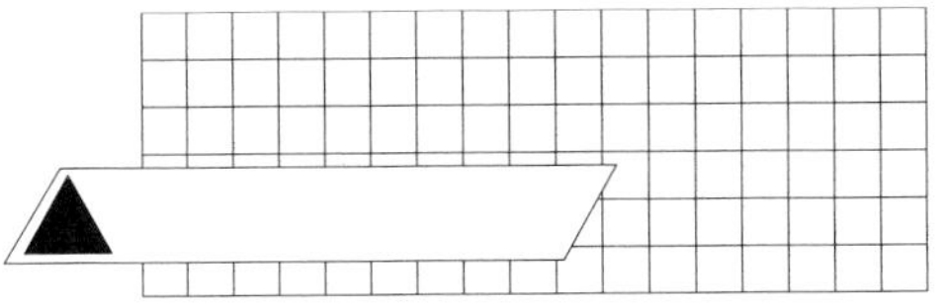

Preface

Fourth-year medical students, interns, and residents are chronically sleep deprived, have little time to study due to their clinical duties, and have a low tolerance for medical literature that is not clear and to the point. All too often as a medical student, and now as a resident, I have heard my colleagues bemoan the fact that there is no succinct, clinical text on each of the core subjects tested on the USMLE Steps 2 & 3. These trainees need review materials they can digest quickly, perhaps a subject in a weekend, which will enable them to answer correctly the majority of questions in each discipline. This attitude is especially evident for the USMLE Step 3, for example, where surgical residents are tested on pediatrics although they have not completed a clinical rotation in the discipline for two years.

Our goal in writing *Blueprints in Obstetrics and Gynecology* was to enable the reader to review the core material quickly and efficiently. The topics were chosen after analyzing over 2,000 review questions, which we believed were representative of the ob/gyn questions on the USMLE Steps 2 & 3 exams. This book is not meant to be comprehensive, but rather it is composed of the "high-yield" topics that consistently appear on these exams.

The questions on the USMLE Steps 2 & 3 are now crafted into clinical vignettes. To assist you in studying for this new format, the material in this book is presented either as the workup of a symptom or as a discussion of a particular disease or pathological process. Although this series is designed for the medical student or resident reviewing for the USMLE, we believe the books will be equally useful to all medical students during their clerkships or subinternships.

We hope that you find *Blueprints in Obstetrics and Gynecology* informative and useful. We welcome any feedback you may have about this text or any others in the Blueprints series.

Bradley S. Marino, MD, MPP
Blueprints Series Editor
c/o Blackwell Science, Inc.
Commerce Place
350 Main Street
Malden, MA 02148

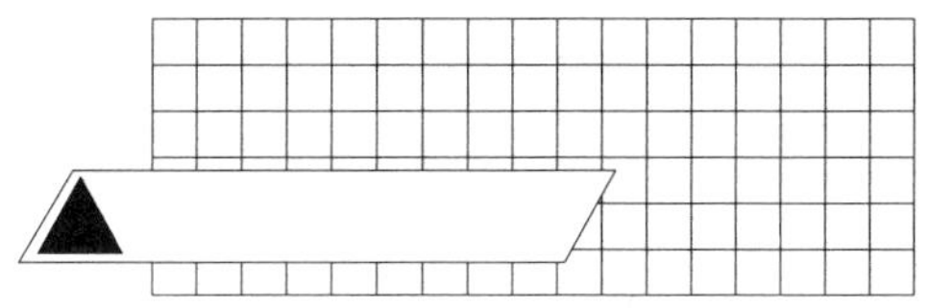

Acknowledgments

I would like to thank Dr. Linda Heffner for her invaluable advice and encouragement in the design and execution of this project. I would also like to express our sincere and deep appreciation to Dr. Annette Chen and Dr. Bruce Feinberg who gave liberally of their time and editing expertise. Without the extraordinary talent and commitment of these physicians, this project would not have been possible. And lastly, I would like to thank my family and friends for their unrelenting confidence and support throughout this exciting journey.

Tamara L. Callahan, MD, MPP

I would like to thank a great many people that were instrumental in my life and in the creation of this book. First, my coauthor, editors, and publisher: Tamara, thanks for being so organized, it's Miller time; Bruce and Annette, thanks for stepping in to edit and re-edit my wandering prose; Joy and Francine, thanks for your patience—could I put in one more picture. Second, thanks to the residents, staff, faculty, and medical students in Obstetrics and Gynecology at the Brigham and Women's Hospital, Massachusetts General Hospital, and Harvard Medical School who have been inspirational and instrumental in my education over the past 6 years—MAC, Blatman, Repke, Peggy & my resident class in particular. Finally, my family and friends, Bill, Carol, Samara, Ethan, Big Guy, Maroobie, Annie, PatnKellie, Crisco, Ted, Alice, Lib, Marty, JimnLynn, Maika, Joan, Timmy and The Mikes, Jackie, and everyone else who have always been so supportive and encouraging—I couldn't have come so far without you.

Aaron B. Caughey, MD, MPP

Figure Credits

The following figures were modified with permission from the publisher.

Figure 1-1. Gabbe SG, Niebyl JR, Simpson JL. Obstetrics: Normal and Problem Pregnancies. 2nd ed. New York: Churchill Livingstone, 1991:128.

Figure 1-2. Gabbe SG, Niebyl JR, Simpson JL. Obstetrics: Normal and Problem Pregnancies. 2nd ed. New York: Churchill Livingstone, 1991:294.

Figure 3-1. Benson RC, Pernoll ML. Handbook of Obstetrics and Gynecology. 9th ed. New York: McGraw-Hill, 1994:157.

Figure 3-2. Hacker N, Moore JG. Essentials of Obstetrics and Gynecology. Philadelphia: Saunders, 1992:120.

Figure 3-3. Creasy R. Management of Labor and Delivery. Cambridge: Blackwell Science, 1997:

Figure 3-4. Repke JT. Intrapartum Obstetrics. New York: Churchill Livingstone, 1996:80-81.

Figure 3-5. DeCherney A, Pernow M. Current Obstetrics and Gynecologic Diagnosis and Treatment. Norwalk, CT: Appleton & Lange, 1994:299.

Figure 3-6. DeCherney A, Pernow M. Current Obstetrics and Gynecologic Diagnosis and Treatment. Norwalk, CT: Appleton & Lange, 1994:299.

Figure 3-7. Hacker N, Moore JG. Essentials of Obstetrics and Gynecology. Philadelphia: Saunders, 1992:252.

Figure 3-8. Hacker N, Moore JG. Essentials of Obstetrics and Gynecology. Philadelphia: Saunders, 1992:258.

Figure 3-9. Beckman CC, et al. Obstetrics and Gynecology for Medical Students. 2nd ed. Baltimore: Williams & Wilkins, 1995:176.

Figure 3-10. DeCherney A, Pernow M. Current Obstetrics and Gynecologic Diagnosis and Treatment. Norwalk, CT: Appleton & Lange, 1994:211.

Figure 3-11. DeCherney A, Pernow M. Current Obstetrics and Gynecologic Diagnosis and Treatment. Norwalk, CT: Appleton & Lange, 1994:212.

Figure 3-12. DeCherney A, Pernow M. Current Obstetrics and Gynecologic Diagnosis and Treatment. Norwalk, CT: Appleton & Lange, 1994:212.

Figures 3-13, 3-14, and 3-15 Creasy R. Management of Labor and Delivery. Cambridge: Blackwell Science, 1997.

Figure 3-16. Cunningham FG, et al. Williams Obstetrics. 19th ed. Norwalk, CT: Appleton and Lange, 1993:618.

Figure 3-17. Benson RC, Pernoll ML. Handbook of Obstetrics and Gynecology. 9th ed. New York: McGraw-Hill, 1994: 180.

Figure 3-18A. Creasy R. Management of Labor and Delivery. Cambridge: Blackwell Science, 1997.

Figure 3-18B. Cunningham FG, et al. Williams Obstetrics. 19th ed. Norwalk, CT: Appleton and Lange, 1993:391.

Figure 3-19. Hacker N, Moore JG. Essentials of Obstetrics and Gynecology. Philadelphia: Saunders, 1992,142.

Figure 4-1. Hacker N, Moore JG. Essentials of Obstetrics and Gynecology. Philadelphia: Saunders, 1992:156.

Figure 4-2. DeCherney A, Pernow M. Current Obstetrics and Gynecologic Diagnosis and Treatment. Norwalk, CT: Appleton and Lange, 1994:400.

Figure 5-1. Gabbe SG, Niebyl JR, Simpson JL. Obstetrics: Normal and Problem Pregnancies. 2nd ed. New York: Churchill Livingstone, 1991:844

Figure 5-2. DeCherney A, Pernow M. Current Obstetrics and Gynecologic Diagnosis and Treatment. Norwalk, CT: Appleton and Lange, 1994:204.

Figure 5-3. Creasy R. Management of Labor and Delivery. Cambridge: Blackwell Science, 1997.

Figure 5-4A. Cunningham FG, et al. Williams Obstetrics. 19th ed. Norwalk, CT: Appleton and Lange, 1993:502.

Figure 5-4B. Chamberlain G. Lecture Notes on Obstetrics. 7th ed. Oxford: Blackwell Science, 1996:178.

Figure 5-5. Chamberlain G. Lecture Notes on Obstetrics. 7th ed. Oxford: Blackwell Science, 1996:181.

Figure 5-6. Cunningham FG, et al. Williams Obstetrics. 19th ed. Norwalk, CT: Appleton and Lange, 1993:506.

Figure 5-7. Gabbe SG, Niebyl JR, Simpson JL. Obstetrics: Normal and Problem Pregnancies. 2nd ed. New York: Churchill Livingstone, 1991:566.

Figure 5-8. Gabbe SG, Niebyl JR, Simpson JL. Obstetrics: Normal and Problem Pregnancies. 2nd ed. New York: Churchill Livingstone, 1991:568.

Figure 5-9. Cunningham FG, et al. Williams Obstetrics. 19th ed. Norwalk, CT: Appleton and Lange, 1993:514.

Figure 6-1. Beckman CC, et al. Obstetrics and Gynecology for Medical Students. 2nd ed. Baltimore: Williams & Wilkins, 1995:147.

Figure 9-1. Clark SL, et al. Critical Care Obstetrics. 2nd ed. Cambridge: Blackwell Science, 1991:162.

Figure 9-2. Clark SL, et al. Critical Care Obstetrics. 2nd ed. Cambridge: Blackwell Science, 1991:163.

Figure 10-1. Gabbe SG, Niebyl JR, Simpson JL. Obstetrics: Normal and Problem Pregnancies. 2nd ed. New York: Churchill Livingstone, 1991:601.

Figure 11-1. Champion RH. Textbook of Dermatology. 5th ed. Oxford: Blackwell Science, 1992, 2852.

Figure 12-1. Hacker N, Moore JG. Essentials of Obstetrics and Gynecology. Philadelphia: Saunders, 1992:325.

Figure 12-2. Beckman CC, Ling F. Obstetrics and Gynecology for Medical Students. Baltimore: Williams & Wilkins, 1992:398.

Figure 12-3. Beckman CC, Ling F. Obstetrics and Gynecology for Medical Students. Baltimore: Williams & Wilkins, 1992:407.

Figure 13-1. Beckman CC, Ling F. Obstetrics and Gynecology for Medical Students. Baltimore: Williams & Wilkins, 1992:306.

Figure 14-1. Champion RH. Textbook of Dermatology. 5th ed. Oxford: Blackwell Science, 1992, 2852.

Figure 14-2. Champion RH. Textbook of Dermatology. 5th ed. Oxford: Blackwell Science, 1992, 2852.
Figure 14-3. Blackwell RE. Women's Medicine. 1996:317.
Figure 14-5. Clarke-Pearson DL, Dawood MY. Green's Gynecology. 4th ed. Boston: Little, Brown, 1990:280.
Figure 14-6. Clarke-Pearson DL, Dawood MY. Green's Gynecology. 4th ed. Boston: Little, Brown, 1990:280.
Figure 14-7. Crissey JT. Manual of Medical Mycology. Boston: Blackwell Science, 1995:90.
Figure 14-8. Cox FEG. Modern Parasitology: A Textbook of Parasitology. 2nd ed. Oxford: Blackwell Science, 1993:9.
Figure 15-1. Clarke-Pearson DL, Dawood MY. Green's Gynecology. 4th ed. Boston: Little, Brown, 1990:309.
Figure 15-2. DeCherney A, Pernoll, M. Current Obstetric and Gynecologic Diagnosis and Treatment. Norwalk, CT: Appleton & Lange, 1994:755.
Figure 16-1. Creasy R. Management of Labor and Delivery. Boston: Blackwell Science, 1997.
Figure 16-2. Hacker N, Moore JG. Essentials of Obstetrics and Gynecology. Philadelphia: Saunders, 1992:397.
Figure 16-3. DeCherney A, Pernoll, M. Current Obstetric and Gynecologic Diagnosis and Treatment. Norwalk, CT: Appleton & Lange, 1994:810.
Figure 16-4. DeCherney A, Pernoll, M. Current Obstetric and Gynecologic Diagnosis and Treatment. Norwalk, CT: Appleton & Lange, 1994:814.
Figure 16-5. Parsons L, Sommers SC. Gynecology. 2nd ed. Philadelphia: Saunders, 1978:1428.
Figure 17-1. Retzky SS, Rogers RM. Clinical symposia: Urinary incontinence in Women. Summit: Ciba Geigy. 1995;47:4.
Figure 17-2. Retzky SS, Rogers RM. Clinical symposia: Urinary incontinence in Women. Summit: Ciba Geigy. 1995;47:5.
Figure 17-3. Whitfield CR. Dewhurst's Textbook of Obstetrics and Gynaecology for Postgraduates. 5th ed. Oxford: Blackwell Science, 1995:656.
Figure 17-4. DeCherney A, Pernoll, M. Current Obstetric and Gynecologic Diagnosis and Treatment. Norwalk, CT: Appleton & Lange, 1994:833.
Figure 17-5. Retzky SS, Rogers RM. Clinical symposia: Urinary incontinence in Women. Summit: Ciba Geigy. 1995;47:12.
Figure 17-6. Retzky SS, Rogers RM. Clinical symposia: Urinary incontinence in Women. Summit: Ciba Geigy. 1995;47:15.
Figure 17-7. Retzky SS, Rogers RM. Clinical symposia: Urinary incontinence in Women. Summit: Ciba Geigy. 1995;47:15.
Figure 17-8. Retzky SS, Rogers RM. Clinical symposia: Urinary incontinence in Women. Summit: Ciba Geigy. 1995;47:15.
Figure 18-1. Speroff L, Glass RH, Kase NG. Clinical Gynecologic Endocrinology and Infertility. 5th ed. Baltimore: Williams and Wilkins, 1994:370.
Figure 18-2. . Speroff L, Glass RH, Kase NG. Clinical Gynecologic Endocrinology and Infertility. 5th ed. Baltimore: Williams and Wilkins, 1994:378.
Figure 18-3. Speroff L, Glass RH, Kase NG. Clinical Gynecologic Endocrinology and Infertility. 5th ed. Baltimore: Williams and Wilkins, 1994:379.
Figure 18-4. Clarke-Pearson DL, Dawood MY. Green's Gynecology. 4th ed. Boston: Little, Brown, 1990:166.
Figure 18-5. Sadler TW. Langman's Medical Embryology. 6th ed. Baltimore: Williams & Wilkins, 1990:21.
Figure 18-6. Sadler TW. Langman's Medical Embryology. 6th ed. Baltimore: Williams & Wilkins, 1990:22.
Figure 19-1. DeCherney A, Pernoll, M. Current Obstetric and Gynecologic Diagnosis and Treatment. Norwalk, CT: Appleton & Lange, 1994:1010.
Figure 19-2. DeCherney A, Pernoll, M. Current Obstetric and Gynecologic Diagnosis and Treatment. Norwalk, CT: Appleton & Lange, 1994:1011.
Figure 19-3. DeCherney A, Pernoll, M. Current Obstetric and Gynecologic Diagnosis and Treatment. Norwalk, CT: Appleton & Lange, 1994:1012.
Figure 21-1. Mishell DR, et al. Infertility, Contraception, and Reproductive Endocrinology. 3rd ed. Cambridge: Blackwell Science, 1991.
Figure 22-1. DeCherney A, Pernoll, M. Current Obstetric and Gynecologic Diagnosis and Treatment. Norwalk, CT: Appleton & Lange, 1994:674.
Figure 22-3. Speroff L, Darney PA. A Clinical Guide for Contraception. 2nd ed. Baltimore: Williams & Wilkins, 1996:257.
Figure 22-4. Kopenski S. Vaginal Contraception. New York: GK Hall.
Figure 22-5. Speroff L, Darney PA. A Clinical Guide for Contraception. 2nd ed. Baltimore: Williams & Wilkins. 1996:247.
Figure 22-6. Speroff L, Darney PA. A Clinical Guide for Contraception. 2nd ed. Baltimore: Williams & Wilkins, 1996:195.
Figure 22-7. Speroff L, Darney PA. A Clinical Guide for Contraception. 2nd ed. Baltimore: Williams & Wilkins, 1996:680.
Figure 22-8. Speroff L, Darney PA. A Clinical Guide for Contraception. 2nd ed. Baltimore: Williams & Wilkins. 1996:675.
Figure 22-9. Speroff L, Darney PA. A Clinical Guide for Contraception. 2nd ed. Baltimore: Williams & Wilkins. 1996:675.
Figure 22-10. Speroff L, Darney PA. A Clinical Guide for Contraception. 2nd ed. Baltimore: Williams & Wilkins. 1996:150.
Figure 22-11. Hacker N, Moore JG. Essentials of Obstetrics and Gynecology. Philadelphia: Saunders, 1992:466.
Figure 22-12. Hacker N, Moore JG. Essentials of Obstetrics and Gynecology. Philadelphia: Saunders, 1992:466.
Figure 22-13. Hacker N, Moore JG. Essentials of Obstetrics and Gynecology. Philadelphia: Saunders, 1992:466.

Figure 22-14. DeCherney A, Pernoll, M. Current Obstetric and Gynecologic Diagnosis and Treatment. Norwalk, CT: Appleton & Lange, 1994:897.

Figure 23.1. DeCherney A, Pernoll, M. Current Obstetric and Gynecologic Diagnosis and Treatment. Norwalk, CT: Appleton & Lange, 1994:683.

Figure 23.2. DeCherney A, Pernoll, M. Current Obstetric and Gynecologic Diagnosis and Treatment. Norwalk, CT: Appleton & Lange, 1994:684.

Figure 25-1. Singer A. Lower Genital Tract Precancer: Colposcopy, Pathology, and Treatment. Oxford: Blackwell Science, 1994:181.

Figure 26.1. DeCherney A, Pernoll, M. Current Obstetric and Gynecologic Diagnosis and Treatment. Norwalk, CT: Appleton & Lange, 1994:922.

Figure 28-1. Robbins, Cotran R, Kumar V. Robbins Pathologic Basis of Disease. Philadelphia: Saunders, 1991:1165.

Figure 28-2. Robbins, Cotran R, Kumar V. Robbins Pathologic Basis of Disease. Philadelphia: Saunders, 1991:1165.

Figure 29-1. Szulman AE. J. Reprod. Med. 29:288, 1984.

Figure 29-2. Chamberlain G. Lecture Notes on Obstetrics. 7th ed. Oxford: Blackwell Science, 1996.

Figure 29-3. Hacker N, Moore JG. Essentials of Obstetrics and Gynecology. Philadelphia: Saunders, 1992:627.

Figure 29-4. DeCherney A, Pernoll, M. Current Obstetric and Gynecologic Diagnosis and Treatment. Norwalk, CT: Appleton & Lange, 1994:974.

Figure 29-5. Hacker N, Moore JG. Essentials of Obstetrics and Gynecology. Philadelphia: Saunders, 1992:631.

Notice: The indications and dosages of all drugs in this book have been recommended in the medical literature and conform to the practices of the general medical community. The medications described do not necessarily have specific approval by the Food and Drug Administration for use in the diseases and dosages for which they are recommended. The package insert for each drug should be consulted for use and dosage as approved by the FDA. Because standards of usage change, it is advisable to keep abreast of revised recommendations, particularly those concerning new drugs.

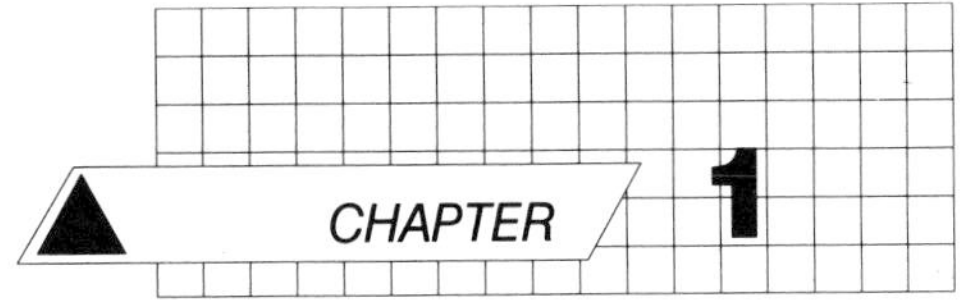

Pregnancy and Prenatal Care

PREGNANCY

Pregnancy is the state of having implanted an embryo in the uterus until such a time that the pregnancy is terminated by spontaneous or elective abortion or delivery. There are a myriad of physiologic changes that occur in a pregnant woman that include every organ system. As physicians, it is imperative to understand these changes and simultaneously incorporate this knowledge into the clinical arena.

Diagnosis

In a patient who has regular menstrual cycles and is sexually active, a period delayed by more than a few days to a week is indicative of pregnancy. Even at this early stage, patients may exhibit signs and symptoms of pregnancy. The classic finding of "morning sickness" can begin this early and often continues until 12 to 16 weeks. On physical examination, there are a variety of physical findings during pregnancy (Table 1-1).

There are many home pregnancy tests that have a high sensitivity and will be positive at or around the time of the missed menstrual cycle. These tests and the hospital laboratory assays test for the beta subunit of human chorionic gonadotropin (β-hCG). This hormone produced by the placenta will rise to a level of 100,000 by 10 weeks gestation and then level off to approximately 20,000 to 30,000 in the third trimester.

A viable pregnancy can be confirmed by ultrasound, which may show the gestational sac as early as 5 weeks, or at a β-hCG of 1,500 to 2,000, and the fetal heart as soon as 6 weeks, or a β-hCG of 5,000 to 6,000.

Terms and Definitions

From the time of fertilization until the pregnancy is 8 weeks old (10 weeks gestational age [GA]), the conceptus is called an **embryo**. After 8 weeks until the time of birth, it is a **fetus**. The term **infant** is used for the period between delivery and 1 year of age. Pregnancy is divided into trimesters. The **first trimester** lasts until 14 weeks GA, the **second trimester** from 14 until 28 weeks GA, and the **third trimester** from 28 weeks GA until delivery. An infant delivered before 24 weeks is considered to be **previable**, from 24 to 37 weeks is considered **preterm**, and from 37 to 42 weeks is **term**. (A pregnancy carried after 42 weeks is considered postdates or **post-term**.)

Gravidity refers to the number of times a woman has been pregnant and **parity** refers to the number of pregnancies that led to a birth after 20 weeks gestation or of a greater than 500-g infant. Parity is further subdivided into term and preterm deliveries, number of abortuses, and number of living children. A woman having given birth to one set of preterm twins, one term infant, and with two miscarriages would be a G4 P1-1-2-3. A multiple gestation is just one delivery but obviously may change the number living by more than one.

Dating of Pregnancy

The GA of a fetus is the age in days or weeks and is measured from the last menstrual period. **Developmental age** (DA) is the number of days or weeks since fertilization has occurred. Because fertilization usually occurs 2 weeks after the menstrual period, the GA is 2 weeks more than the DA.

Classically, Nagele's rule to calculate the estimated date of confinement (EDC) is to subtract 3 months from the last menstrual period (LMP) and add 7 days. Thus, a pregnancy with an LMP of 9/2/96 would have an EDC of 6/9/97. Exact dating uses an EDC calculated as 280 days after a certain LMP. If there is knowledge as to the date of ovulation, the EDC can be calculated by adding 266 days. This dating should be consistent with the initial examination of the uterus.

With an uncertain LMP, ultrasound is often used to determine the EDC. Ultrasound has a level of uncertainty that increases during the pregnancy. A safe rule of thumb is that the ultrasound is rarely off by more than 1 week in the first trimester, 2 weeks in the second trimester, and 3 weeks in the third trimester. The dating done with crown-rump length in the first half of the first trimester is probably even more accurate to within 3 to 5 days.

Other measures used to estimate gestational age include nonelectronic fetoscopy, which can hear the fetal heart (FH) at 20 weeks; Doppler ultrasound, which can appreciate the FH at 10 weeks; and maternal awareness of fetal movement, "quickening," which occurs between 16 and 20 weeks.

TABLE 1-1

Signs and Symptoms of Pregnancy

Signs and Symptoms of Pregnancy
Signs
Chadwick's sign: Bluish discoloration of vagina and cervix
Goodell's sign: Softening and cyanosis of the cervix at or after 4 weeks
Ladin's sign: Softening of the uterus after 6 weeks
Breast swelling and tenderness
Development of the linea nigra from umbilicus to pubis
Telangiectasias
Palmar erythema
Symptoms
Amenorrhea
Nausea and vomiting
Breast pain
Quickening—fetal movement

Physiology

Cardiovascular

During pregnancy, cardiac output increases by 30 to 50%. Most increases occur during the first trimester, with the maximum being reached between 20 and 24 weeks gestation and maintained until delivery. Systemic vascular resistance decreases during pregnancy, resulting in a fall in arterial blood pressure. This decrease is most likely due to the elevated progesterone leading to smooth muscle relaxation. There is a decrease in systolic blood pressure of 5 to 10 mm Hg and in diastolic blood pressure of 10 to 15 mm Hg that nadirs at 24 weeks. Between 24 weeks gestation and term, blood pressure slowly returns to prepregnancy levels but should never exceed them.

Pulmonary

There is an increase of 30 to 40% in tidal volume (V_T) during pregnancy (Fig. 1-1) despite the fact that the total lung capacity is decreased by 5% due to the elevation of the diaphragm. This increase in V_T decreases the expiratory reserve volume by about 20%. The increase in V_T with a constant respiratory rate leads to an increase in minute ventilation of 30 to 40%. This leads to an increase in alveolar (PA_{O_2}) and arterial (Pa_{O_2}) P_{O_2} levels and a decrease in PA_{CO_2} and Pa_{CO_2} levels.

Pa_{CO_2} decreases to approximately 30 mm Hg by 20 weeks gestation from 40 mm Hg prepregnancy. This change leads to an increased CO_2 gradient between mother and fetus and is likely caused by elevated progesterone levels that either increases the responsiveness to CO_2 of the respiratory center or acts as a primary stimulant. Dyspnea of pregnancy occurs in 60 to 70% of patients. It is likely secondary to decreased Pa_{CO_2} levels, increased V_T, or possibly decreased total lung capacity (TLC).

Gastrointestinal

There is nausea and vomiting, termed "morning sickness," in greater than 70% of pregnancies. These symptoms are attributed to the elevation in estrogen, progesterone, and hCG. The nausea and vomiting should routinely resolve by 14 to 16 weeks gestation. During pregnancy, the stomach is noted to have increased gastric emptying times, and the gastroesophageal sphincter has decreased tone. These changes together lead to reflux and possibly combine with decreased esophageal tone to cause ptyalism, or spitting,

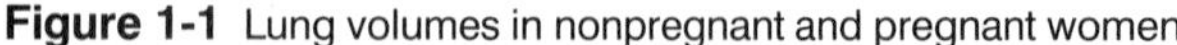

Figure 1-1 Lung volumes in nonpregnant and pregnant women.

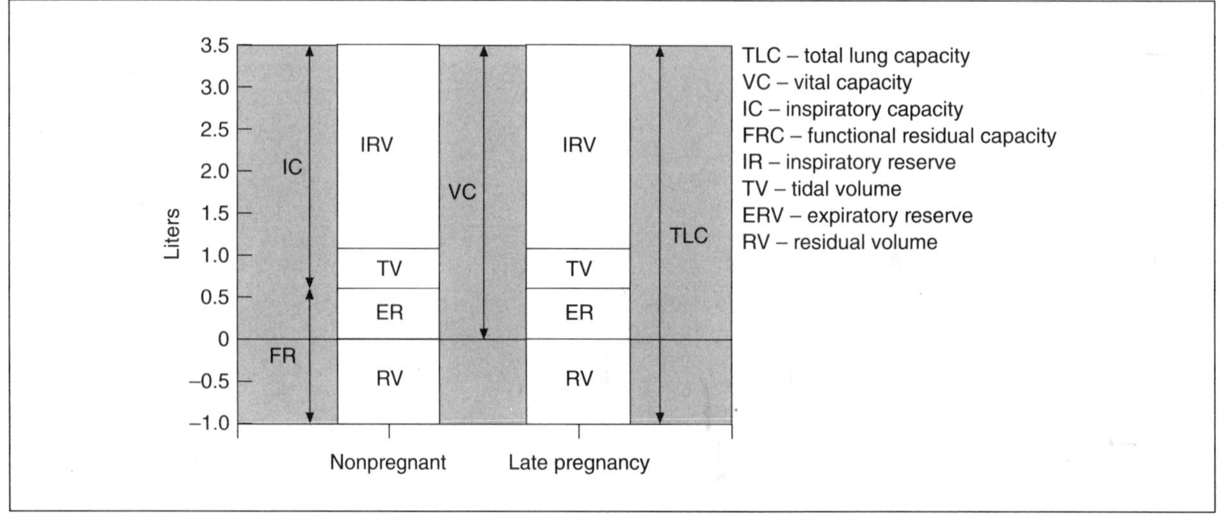

during pregnancy. The large bowel also has decreased motility, which leads to increased water absorption and constipation.

Renal

The kidneys actually increase in size and the ureters dilate during pregnancy, which may lead to increased rates of pyelonephritis. The glomerular filtration rate (GFR) increases by 50% early in pregnancy and is maintained until delivery. As a result of increased GFR, blood urea nitrogen and creatinine decrease by about 25%. There is an increase in the renin-angiotensin system that leads to increased levels of aldosterone. This ultimately results in increased sodium resorption. This does not increase plasma levels of sodium, because there is a simultaneous increase in GFR.

Hematology

Although the plasma volume increases by 50% in pregnancy, the red blood cell volume increases by only 20 to 30%, which leads to a decrease in the hematocrit. The white blood count (WBC) increases during pregnancy to a mean of 10.5 million/mL with a range of 6 to 16. During labor, the WBC may rise due to the stress to over 20 million/mL. There is a slight decrease in the concentration of platelets, probably secondary to increased plasma volume and increase in peripheral destruction. Although a small percentage of patients may have platelets less than 150 million/mL, a drop in the platelet count over a short time is not normal and should be investigated.

Pregnancy is considered to be a hypercoagulable state, and the number of thromboembolic events increases. There are elevations in the levels of fibrinogen and factors VII through X. However, the actual clotting time and bleeding time does not change. The increased rate of thromboembolic events in pregnancy may be secondary to venous stasis and vessel endothelial damage.

Endocrine

Pregnancy is a hyperestrogenic state. Most estrogen is produced in the placenta with decreased production by the ovaries. Unlike estrogen production in the ovaries, where estrogen precursors are produced in ovarian theca cells and transferred to the ovarian granulosa cell, estrogen in the placenta is derived from circulating plasma-borne precursors produced by the maternal adrenal glands. Fetal well-being has been correlated with estrogen levels and low maternal estrogen levels have been associated with conditions such as fetal death and anencephaly.

hCG is composed of two dissimilar alpha and beta subunits. The alpha subunit of hCG is identical to the alpha subunit of luteinizing hormone, follicle-stimulating hormone, and thyroid stimulating hormone whereas the beta subunit differs. The placenta produces hCG, which acts to maintain progesterone production by the corpus luteum. Levels of hCG double approximately every 48 hours during early pregnancy, reaching a peak at approximately 10 to 12 weeks, thereafter declining and reaching steady state after week 15.

Human placental lactogen (hPL), also known as human chorionic somatomammotropin, is produced in the placenta and is important for ensuring a constant nutrient supply to the fetus. Lipolysis with a concomitant increase in circulating free fatty acids is caused by hPL. hPL also acts as an insulin antagonist, along with a variety of other placental hormones, thereby having a diabetogenic effect. This leads to increased levels of insulin and protein synthesis.

Progesterone is produced by the corpus luteum during early pregnancy, after which biosynthesis occurs primarily in the placenta. Progesterone precursors are derived from low-density-lipoprotein cholesterol. Levels of progesterone increase over the course of pregnancy. Progesterone causes relaxation of smooth muscle, which leads to multiple effects on the gastrointestinal, cardiovascular, and genitourinary systems.

High estrogen levels cause an increase in thyroid binding globulin. Placental hormones such as hCG may also have thyroid-stimulating properties, which lead to an elevation in total T3 and T4. Together, these changes lead to a relatively euthyroid state, although free T3 and T4 levels may decrease slightly in pregnancy. Levels of prolactin are markedly increased during pregnancy. Levels paradoxically decrease after delivery but later increase in response to suckling.

Musculoskeletal and Dermatologic

The obvious change in the center of gravity during pregnancy can lead to a shift in posture and lower back strain. There are numerous changes in the skin in pregnancy, including spider angiomata and palmar erythema secondary to increased estrogen levels and hyperpigmentation of the nipples, umbilicus, abdominal midline (the **linea nigra**), the perineum, and the face (**melasma** or **chloasma**) secondary to increased levels of alpha-melanocyte stimulating hormone and the steroid hormones.

Nutrition

During pregnancy and breastfeeding, the nutritional requirements increase. The average woman requires 2,000 to 2,500 kcal/day. The caloric requirement is increased by 300 kcal/day during pregnancy and by 500 kcal/day when breastfeeding. Most patients should gain between 20 and 30 pounds during pregnancy. Obese women are advised to gain less, between 15 and 20 pounds, and thin women are advised to gain slightly more, 25 to 35 pounds, during pregnancy.

In addition to the increased caloric requirements, there are increased nutritional requirements for protein, iron, folate, calcium, and other vitamins and minerals. The protein requirement increased from 60 g/day to 70 or 75 g/day. Recommended calcium intake is 1.5 g/day. Many patients develop iron deficiency anemia because of the increased demand of hematopoiesis by both the mother and the fetus. Folate requirements increase from 0.4 to 0.8 mg/day and are important in preventing neural tube defects.

All patients are advised to take prenatal vitamins during pregnancy. These are designed to compensate for the increased nutritional demands of pregnancy. Furthermore, any patient whose hematocrit falls during the third trimester is advised to increase iron intake with supplementation (Table 1-2).

Key Points

1. A urine pregnancy test will often be positive at the time of the missed menstrual cycle.
2. Physiologic changes during pregnancy, mediated by the placental hormones, affect every organ system.
3. Cardiovascular changes include a 50% rise in blood volume and decrease in systemic vascular resistance.
4. Pulmonary changes include a >30% increase in V_T leading to a decrease in $Paco_2$ to 30 mm Hg and increase in blood pH to 7.45.

▶ PRENATAL CARE

Prenatal visits are designed to screen for a variety of complications of pregnancy while educating the patient

TABLE 1-2

Recommended Daily Dietary Allowances for Nonpregnant, Pregnant, and Lactating Women

	Nonpregnant Women (yr)						
	11–14	15–18	19–22	23–50	51+	Pregnant Women	Lactating Women
Energy (kcal)	2,400	2,100	2,100	2,000	1,800	+300	+500
Protein (g)	44	48	46	46	46	+30	+20
Fat-soluble vitamins							
Vitamin A activity (RE)	800	800	800	800	800	1,000	1,200
(IU)	4,000	4,000	4,000	4,000	4,000	5,000	6,000
Vitamin D (IU)	400	400	400	...	...	400	400
Vitamin E activity (IU)	12	12	12	12	12	15	15
Water-soluble vitamins							
Ascorbic acid (mg)	45	45	45	45	45	60	80
Folate (μg)	400	400	400	400	400	800	600
Niacin (mg)	16	14	14	13	12	+2	+4
Riboflavin (mg)	1.3	1.4	1.4	1.2	1.1	+0.3	+0.5
Thiamin (mg)	1.2	1.1	1.1	1	1	+0.3	+0.3
Vitamin B_6 (mg)	1.6	2	2	2	2	2.5	2.5
Vitamin B_{12} (μg)	3	3	3	3	3	4	4
Minerals							
Calcium (mg)	1,200	1,200	800	800	800	1,200	1,200
Iodine (μg)	115	115	100	100	80	125	150
Iron (mg)	18	18	18	18	10	+18	18
Magnesium (mg)	300	300	300	300	300	450	450
Phosphorus (mg)	1,200	1,200	800	800	800	1,200	1,200
Zinc (mg)	15	15	15	15	15	20	25

From Gabbe SG, Niebyl JR, Simpsen JL. Obstetrics: normal and problem pregnancies. 2nd ed. New York: Churchill Livingstone, 1991:196.

during her pregnancy. They include a series of outpatient office visits that involve routine physical examinations and a variety of screening tests that occur at different points during the pregnancy. Important issues of prenatal care include initial evaluation of patient, routine evaluation of the patient, nutrition, disease states during the pregnancy, and preparing for the delivery.

Initial Visit

Often this is the longest of the prenatal visits because it involves a complete history and physical as well as a battery of initial laboratory tests. It should occur early in the first trimester, although occasionally patients will not present for their initial prenatal visit until later in the pregnancy.

History

The patient's history includes the present pregnancy, the last menstrual period, and symptoms during the pregnancy. After this, an obstetric history of prior pregnancies including when, the outcome, mode of delivery, length of time in labor and second stage, birthweight, and any complications. Finally, a complete medical, surgical, family, and social history should be taken because these can have an impact on the pregnancy.

Physical Examination

A routine physical examination is performed, paying particular attention to the patient's prior medical and surgical history. The pelvic examination includes a Pap smear, unless one has been done in the past 6 months, and cultures for gonorrhea and chlamydia. On bimanual examination, the size of the uterus should be compared with the gestational age from the LMP.

Diagnostic Evaluation

The panel of tests in the first trimester include a complete blood count, blood type, antibody screen, rapid plasma reagin (RPR), rubella antibody screen, hepatitis B surface antigen, urinalysis, and urine culture. A PPD is usually planted during the first trimester. A urine pregnancy test should be sent if the patient is not entirely certain she is pregnant. If there has been any bleeding or cramping, a β-hCG level should be obtained. There is some debate over the use of routine toxoplasma titers; they are often sent as well. Human immunodeficiency virus testing should be offered but is not routinely performed (Table 1-3).

Routine Prenatal Visits

On each follow-up prenatal care visit, there are routine events. Maternal blood pressure decreases during the first and second trimester and slowly returns to baseline during the third trimester; if it is elevated this may be a sign of pre-eclampsia. Maternal weight is followed serially throughout the pregnancy to determine if the patient is gaining adequately. Measurement of the fundal height is taken, which roughly correlates in centimeters to the weeks of gestation. If the fundal height is progressively decreasing or 3 cm less or more than gestational age, an ultrasound scan is done for fetal growth. After 10 to 14 weeks, the doptone is used to listen for the fetal heart rate. Urine is routinely dipped for protein, glucose, blood, and leukocyte esterase. Protein may be indicative of pre-eclampsia, glucose of diabetes, and leukocyte esterase of urinary infection.

TABLE 1-3

Routine Tests in Prenatal Care

Initial Visit and First Trimester	Second Trimester	Third Trimester
Hematocrit	MSAFP	Hematocrit
Blood type and screen	Ultrasound	RPR
RPR	Amniocentesis in AMA patients	GLT
Rubella antibody screen		Repeat gonorrhea and chlamydia
Hepatitis B surface antigen		Chest X-ray if PPD +
Gonorrhea culture		Group B strep culture
Chlamydia culture		
PPD		
Pap smear		
Urinalysis and culture		
Human immunodeficiency virus offered		

In the third trimester, Leopolds (see Fig. 3-1, p. 17) are performed to determine the presentation.

First Trimester Visits

During the first trimester, the patient needs to be familiarized with pregnancy, particularly nulliparous women. At the visit after the initial visit, all labs can be reviewed. The symptoms of pregnancy can be reviewed as well. Patients with poor weight gain or c/o decreased caloric intake secondary to her nausea and vomiting can be referred to a nutritionist. If patients were treated for infections noted at the initial prenatal visit, they should be cultured for test of cure.

Second Trimester Visits

During the second trimester, much of the screening for congenital abnormalities is done. This enables a patient to still obtain an elective termination if there are abnormalities. The fetal heart is usually first heard during the second trimester and the first fetal movement, or **"quickening,"** is felt in the late second trimester. Because the risk of spontaneous abortions is now decreased, childbirth classes and tours of the labor floor should now be discussed.

Maternal serum alpha fetal protein (MSAFP) is measured between 16 and 18 weeks. Elevation is correlated with increased risk for neural tube defects. Decreased levels are correlated with Down's syndrome. Between 18 and 20 weeks gestation, most patients are offered a screening ultrasound. This is done to do a fetal anatomic survey. Also noted is the amniotic fluid volume and placental location. For patients with an abnormal MSAFP or patients over the age of 35, a 16- to 18-week amniocentesis is offered to obtain fetal cells for karyotype.

Third Trimester Visits

During the third trimester, the fetus attains viability. Patients will begin to have occasional Braxton Hicks contractions. The prenatal visits increase to every 2 to 3 weeks from 28 to 36 weeks and then to every week after 36 weeks. In addition, patients who are Rh negative should receive RhoGAM at 28 weeks.

Third Trimester Labs

At 27 to 29 weeks, the third trimester labs are ordered. They consist of the hematocrit, RPR, and **glucose loading test** (GLT). The hematocrit is getting close to its nadir. Patients in the low thirties should be started on iron supplementation. Because this will cause further constipation, stool softeners are given in conjunction with iron. The GLT is a screening test for gestational diabetes. This consists of a 50-g oral loading dose and a serum glucose 1 hour later. If this value is greater than or equal to 140 mg/dL, a **glucose tolerance test** (GTT) is administered.

The GTT consists of a fasting serum glucose and then administration of a 100-g oral glucose loading dose. The serum glucose is then measured at 1, 2, and 3 hours after the oral dose is given. The test is indicative of gestational diabetes if the fasting glucose is over 105 mg/dL or if any two of three values are over 190, 165, or 145 mg/dL, respectively.

In high risk populations, vaginal cultures for gonorrhea and chlamydia are repeated late in the third trimester. These infections are transmitted vertically during birth and should be treated if cultures or DNA tests return positive. At 36 weeks, screening for group B streptococcus is performed. Patients that have a positive culture can be treated with intravenous penicillin when they present in labor.

Key Points

1. Good nutrition in pregnancy is important; in particular folate supplementation has been shown to decrease neural tube defects.
2. Prenatal care is divided into a series of visits, with routine tests performed at each visit depending on the gestation of the pregnancy.
3. It is imperative to verify dating of the pregnancy at the first prenatal visit

▶ ROUTINE PROBLEMS OF PREGNANCY

Back Pain

Low back pain in pregnancy is quite common, particularly as the pregnancy gets to advanced ages where the patient's center of gravity has shifted and there is increased strain on the lower back. Mild exercise, particularly stretching, may release endorphins and reduce the amount of back pain. Tylenol can be used for mild pain. For patients near term with severe back pain, muscle relaxants or occasionally narcotics can be used.

Constipation

The decreased bowel motility secondary to elevated progesterone level leads to increased transit time in the large bowel. In turn, there is greater reabsorption of water from the gastrointestinal tract. The result can be constipation. Increased fluids, particularly water, should be recommended. In addition, stool softeners or laxatives may help.

Contractions

Occasional irregular contractions are considered Braxton Hicks contractions and will occur several times per day. Patients should be warned about these and assured that they are perfectly normal. Dehydration may cause increased contractions, and patients should be advised to drink many (10 to 14) glasses of water and juice per day. Regular contractions, every 10 to 15 minutes or less, should be considered a sign of preterm labor and should result in a cervical examination. If a patient has had several days of contractions and no documented cervical change, this is reassuring to both the obstetrician and the patient that delivery is not imminent.

Dehydration

Because of the expanded intravascular space and increased third spacing of fluid, patients have a difficult time maintaining their intravascular volume status. Dietary recommendations should include increased fluids.

Edema

Compression of the inferior vena cava (IVC) can lead to increased hydrostatic pressures in the lower extremities and eventually edema in the feet and ankles. The patient can lay on her side or she can elevate her lower extremities above her heart. Severe edema of the face and hands may be indicative of pre-eclampsia and further evaluation is needed.

Gastroesophageal Reflux Disease

Relaxation of the lower esophageal sphincter and increased transit time in the stomach can lead to reflux and nausea. Patients should be started on antacids, advised to eat multiple small meals per day, and not to lay down within an hour of eating. For patients with continued symptoms, H_2 blockers can be given.

Hemorrhoids

Patients will have increased venous stasis and IVC compression that leads to increased venous pressures. This backup in pelvic veins and pressures combined with increased abdominal pressure with bowel movements secondary to constipation can lead to hemorrhoids. Hemorrhoids are treated symptomatically with topical anesthetics and steroids for pain and swelling. Prevention of constipation with increased fluids, increased fiber in the diet, and stool softeners may prevent or decrease the exacerbation of hemorrhoids.

Pica

Rarely, a patient will have cravings for nonedible items like dirt or clay. As long as they are nontoxic, the patient is advised to maintain adequate nutrition. However, if patients have been consuming toxic substances, immediate cessation along with a toxicology consult is advised.

Round Ligament Pain

Usually late in the second trimester or early in the third trimester, there may be some pain in the adnexa or lower abdomen. This pain is likely secondary to the rapid expansion of the uterus and stretching of the ligamentous attachments, such as the round ligaments. This is often self-limiting but may be benefited by Tylenol.

Urinary Frequency

Increased intravascular volumes and elevated GFR can lead to increased urine production during pregnancy. However, the most likely cause of urinary frequency during pregnancy is the uterus, which is increasingly compressing the bladder as it expands. A urinary tract infection may also present with isolated urinary frequency but will often have concomitant dysuria. A urinalysis and culture is sent to rule out infection. If there is no infection, patients can be assured that the increasing voiding is normal. Patients should be advised to keep up PO hydration despite urinary frequency.

Varicose Veins

The lower extremities or the vulva may develop varicosities during the pregnancy. The relaxation of the venous smooth muscle and increased venous pressures both probably contribute to the pathogenesis of these varicosities. Elevation of the lower extremities or the use of pressure stockings may help reduce current varicosities or prevent more from developing. If they do not resolve by 6 months postpartum, patients may be referred for surgical therapy.

Key Points

1. Many of the routine problems of pregnancy are related to hormonal effects of the placenta.
2. It is important to discuss the side effects of pregnancy in order to best prepare the patient.

▶ PRENATAL ASSESSMENT OF THE FETUS

Ultrasound

Ultrasound can be used for dating a pregnancy with an unknown or uncertain LMP. Furthermore, it is used for monitoring at-risk infants with biophysical profiles and fetal growth. In the setting of prenatal diagnosis of fetal malformations, most patients undergo a routine screening ultrasound at 18 weeks for fetal survey. Routinely, an attempt is made to identify all internal organs and any obvious malformations.

Maternal Serum AFP

AFP is produced by the placenta and is present in the amniotic fluid. A certain amount crosses into the maternal circulation and can be measured as MSAFP (Fig. 1-2). Elevation of the MSAFP is correlated with neural tube defects, abdominal wall defects (gastroschisis and omphalocele), multiple gestations, fetal death, and placental abnormalities like abruption.

Decreased levels of MSAFP can be correlated with some chromosomal abnormalities, particularly Down's syndrome. This screening test is augmented with levels of estriol and hCG, which are elevated in the setting of Down's. This is called the triple screen (Table 1-4) and can also be used to screen for Edward's syndrome (Trisomy 18). Patau's syndrome (Trisomy 13) is associated with birth defects that can make the screen unpredictable.

Amniocentesis

Once a fetal anomaly is suspected on ultrasound, the MSAFP is aberrant, or there is a family history of congenital abnormalities, an amniocentesis may be performed to obtain a fetal karyotype. Amniocentesis is also offered to any patient of advanced maternal age (AMA). Patients over the age of 35 at delivery are considered AMA because the risk of chromosomal abnormalities increases to 1 in 200.

Usually the risk of complication secondary to amniocentesis ranges from 1 in 200 to 250. The common risks are of rupture of membranes, preterm labor, and fetal injury. Because the risk of a chromosomal abnormality in patients of AMA is greater than 1 in 200, amniocentesis is routinely offered to these patients.

TABLE 1-4
Triple Screen Table

	Trisomy 21	Trisomy 18	Trisomy 13
MSAFP	Decreased	Decreased	Depends on defects
Estriol	Decreased	Decreased	Depends on defects
β-hCG	Elevated	Decreased	Depends on defects

Chorionic Villous Sampling

Chorionic villous sampling (CVS) can obtain a fetal karyotype sooner than amniocentesis because it can be

Figure 1-2 Median maternal serum |ga-fetoprotein levels throughout gestation. Increasing values with increasing gestational age require accurate dating to interpret low or high MSAFP

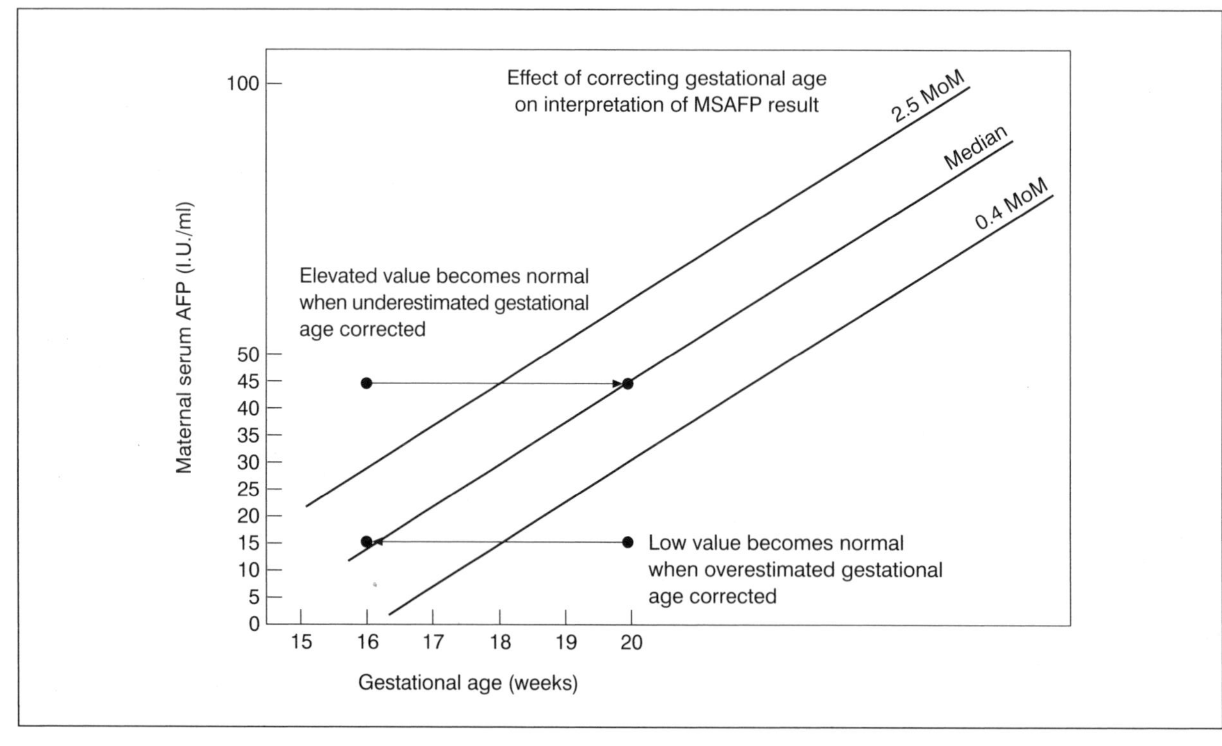

performed at 9 to 11 weeks. This involves the placement of a catheter in the intrauterine cavity and aspirating a small quantity of chorionic villi from the placenta. The risk of CVS is slightly higher than the amniocentesis rate of 1 in 200 complications including preterm, premature rupture of membranes, previable delivery, and fetal injury.

Fetal Blood Sampling

Percutaneous umbilical blood sampling is performed by placing a needle transabdominally into the uterus and phlebotomizing the umbilical cord. This may be used when the fetal hematocrit needs to be obtained, particularly in the setting of Rh isoimmunization, concern for fetal anemia, and hydrops.

Fetal Lung Maturity

There are many different tests for fetal lung maturity. Classically, the lecithin to sphingomyelin (L/S) ratio has been used as a predictor of fetal lung maturity. The type II pneumocytes secrete surfactant that uses phospholipids in its synthesis. Commonly, lecithin increases as the pregnancy matures, whereas sphingomyelin remains constant. Thus, the L/S ratio should increase as the pregnancy progresses. It has been shown in repetitive studies that an L/S ratio of greater than 2 is associated with only rare cases of **respiratory distress syndrome** (RDS). With an L/S ratio below 1.5, the risk of RDS is 70%. There are many other fetal lung maturity tests that are performed that involve screening for phospholipids in the amniotic fluid. Examples of these include the fetal lung maturity (FLM) screen and measuring of **saturated phosphatidyl choline (SPC).**

Formal Testing

Forms of formal testing include the nonstress test (NST), the oxytocin challenge test (OCT), and the biophysical profile (BPP). An NST is considered formally reactive if there are two accelerations in 20 minutes that are at least 15 beats above the baseline heart rate and last for at least 15 seconds. An OCT or contraction stress test (CST) is obtained by getting at least three contractions in 10 minutes and analyzing the fetal heart rate (FHR) tracing during that time. The reactivity is the same as the NST. In addition, it is considered nonreassuring if there are late decelerations with any of the contractions. Ultrasound is used to perform a BPP. The BPP looks at five categories and gives a score of either 0 or 2 for each. The categories include amniotic fluid volume, fetal tone, fetal activity, fetal breathing movements, and the NST. A BPP of 8/10 or better is reassuring. Ultrasound can also be used to assess the blood flow velocity in the umbilical cord and the presence or absence of diastolic flow.

Key Points

1. The fetus can be assessed with ultrasound, nonstress test, and oxytocin challenge test.
2. Common screening tests for fetal abnormalities include MSAFP, the triple screen, screening ultrasound, and amniocentesis.

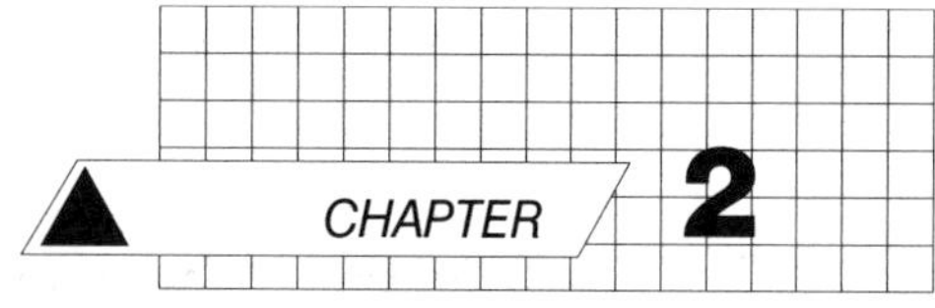

Early Pregnancy Complications

▶ ECTOPIC PREGNANCY

An ectopic pregnancy is one that implants outside the uterine cavity. They implant in the fallopian tube in over 99% of the cases (Fig. 2-1). Implantation may also occur on the ovary, the cervix, the outside of the fallopian tube, the abdominal wall, or the bowel. The incidence of ectopic pregnancies has been increasing over the past 10 years, and now occurs in greater than 1 of every 100 pregnancies. This is thought to be secondary to the increase in assisted fertility, sexually transmitted infections, and pelvic inflammatory disease (PID). Patients who present with vaginal bleeding and abdominal pain should always be evaluated for ectopic pregnancy because a ruptured ectopic pregnancy is a true emergency. It can result in rapid hemorrhage, leading to shock and eventually death.

Risk Factors

There are several risk factors that predispose patients to extrauterine implantation of their pregnancy (Table 2-1. Many have effects on the fallopian tubes either to cause tubal scarring or to cause decreased peristalsis of the tube. Use of an intrauterine device (IUD) for birth control leads to an increased rate of ectopic pregnancy in those patients who become pregnant, because the IUD prevents intrauterine implantation.

Diagnosis

The diagnosis of ectopic pregnancy is made by history, physical examination, laboratory tests, and ultrasound. On history, patients often complain of unilateral pelvic or lower abdominal pain and vaginal bleeding. Physical examination may reveal an adnexal mass, often tender; a uterus that is small for gestational age; and bleeding from the cervix. Patients with ruptured ectopic pregnancies may be hypotensive, unresponsive, or show peritoneal signs.

On laboratory studies, the classic finding is a beta human chorionic gonadotropin (β-hCG) level that is low for gestational age and does not increase at the expected rate. In patients with a normal intrauterine pregnancy (IUP), the trophoblastic tissue secretes β-hCG, which doubles approximately every 48 hours. An ectopic pregnancy has a poorly implanted placenta, and the level of β-hCG does not double every 48 hours. The hematocrit may be low or drop in patients with ruptured ectopic pregnancies.

Ultrasound may show an adnexal mass or an extrauterine pregnancy. A gestational sac and yolk seen in the uterus on ultrasound rules in an intrauterine pregnancy. However, there is always a small risk for heterotopic pregnancy, which is a multiple gestation with at least one IUP and at least one ectopic pregnancy. At early gestations, neither an IUP or an adnexal mass can be seen.

Patients who cannot be diagnosed with ectopic pregnancy because they do not have an adnexal mass on physical examination or ultrasound and are seemingly stable may be followed with serial β-hCG levels every 48 hours to assess the possibility of ectopic pregnancy. Each 48 hours, the level should double. An IUP should be seen on transvaginal ultrasonography with a β-hCG between 1,500 and 2,000. A fetal heart beat should be seen with β-hCG > 5,000.

Treatment

If an unstable patient presents with a ruptured ectopic pregnancy, the first priority is to stabilize with intravenous fluids, blood products, and pressors if necessary. The patient should then be taken to the operating room where exploratory laparotomy can be performed, the bleeding stabilized, and the ectopic pregnancy removed.

Patients who present with an unruptured ectopic pregnancy should be monitored for signs of rupture—increased abdominal pain, bleeding, or signs of shock. These patients are often treated surgically with laparoscopic resection of the ectopic pregnancy. Methotrexate therapy for treatment of the ectopic pregnancy is being used in some institutions for uncomplicated, nonthreatening ectopic pregnancies.

Key Points

1. Ectopic pregnancy is implantation of the pregnancy outside the uterine cavity.
2. Ectopic pregnancy occurs in approximately 1% of pregnancies.
3. Patients present with bleeding and unilateral pelvic pain, and diagnosis is made with palpation of

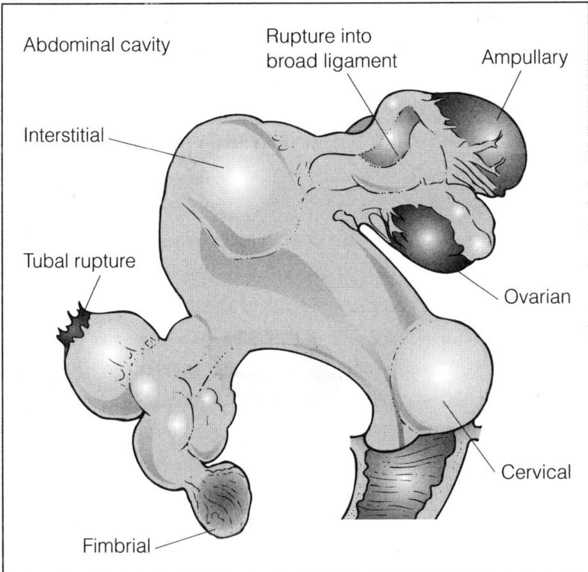

Figure 2-1 Sites of ectopic pregnancies

an adnexal mass or visualization of an extrauterine pregnancy on ultrasound.

4. Treatment is often surgical and includes stabilizing the patient and removal of the pregnancy; methotrexate therapy is used for certain ectopic pregnancies.

TABLE 2-1

Risk Factors for Ectopic Pregnancy

History of sexually transmitted infections or PID
Prior ectopic pregnancy
Previous tubal surgery
Prior pelvic or abdominal surgery resulting in adhesions
Endometriosis
Current use of exogenous hormones including progesterone or estrogen
In vitro fertilization and other assisted reproduction
DES-exposed patients with congenital abnormalities
Congenital abnormalities of the fallopian tubes
Use of an IUD for birth control

► SPONTANEOUS ABORTION

A spontaneous abortion (SAB), or miscarriage, is a pregnancy that ends before 20 weeks gestation. SABs are estimated to occur in 15 to 25% of all pregnancies. This number may even be higher because losses that occur at 4 to 6 weeks gestational age are often confused with menses. The type of SAB is defined by whether any or all of the **products of conception** (POCs) have passed and whether the cervix is dilated or not. Definitions are as follows:

- ▲ **Abortus:** fetus lost before 20 weeks gestation, less than 500 g, or less than 25 cm.
- ▲ **Complete abortion:** complete expulsion of all POCs before 20 weeks gestation (Fig. 2-2).
- ▲ **Incomplete abortion:** partial expulsion of some but not all POCs, before 20 weeks gestation (Fig. 2-2).
- ▲ **Inevitable abortion:** no expulsion of products, but bleeding and dilation of the cervix such that a viable pregnancy is unlikely.
- ▲ **Threatened abortion:** any intrauterine bleeding before 20 weeks, without dilatation of the cervix or expulsion of any POCs.
- ▲ **Missed abortion:** death of the embryo or fetus before 20 weeks with complete retention of POCs; these often proceed to complete abortions in 1 to 3 weeks but occasionally are retained much longer.

First Trimester Abortions

It is estimated that 60% of all SABs in the first trimester (early abortions are at <12 weeks gestational age) are associated with abnormal chromosomes. This percentage may be higher because many abortions likely occur before implantation. Other factors associated with spontaneous early abortions include infections, maternal anatomic defects, immunologic factors, and endocrine factors. A large number of first trimester abortions have no obvious cause.

Diagnosis

Most patients present with bleeding per vagina (Table 2-2). Other findings include cramping, abdominal pain, and decreased symptoms of pregnancy. The physical examination should include vital signs to rule out shock and febrile illness. The pelvic examination can be performed to look for sources of bleeding other than uterine and for changes in the cervix suggestive of an inevitable abortion. The laboratory tests ordered include a quantitative level for β-hCG, complete blood count, blood type, and antibody screen. An ultrasound can assess fetal viability and placentation.

Because ectopic pregnancy also presents with vaginal bleeding, it needs to be ruled out of the differential diagnosis. An ultrasound showing a viable IUP or serial β-hCG levels doubling every 48 hours in early pregnancy are consistent with IUP.

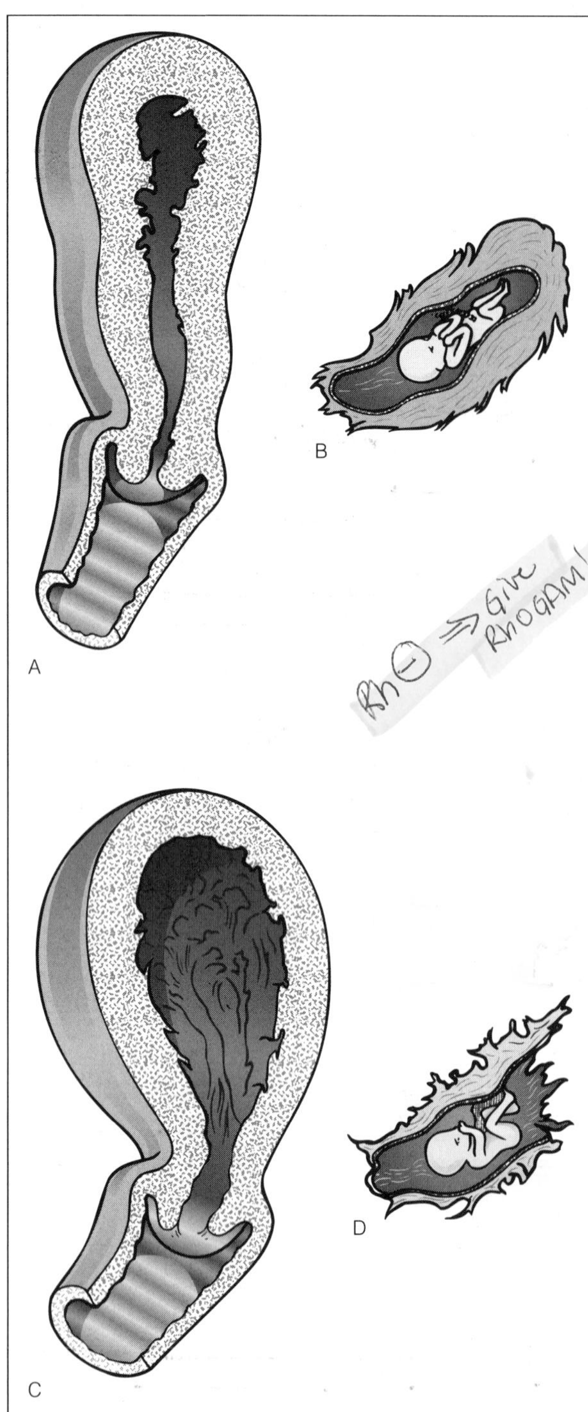

Figure 2-2 A. Complete abortion. B. Product of complete abortion. C. Incomplete abortion. D. Product of incomplete abortion.

Treatment

The treatment plan is based on specific diagnosis and dependent on the decisions made by the patient and her caregivers. Initially, all patients pregnant and bleeding need to be stabilized if hypotensive. A **complete abortion** can be followed for recurrent bleeding and elevated temperature. Any tissue that the patient may have passed at home and at the hospital should be sent to pathology, both to assess that POCs have passed and for chromosome analysis.

An **incomplete abortion** can be allowed to finish on its own but is often taken to completion with a dilation and evacuation (D&E). Any tissue that has passed or been evacuated needs to be sent to pathology. **Inevitable abortions** and **missed abortions** are similar to incomplete abortions.

Someone with a **threatened abortion** should be followed for continued bleeding and placed on pelvic rest with nothing per vagina. Often, the bleeding will resolve; however, these patients are at increased risk for preterm labor. If patients are Rh negative, a Kleihauer-Behtke can be sent to assess the amount of fetal blood that may have passed into the maternal circulation. All Rh-negative patients should receive RhoGAM whenever there is vaginal bleeding.

Key Points

1. The most common cause of first trimester abortions is fetal chromosomal abnormalities.
2. It is important to rule out ectopic pregnancy with history, physical examination, laboratory studies, and ultrasound.
3. Incomplete, inevitable, and missed abortions are usually completed with a D&E, although expectant management has been used.
4. RhoGAM should be given to all Rh-negative patients with bleeding.

Second Trimester Abortions

Second trimester abortions (12 to 20 weeks gestational age) have multiple etiologies. Infection, maternal uterine or cervical anatomic defects, maternal systemic disease, exposure to fetotoxic agents, and trauma are all associated with late abortions. Abnormal chromosomes are not a frequent cause of late abortions. Late second trimester abortions and periviable deliveries are also seen with preterm labor and incompetent cervix.

Diagnosis

Patients commonly present with bleeding per vagina. Other findings include cramping, abdominal pain, and

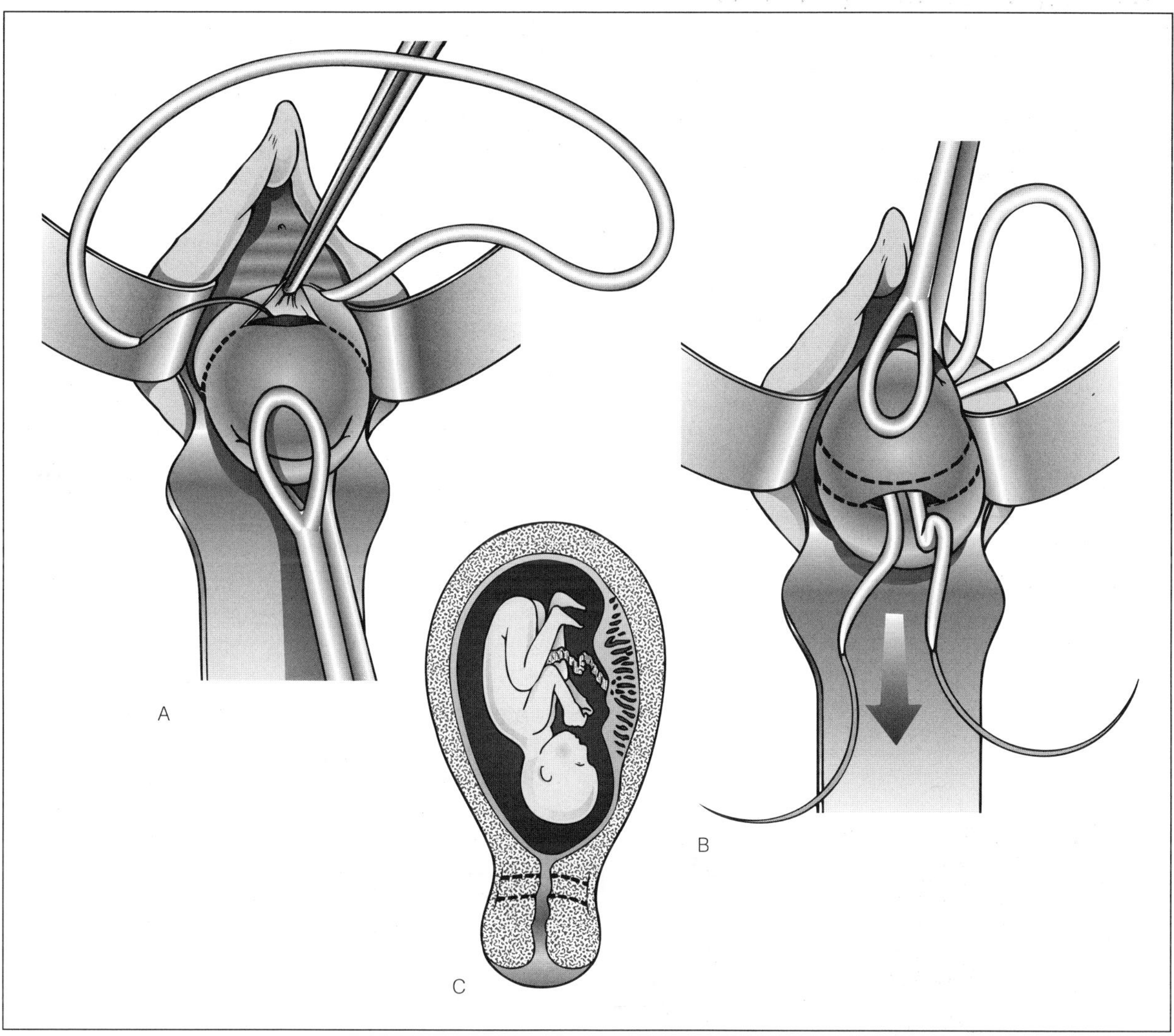

Figure 2-3 Cerclage of the cervix (Shirodkar) with incompetent cervix in pregnant patient. A. Placement of the suture. B. Cinching the suture down to tie the knot posterior. C. The tightened cerclage almost at the internal os.

TABLE 2-2

Differential Diagnosis of First Trimester Bleeding

Spontaneous abortion
Postcoital bleeding
Ectopic pregnancy
Vaginal or cervical lesions or lacerations
Extrusion of molar pregnancy
Nonpregnant causes of bleeding

decreased symptoms of pregnancy. Occasionally, patients will notice no fetal movement in a previously active fetus. The physical examination, laboratory studies, and ultrasound are similar to those for a first trimester abortion.

Treatment

As in first trimester abortions, once the diagnosis of ectopic pregnancy has been eliminated, the treatment plan is based on the specific clinical scenario. All hypotensive or hemorrhaging patients need to be stabilized. A **complete abortion** can be followed for recurrence of bleeding and elevated temperature. If there is any concern for retained POCs, a D&E can be used to ensure completion of the abortion.

Incomplete and **missed abortions** can be allowed to finish on their own but are often taken to completion with a D&E. Commonly, between 16 and 20 weeks and beyond, labor may be induced with high doses of oxytocin or prostaglandins. This allows completion of the abortion without instrumentation. Great care should be taken to ensure the complete extrusion of all POCs.

In the second trimester, the diagnoses of **preterm labor** and **incompetent cervix** need to be ruled out. Particularly in the setting of **inevitable abortions** or **threatened abortions,** the etiology is likely to be related to the inability of the uterus to maintain the pregnancy. Preterm labor begins with contractions leading to cervical change, whereas an incompetent cervix is characterized by painless dilatation of the cervix. In the setting of incompetent cervix, an emergent cerclage may be offered. Preterm labor can be managed with tocolysis.

Key Points

1. Most second trimester abortions are secondary to uterine or cervical abnormalities, trauma, systemic disease, or infection.
2. D&E or oxytocic agents can be used for the management of spontaneous abortions in the second trimester that need assistance to completion.
3. The risk of uterine perforation from D&E is greater in the second trimester than the first, although it is always a risk.

▶ INCOMPETENT CERVIX

Patients with an **incompetent cervix** present with painless dilatation and effacement of the cervix, often in the second trimester of pregnancy. As the cervix dilates, the fetal membranes are exposed to vaginal flora and increased trauma. Thus, rupture of the membranes or infection are common findings in the setting of incompetent cervix. Patients may also present with cramping or contracting for a short while, leading to advanced cervical examinations or pressure in the vagina with the chorionic and amnionic sacs bulging through the cervix. Cervical incompetence is estimated to cause approximately 15% of all second trimester losses.

Risk Factors

Surgery or other cervical trauma is the most common cause of cervical incompetence (Table 2-3). The other possible cause is a congenital disturbance of the cervix as in diethylstilbestrol (DES) exposed women. However, there are those individuals who present with cervical incompetence without any known risk factors.

TABLE 2-3

Risk Factors for Cervical Incompetence

History of cervical surgery, such as a cone biopsy or dilation of the cervix
History of cervical lacerations during prior vaginal delivery
Uterine anomalies
History of DES exposure

Diagnosis

Patients with incompetent cervix often present with an advanced cervical examination noted on routine examination, ultrasound, or in the setting of bleeding or rupture of membranes. Occasionally, patients have small amounts of cramping or pressure in the lower abdomen or vagina. On examination they have a cervix that is dilated more than expected with the amount of contractions experienced. In this setting, it is difficult to differentiate between incompetent cervix and preterm labor. However, patients who present with mild cramping and have an advanced cervical examination and/or a bulging amniotic sac through the cervix are more likely to have incompetent cervix, with the cramping being instigated by the dilated cervix and exposed membranes.

Treatment Key Points

Individual obstetric issues should be treated accordingly. If the fetus is previable, expectant management versus elective termination are options. Patients with viable pregnancies are treated with beta-methasone to decrease the risk of prematurity and managed expectantly with strict bedrest. If there is a component of preterm contractions or preterm labor, tocolysis may be used with viable pregnancies.

One alternative course of management for incompetent cervix in a previable pregnancy is the placement of an emergent cerclage. The cerclage is a suture placed around the cervix either at the cervical-vaginal junction (McDonald) or the internal os (Shirodkar). The intent of a cerclage is to close the cervix. Complications include rupture of membranes and preterm labor.

If incompetent cervix was the suspected diagnosis in a previous pregnancy, a patient may receive an elective cerclage (see Fig. 2-3). Placement of the elective cerclage is similar to the emergent cerclage with either the McDonald or Shirodkar being used, usually at 13 to 14 weeks gestation.

Key Points

1. Incompetent cervix is painless dilation of the cervix. However, once the cervix is dilated, it may lead to infection, preterm premature rupture of membranes (PPROM), or preterm labor (PTL).

2. Incompetent cervix in the previable infant is treated with expectant management, elective termination, or emergent cerclage.
3. Patients with a history of incompetent cervix should be offered an elective prophylactic cerclage at 13 to 14 weeks gestational age.

▶ RECURRENT ABORTIONS

A recurrent or habitual aborter is someone with three or more consecutive SABs. Less than 1% of the population is diagnosed with recurrent abortions. The risk of a SAB after 1 prior SAB is 20 to 25%, after two consecutive SABs 25 to 30%, and after three consecutive SABs it goes up to 30 to 35%.

Pathogenesis

The etiologies of recurrent abortions are similar to those of SABs in general. They include chromosomal abnormalities, maternal systemic disease, maternal anatomic defects, and infection. Fifteen percent of patients with recurrent abortions have the antiphospholipid antibody (APA) syndrome. Another group of patients are thought to have a luteal phase defect and lack the level of progesterone to maintain the pregnancy.

Diagnosis

Patients who are habitual aborters should be worked up for the etiology. Patients with only two consecutive SABs are occasionally worked-up as well, particularly in patients with advancing maternal age or if continued fertility may be an issue. Patients are often screened in the following manner. First, a karyotype of both parents is obtained as well as the karyotypes of the POCs from each of the SABs. Second, the anatomy should be examined first with a hysterosalpingogram (HSG). If the HSG is abnormal or nondiagnostic, a hysteroscopic or laparoscopic exploration may be performed. Third, screening tests for hypothyroidism, diabetes mellitus, APA syndrome, and lupus should be performed. Fourth, a level of serum progesterone should be obtained in the luteal phase of the menstrual cycle. Finally, cultures of the cervix, vagina, and endometrium can be taken to rule out infection. Furthermore, the endometrial biopsy can be done during the luteal phase as well to look for proliferative endometrium.

Treatment

Treatment of habitual aborters depends on the etiology of the SABs. For many (approximately 30%), no etiology is ever found. For others, the etiology itself needs to be diagnosed as above and often can be treated on an individual basis. For patients with chromosomal abnormalities such as balanced translocations, in vitro fertilization can be done with donor sperm or ova. Patients with anatomic abnormalities may or may not be able to have these corrected. If incompetent cervix is suspected, a cerclage may be placed. If a luteal phase defect is suspected, progesterone may be given. Patients with APA syndrome are treated with low-dose aspirin. Maternal diseases should be treated with the appropriate therapy (e.g., hypothyroidism with thyroid hormone, infection with antibiotics). However, with some systemic disease, treatment may not decrease the risk for SAB. Because even patients with three prior consecutive SABs will have a normal pregnancy two thirds of the time, it is difficult to estimate whether certain treatments of recurrent abortions are effective.

Key Points

1. Habitual abortion is defined as three or more consecutive SABs.
2. Despite extensive workups to diagnose the etiology of SABs, the cause of recurrent SABs is undiagnosed in greater than one third of all cases.
3. Treatment is specific to the etiology but is difficult to measure efficacy because two thirds of subsequent pregnancies would be normal without therapy.

CHAPTER 3

Normal Labor and Delivery

LABOR AND DELIVERY

When a patient first presents to the labor floor, a quick initial assessment is made using the history of present pregnancy, obstetric history, and the standard medical and social history. Beyond the standard physical examination, the obstetric examination includes maternal abdominal examination for contractions and of the fetus (**Leopold maneuvers**), cervical examination, and fetal heart tones.

Obstetric Examination

The physical examination includes determination of fetal lie and presentation and a cervical examination. In addition, if there is a question of rupture of membranes, a sterile speculum examination is performed. The fetal lie and presentation can usually be determined by Leopold maneuvers. The maneuvers involve palpating first at the fundus of the uterus in the maternal upper abdominal quadrants, then on either side of the uterus (maternal left and right), and finally palpation of the presenting part just above the pubic symphysis. **Fetal lie,** that is, whether the infant is longitudinal or transverse within the uterus, is relatively easy to determine with Leopold's (Fig. 3-1. **Fetal presentation,** either breech or vertex (cephalic), can be more difficult, and even the most experienced examiner may require ultrasound.

Rupture of Membranes

In 10% of pregnancies, the membranes surrounding the fetus rupture before labor; this is called premature rupture of membranes (ROM). When ROM occurs more than 18 hours before delivery, it is considered prolonged ROM (PROM) and puts both mother and fetus at increased risk for infection. Often PROM is confused with PPROM, which is preterm premature rupture of membranes, preterm being before 37 weeks gestational age.

Diagnosis

Diagnosis is suspected with a history of a gush or leaking of fluid from the vagina, although sometimes it is difficult to differentiate between stress incontinence and small leaks of amniotic fluid. Diagnosis of ROM can be made by the pool, nitrazine, and fern tests. Ultrasound to examine fluid quantity may be helpful. If uncertain, diagnosis can be confirmed by the amniocentesis dye test.

Using a sterile speculum to examine the vaginal vault, the **pool test** is positive if there is a collection of fluid in the vagina. This can be augmented by asking the patient to cough or bear down and more fluid can be seen escaping from the cervix. Vaginal secretions are normally acidic, whereas amniotic fluid is alkaline; thus, when placed on **nitrazine** paper, it should immediately turn blue. The estrogens in the amniotic fluid cause crystallization of the salts in the amniotic fluid when it is dried. The crystals are visible under low microscopic power and resemble the blades of a fern. Cervical mucus can give false-positive results, so it is important to sample fluid that is not directly from the cervix.

An ultrasound examination can determine the quantity of fluid around the infant. If there previously was normal fluid or there is no reason to suspect low fluid, **oligohydramnios** is indicative of ROM. If these tests are equivocal, the amnio/dye test is performed by injecting a dye directly into the amniotic fluid via amniocentesis. Observation of the dye leaking from the cervix or in any fluid in the vagina confirms ROM. This test is also called the **tampon test,** because often the dye is absorbed into a tampon.

Cervical Examination

The cervical examination enables the obstetrician to determine whether a patient is in labor, the phase of labor, and how labor is progressing. The five components of the cervical examination are dilation, effacement, station, cervical position, and consistency of the cervix. These five aspects of the examination make up the **Bishop score** (Table 3-1). A Bishop score greater than 8 is consistent with a cervix favorable for both spontaneous and, more commonly, induced labor.

Dilation is assessed by using either one or two fingers of the examining hand to assess how open the cervix is at the level of the **internal os.** The measurements are in centimeters and range from closed, or 0 cm, to fully dilated, or 10 cm. On average, 10-cm dilation is necessary to accommodate the term infant's biparietal diameter.

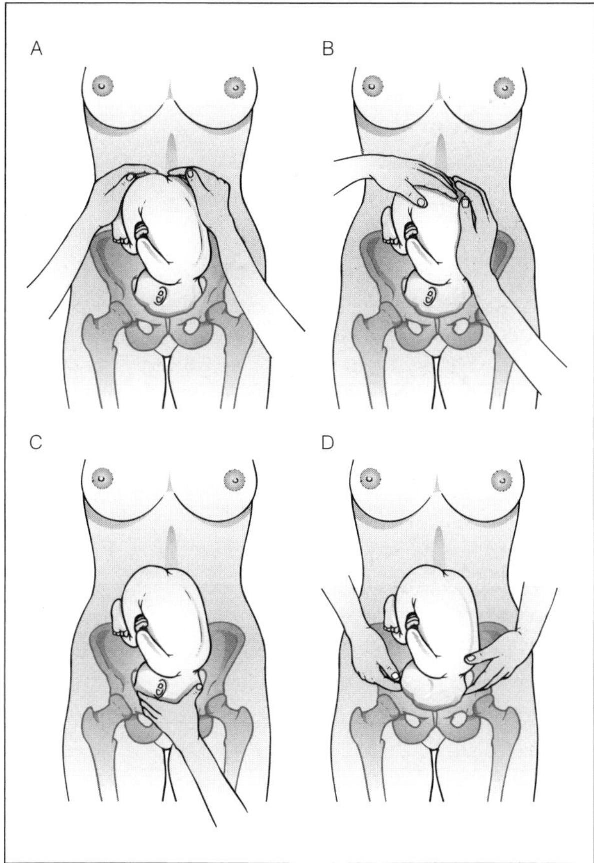

Figure 3-1 Leopold's maneuvers. Determining fetal presentation (A and B), position (C), and engagement (D).

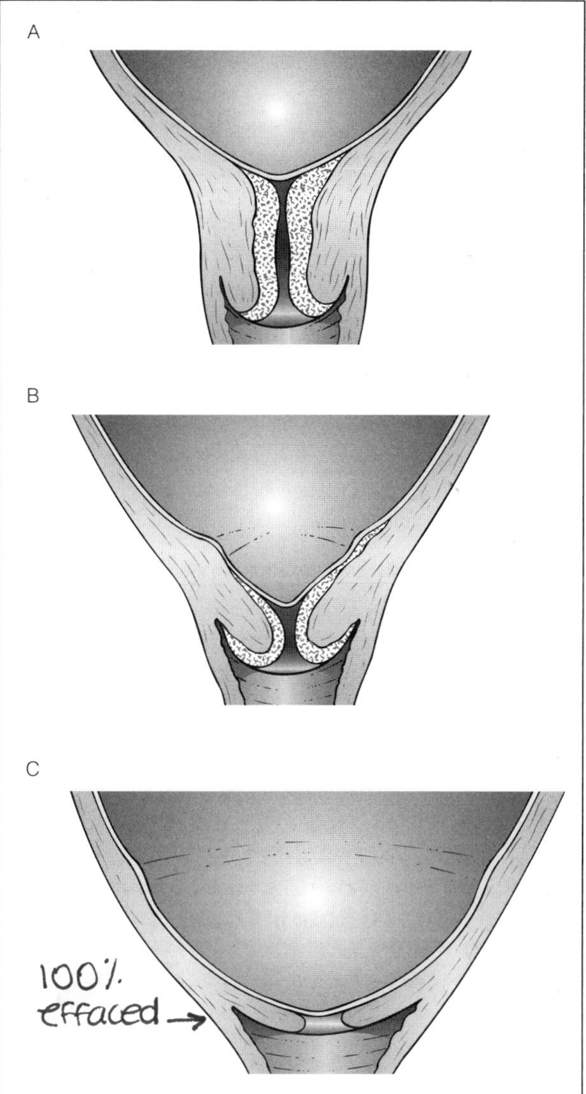

Figure 3-2 (A) CVX is fingertip dilated, not effaced. (B) CVX is fingertip dilated, 50% effaced. (C) CVX is 1 cm dilated, 100% effaced.

Effacement is also a subjective measurement made by the examiner. It is a determination of how much length is left of the cervix or how effaced (thinned out) it is (Fig. 3-2). The typical cervix is 3 to 5 cm in length; thus, if the cervix feels like it is about 2 cm from external to internal os, it is 50% effaced.

TABLE 3-1

The Bishop Score

Score	0	1	2	3
Cervical dilatation (cm)	Closed	1–2	3–4	>5
Cervical (%) effacement	0–30	40–50	60–70	>80
Station	−3	−2	−1, 0	>+1
Cervical consistency	Firm	Medium	Soft	
Cervical position	Posterior	Mid	Anterior	

Complete or 100% effacement occurs when the cervix is as thin as the adjoining lower uterine segment.

The relation of the fetal head to the ischial spines of the female pelvis is known as station (Fig. 3-3). When the most descended aspect of the presenting part is at the level of the ischial spines, that is considered 0 station. Station is negative when the presenting part is above the ischial spines and positive when it is below. There are two systems of measuring how far above and below the presenting part is. One divides the distance

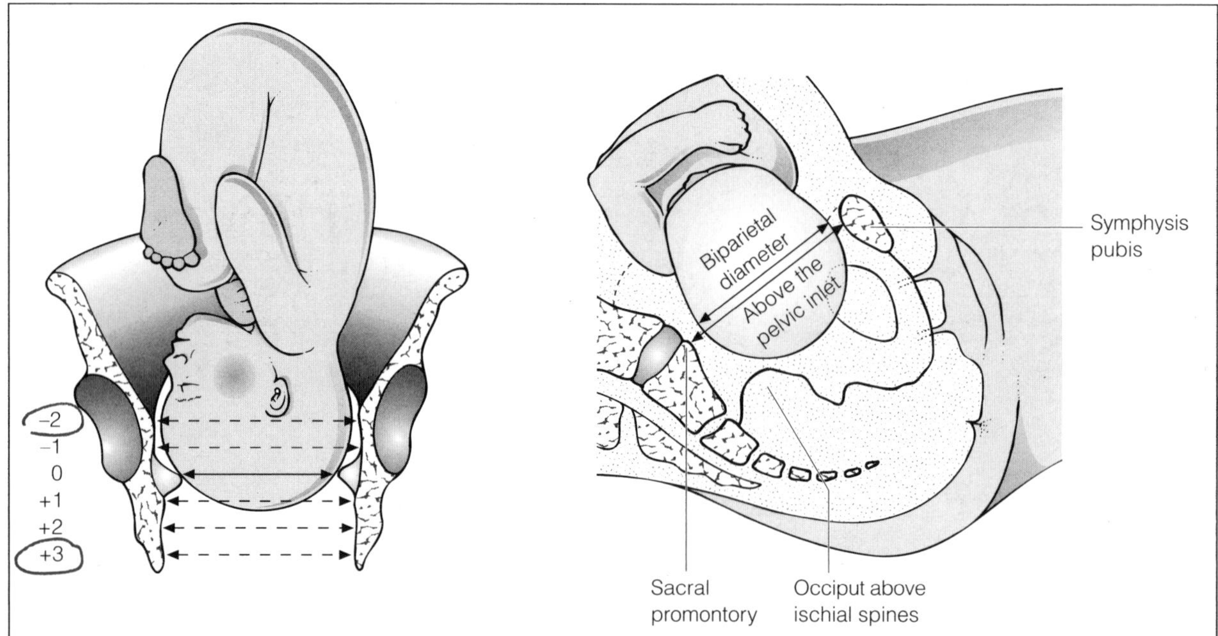

Figure 3-3 The relationship of the leading edge of the presenting part of the ischial spines determines the station. Station 1 is depicted in the frontal view on the left and station −2 to −1 is depicted in the lateral view on the right.

to the pelvic inlet into thirds and thus station is −3 to 0 and then 0 to +3, which is at the level of the introitus. The other commonly used method uses centimeters, which gives stations of −5 to +5. Either system is effective and both are widely used among different institutions.

Cervical **consistency** is self-explanatory. Whether the cervix feels firm or soft or somewhere in between should be noted. Cervical **position** ranges from posterior to mid to anterior. A posterior cervix is high in the pelvis, located behind the fetal head and often quite difficult to reach, let alone examine. The anterior cervix can usually be felt easily when examining is often lower down in the vagina. During early labor, the cervix often changes its consistency to soft and advances position from posterior to mid to anterior.

Fetal Presentation and Position

The fetal **presentation** can be **vertex** (head down), **breech** (butt down), or **transverse** (neither down). Although presentation may already be known from the Leopold maneuvers, it can be confirmed by examination of the presenting part during cervical examination. Assuming that the cervix is somewhat dilated, the fetal presenting part may be palpated as well during this examination. Early on in labor, even this can lead to false determination of presentation. However, palpation of hair or sutures on the fetal vertex or the gluteal cleft or anus on the breech usually leaves little doubt. If the fetus is vertex, further palpation should be made to determine that the fetus is not presenting with either the face or brow.

Fetal **position** in the vertex presentation is usually based on the relationship of the fetal occiput to the maternal pelvis (Fig. 3-3). Presentation is determined by palpation of the sutures. The vault, or roof, of the fetal skull is composed of five bones: two frontal, two parietal, and one occipital. The **anterior fontanelle** is the junction between the two frontal bones and two parietal bones and is generally considered to be diamond-shaped. The **posterior fontanelle** is the junction between the two parietal bones and the occipital bone and is more triangular-shaped. With face presentations, the chin or mentum is the fetal reference point; with breech presentations it is the fetal sacrum.

If fetal presentation cannot be determined with physical examination, ultrasound can confirm presentation. It is also useful in determining whether a breech presentation is frank, complete, or footling. Breech presentations are discussed further in Chapter 5.

Key Points

1. Upon presentation to the labor floor a patient receives a full history and physical.

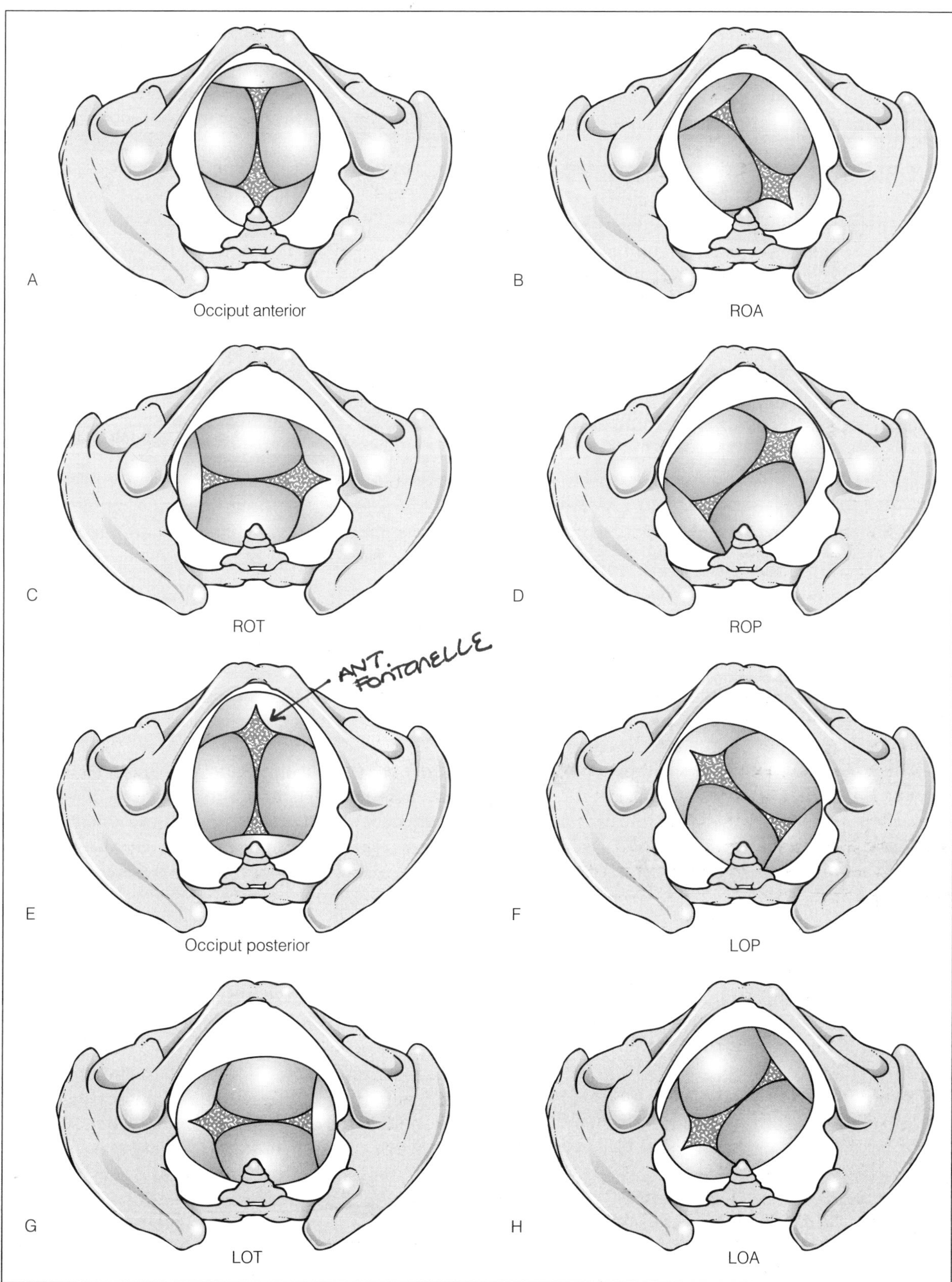

Figure 3-4 (A–H) Various possible positions of the fetal head in the maternal pelvis.

2. The physical exam of a pregnant woman can include Leopold's, a sterile speculum exam, and a cervical exam.
3. It is important to determine both the position of the fetus and status of the cervix.

▶ NORMAL LABOR

Labor is defined as contractions that cause cervical change in either effacement or dilation. **Prodromal labor** or "false labor" is common in the differential diagnosis of labor. These patients usually present with irregular contractions that vary in amount of duration, intensity, and intervals and yield little or no cervical change.

The diagnosis of labor strictly defined seems clear; assessment of contractions and cervical change determine whether a patient is in labor. However, there are many other signs of labor used by clinicians that include patient discomfort, bloody show, nausea and vomiting, and palpability of contractions. These signs and symptoms can all vary from patient to patient, and although they can add to the clinician's assessment, one should rely on an objective definition.

▶ INDUCTION AND AUGMENTATION OF LABOR

Induction of labor is the attempt to begin labor in a nonlaboring patient, whereas **augmentation of labor** is intervening to increase the already present contractions. Labor is induced with **prostaglandins, oxytocic agents,** and/or **artificial rupture of membranes.** The indications for induction are based on either maternal, fetal, or fetoplacental reasons. Common reasons for induction of labor include postterm pregnancy, pre-eclampsia, premature ROM, nonreassuring fetal testing at term, and intrauterine growth restriction. They do not include the patient's desire to end the pregnancy.

Preparing for Induction

When proper indications for induction exist, the situation should be discussed with the patient and a plan for induction made. When the indication is more pressing, induction should be started without significant delay. The success of an induction (defined as achieving vaginal delivery) is often correlated with cervical favorability as defined by the Bishop score. A Bishop score of five or less leads to a failed induction as often as 50% of the time. In these patients, prostaglandin E_2 (PGE_2) gel is often used to "ripen" the cervix.

There are both maternal and obstetric contraindications for the use of PGE_2 gel. Maternal reasons include asthma and glaucoma. The obstetric reasons include having had more than one prior cesarean section and nonreassuring fetal testing. Because PGE_2 gel cannot be turned off with the ease of pitocin, one is concerned about the risk of uterine hyperstimulation and tetanic contractions. In this setting, a biophysical dilator and ripener such as Laminaria can be used. The Laminaria tents are placed inside the cervical canal and over the course of 6 to 12 hours dilate the cervix as they enlarge by absorbing water and expanding.

Induction

Induction may actually begin with the placement of PGE_2 gel. However, induction is usually begun pharmacologically with pitocin. This is a synthesized, but identical, version of the octapeptide oxytocin normally released from the posterior pituitary that causes uterine contractions.

Labor may also be induced by amniotomy. Amniotomy is performed with an amnio hook that is used to tear the amniotic sac around the fetus and release some of the amniotic fluid. After the amniotomy is performed, a careful examination should be performed to ensure that prolapse of the umbilical cord has not occurred. When performing amniotomy, it is important not to elevate the fetal head from the pelvis to release more of the amniotic fluid because this may lead to prolapse of the umbilical cord beyond the fetal head.

Augmentation

Aside from the induction of labor, pitocin and amniotomy are used to augment labor. The indications for augmentation of labor include those for induction and inadequate contractions or a prolonged phase of labor. The adequacy of contractions is indirectly assessed by the progress of cervical change. It may also be measured directly using an intrauterine pressure catheter (IUPC), which determines the absolute change in pressure during a contraction and thus estimates the strength of contractions.

▶ MONITORING OF THE FETUS IN LABOR

It is easy to monitor the mother in labor with vital signs and laboratory studies. Monitoring the infant is indirect and thus more difficult than maternal assessment. Determination of the baseline rate and variations of the heart rate with contractions can be assessed by auscultation. The normal range for the fetal heart rate is between 110 and 160 beats per minute. With baselines above 160, fetal distress secondary to infection or anemia is of concern. Any bradycardia of greater than 3 minutes with a heart rate less than 90 is considered severe and needs immediate attention.

External Electronic Monitors

Since the advent of electronic fetal monitoring, auscultation is rarely used. Continuous fetal heart monitors are the standard in most hospitals in the United States because they afford several advantages over auscultation. The information gathered is more subtle and includes variations in heart rate. Probably the greatest advantage is that the information is easier to gather and record, thus allowing for more time to analyze the data.

The external tocometer has a pressure transducer that is placed against the patient's abdomen, usually near the fundus of the uterus. During uterine contractions, the abdomen becomes firmer, and this pressure is transmitted through the transducer to the tocometer which records the contraction. The relative heights of the tracings on different patients or at different locations on the same patient cannot be used to compare strength of contractions. They are most useful for measuring the frequency of contractions and comparing with the fetal heart rate tracing to determine the type of decelerations occurring.

A fetal heart rate tracing is examined for several characteristics that are considered reassuring. First, the baseline is determined and should be in the normal range. Then the variations from the baseline should be examined. A flat tracing is not reassuring, rather there should be a jagged appearance from the beat-to-beat variability of the heart rate. There should also be at least three to five cycles per minute of the heart rate around the baseline. Finally, a tracing can be considered formally reactive (Fig. 3-5) if there are two accelerations of at least 15 beats per minute over the baseline that last for at least 15 seconds in 20 minutes.

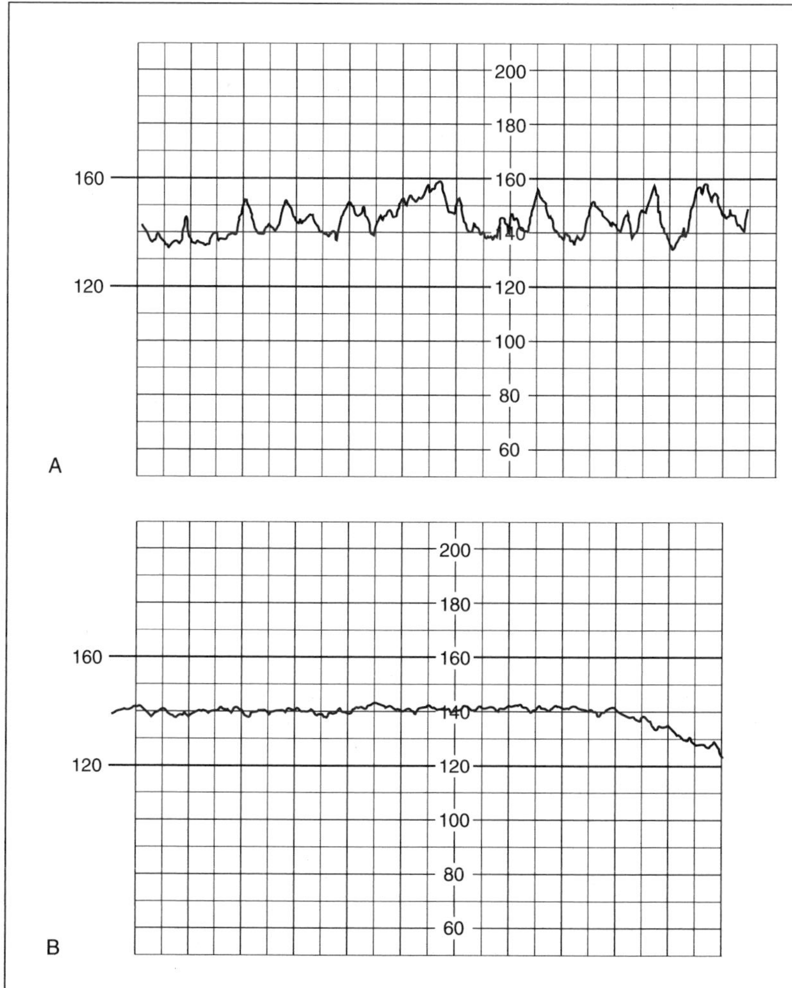

Figure 3-5 (A) Normal short-term and long-term beat-to-beat variability. (B) Reduced variability. This may occur during fetal sleep, following maternal intake of drugs, or with reduced fetal central nervous system function, as in asphyxia.

Decelerations of the Fetal Heart Rate

The fetal heart rate tracing should also be used to examine decelerations (decels) and can be used along with the tocometer to determine the type and severity. There are three types of decelerations: **early, variable, and late.** Early decelerations begin and end approximately at the same time as contractions (Fig. 3-6A). They are a result of increased vagal tone secondary to head compression during a contraction. Variable decelerations can occur at any time and have the characteristic of being a more precipitous drop than either early or late decels (Fig. 3-6C). They are a result of umbilical cord compression. Repetitive variables with contractions can be seen when the cord is entrapped either under a fetal shoulder or around the neck and is compressed with each contraction. Late decelerations begin at the peak of a contraction and slowly return to baseline after the contraction has finished (Fig. 3-6B). These decelerations are a result of uteroplacental insufficiency and are the most worrisome type. They may degrade into bradycardias as labor progresses, particularly with stronger contractions.

Fetal Scalp Electrode

In the setting of repetitive decels or in patients that are difficult to trace externally with Doppler, a **fetal scalp electrode** (FSE) is often used. A small electrode is attached to the fetal scalp and senses the potential differences created by the depolarization of the fetal heart. The information obtained from the scalp electrode is more sensitive in terms of the beat-to-beat variability and is in no danger of being lost during contractions as the fetal position changes. Contraindications include a history of maternal hepatitis or human immunodeficiency virus.

Intrauterine Pressure Catheter

The external tocometer records the onset and end of contractions. The absolute values of the readings mean little and are entirely position dependent. Furthermore, on some patients, particularly those that are obese, the tocometer does not show much in the way of fluctuation from the baseline. If it is particularly important to determine the timing or strength of contractions, an IUPC may be used (Fig. 3-7). This catheter is threaded past the fetal presenting part into the uterine cavity to measure the pressure changes during contractions. The baseline intrauterine pressure is usually between 10 and 15 mm Hg. Contractions during labor will increase by 20 to 30 mm Hg in early labor and by 40 to 60 mm Hg as labor progresses. The most commonly used way of assessing the adequacy of uterine contractions is the Montevideo unit, which is an average of the variation of the intrauterine pressure from the baseline times the number of contractions in a 10-minute period.

Fetal Scalp pH

If a fetal heart rate tracing is nonreassuring, the fetal scalp pH may be obtained to assess fetal hypoxia directly (Fig. 3-8). Fetal blood is obtained by making a small nick in the fetal scalp and drawing up a small amount of fetal blood into capillary tubes. The results are reassuring when the scalp pH is greater than 7.25, indeterminate between 7.20 and 7.25, and nonreassuring when less than 7.20. Care must be taken to avoid contamination of the blood sample with amniotic fluid, which is basic and will falsely elevate the results.

Key Points

1. Labor can be induced or augmented with prostaglandin, pitocin, laminoria, and artificial rupture of membranes.
2. The fetus can be monitored in labor with external fetal monitoring, fetal scalp electrode, ultrasound, and fetal scalp pH.

▶ THE PROGRESSION OF LABOR

Labor is assessed by the progress of cervical effacement, cervical dilatation, and descent of the fetal presenting part. To assess the progress of labor, it is important to understand the cardinal movements or mechanisms of labor.

Cardinal Movements of Labor

The cardinal movements are engagement, flexion, descent, internal rotation, extension, and external rotation or resolution (Fig. 3-9). When the fetal presenting part enters the pelvis, it is said to have undergone **engagement.** The head will then undergo **flexion,** which allows the smallest diameter to present to the pelvis. **Descent** of the vertex will occur with passage of the head down into the pelvis. With descent into the midpelvis, the fetal vertex will **internally rotate** so that the sagittal suture is parallel to the anteroposterior diameter of the pelvis. As the vertex passes beneath and beyond the pubic symphysis, it will **extend** to deliver. Once the head delivers, **externally rotation** occurs and the shoulders may be delivered.

Stages of Labor

Labor and delivery are divided into three stages. Each stage has different concerns and considerations. Stage 1 begins with the onset of labor and lasts until dilatation and effacement of the cervix is completed. Stage 2

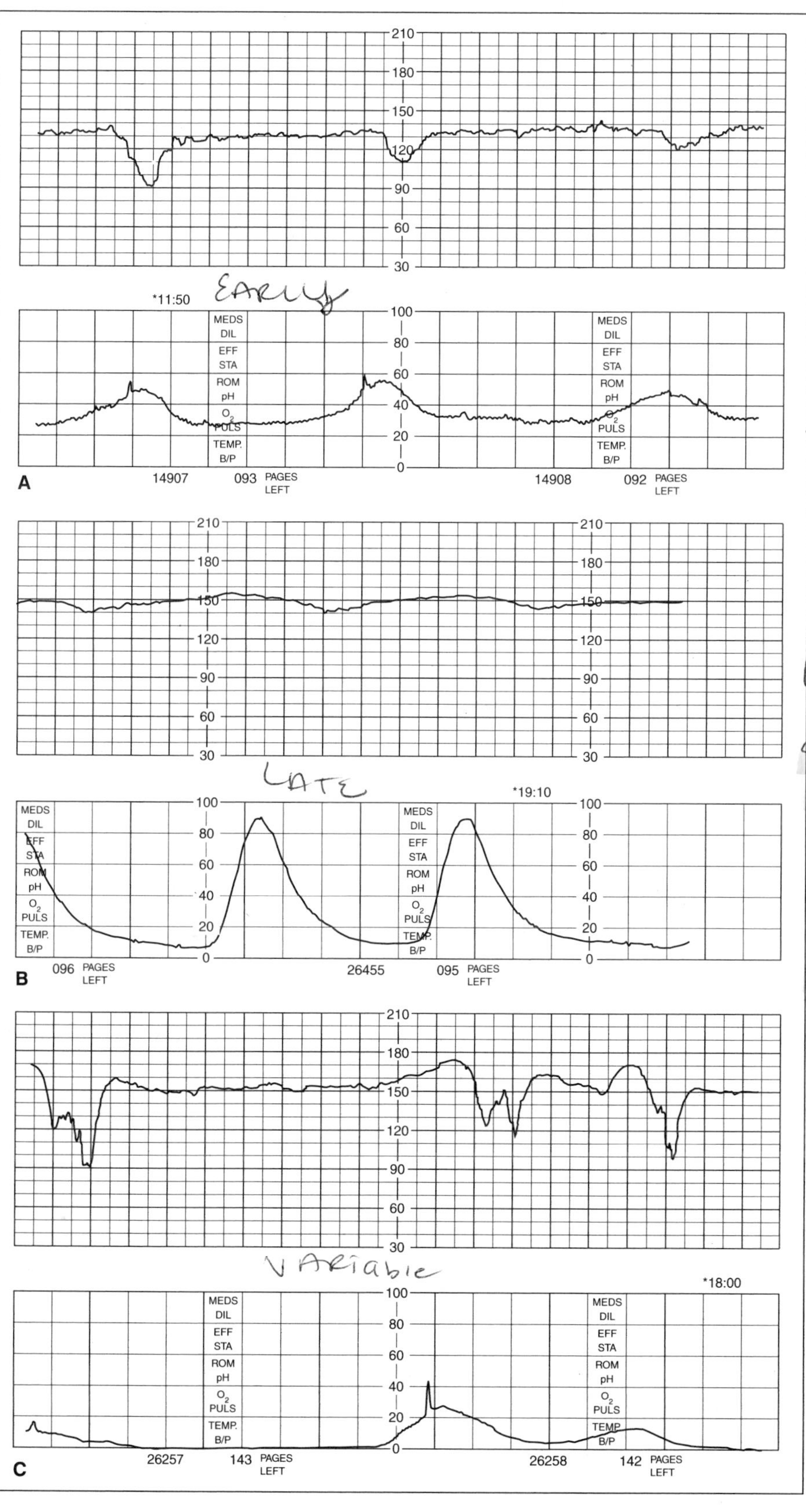

Figure 3-6 (A) An early deceleration pattern is depicted in this fetal heart rate (FHR) tracing. Note that each deceleration returns to baseline before the completion of the contraction. The remainder of the fetal heart rate tracing is reassuring. (B) Repetitive late decelerations in conjunction with decreased variability. (C) Variable decelerations are the most common periodic change of the fetal heart rate during labor. Repetitive mild- to moderate variable decelerations are present. The baseline is normal.

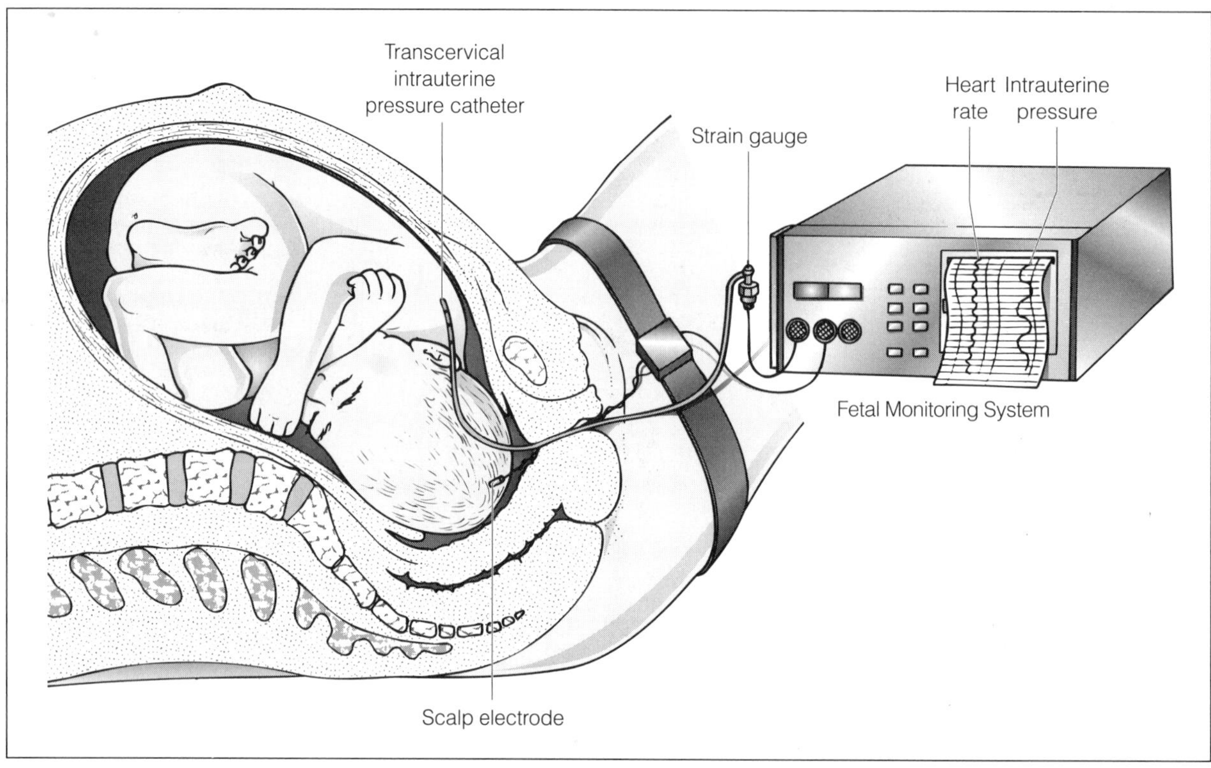

Figure 3-7 Technique for continuous electronic monitoring of fetal heart rate and uterine contractions.

Figure 3-8 Technique of fetal scalp blood sampling via an amnioscope. After making a small stab incision in the fetal scalp, the blood is drawn off through a capillary tube.

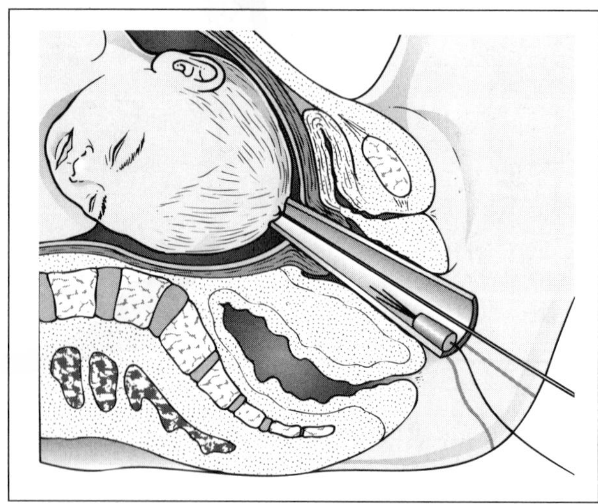

is from the time of full dilatation until delivery of the infant. Stage 3 begins after delivery of the infant and ends with delivery of the placenta.

Stage 1

The first stage of labor ranges from the onset of labor until complete dilatation of the cervix has occurred. It has been approximated that an average first stage of labor lasts 10 to 12 hours in a nulliparous patient and 6 to 8 hours in a multiparous patient. The range of what is considered within normal limits is quite wide, from 6 hours up to 20 hours in a nulliparous patient and from 2 to 12 hours in a multiparous patient. The first stage is divided further into the latent and active phases (Fig. 3-10).

The latent phase generally ranges from the onset of labor until 3 or 4 cm of dilation. The active phase then ranges until greater than 9 cm of dilation. A third phase is often delegated at this point called deceleration or transition phase as the cervix completes dilatation. The latent phase is characterized by slow cervical change. During the active phase, at least 1 cm/hr of

A Before engagement

B Engagement, flexion, descent

C Descent, rotation

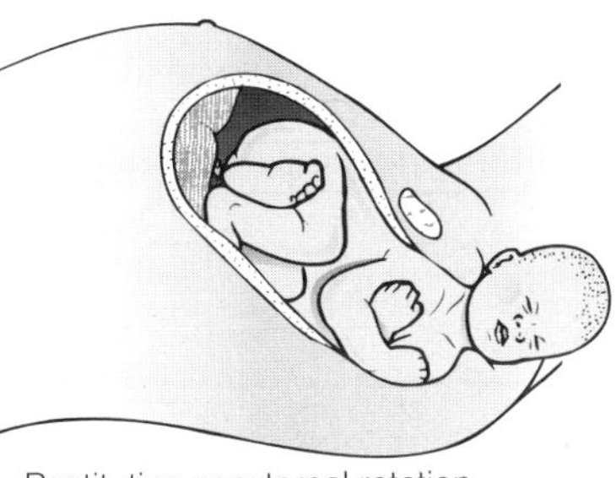

D Complete rotation, early extension

E Complete extension

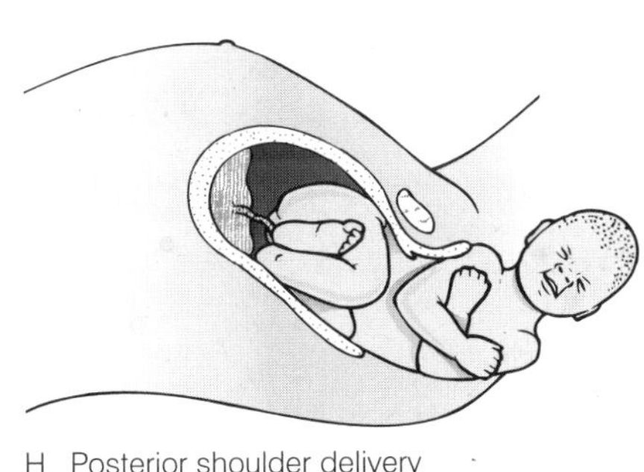

F Restitution or external rotation

G Anterior shoulder delivery

H Posterior shoulder delivery

Figure 3-9 (A–H) Cardinal movements of labor.

dilation is expected in the nulliparous patient and 1.2 cm/hr in the multiparous patient.

The three "Ps," powers, passenger, and pelvis, can all affect the transit time during the active phase of stage 1. The "powers" are determined by the strength and frequency of uterine contractions. The size and position of the infant affects the duration of the active phase as can the size and shape of the maternal pelvis.

Stage 2

When the cervix has completely dilated and the mother begins bearing down or "pushing" during contractions, stage 2 has begun. Stage 2 is completed with delivery of the infant. Stage 2 is considered prolonged if it lasts more than 2 hours in a nulliparous patient, although 3 hours is given in patients with epidurals. In multiparous women, stage 2 is prolonged if it lasts

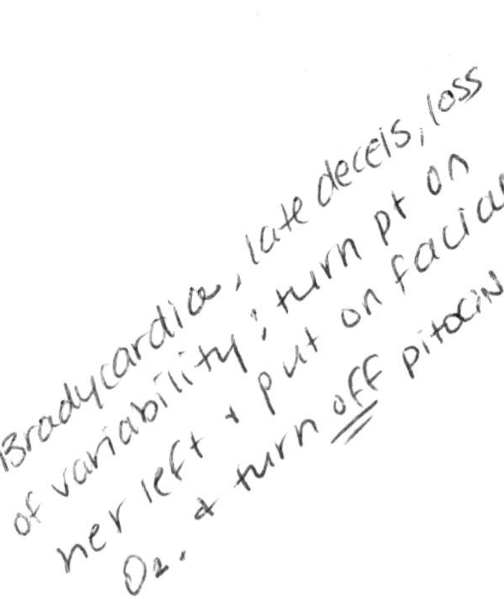

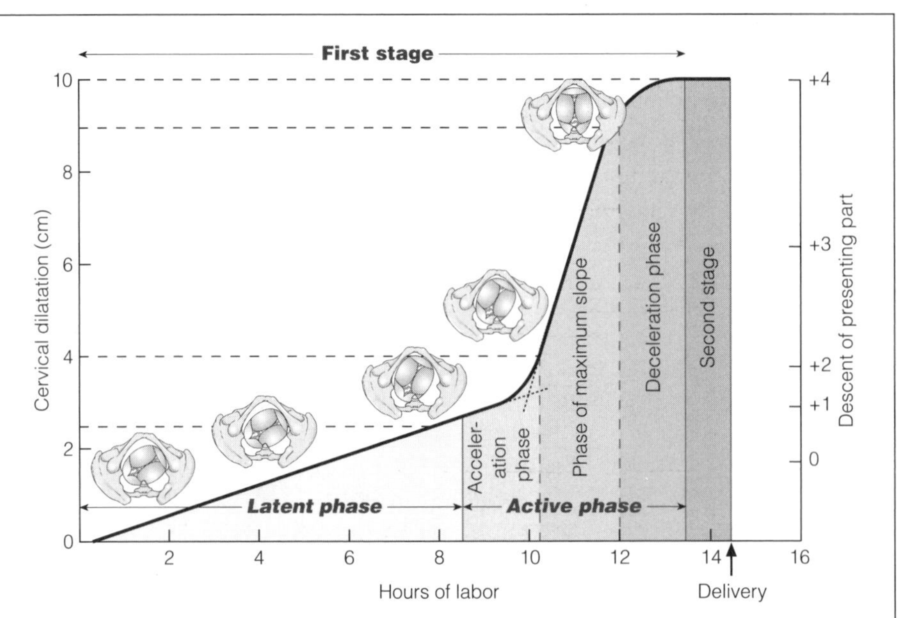

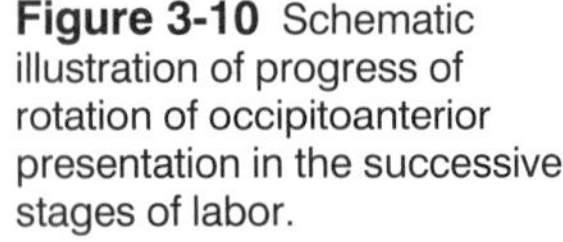

Figure 3-10 Schematic illustration of progress of rotation of occipitoanterior presentation in the successive stages of labor.

longer than 1 hour without an epidural and 2 hours with an epidural. In multiparous women, it is rare for stage 2 to last longer than 30 minutes unless there is macrosomia or malpresentation such as persistent occiput posterior, compound presentation, or asynclitism.

Monitoring Repetitive early and variable decels are common during second stage. The clinician can be reassured if these decels resolve quickly after each contraction and there is no loss of variability in the tracing. Repetitive late decels, bradycardias, and loss of variability are all nonreassuring and signs of fetal distress. With these tracings, the patient should be placed on face mask O_2, turned onto her left side, and, if it is being used, the pitocin should be shut off until the tracing resumes a reassuring pattern.

Vaginal Delivery As the patient begins crowning for a vaginal delivery, the delivering clinician should be dressed with goggles, sterile gown, and sterile gloves (for self-protection rather than prevention of maternal/fetal infection) and have two clamps, scissors, suction bulb, and, in the setting of meconium, a DeLee suction trap. A variety of approaches can be taken to the vaginal delivery, but most clinicians would agree that a smooth controlled delivery leads to less perineal trauma. A modified Ritgen's maneuver (Fig. 3-11) using the heel of the delivering hand to exert pressure on the perineum and to extend the fetal head to hasten delivery and maintain station between contractions may be performed. Simultaneously, the opposite hand should be used to flex the head to keep it from extending too far and causing periurethral and labial lacerations. This hand can also be used to massage the labia over the head during delivery.

Once the head of the infant is delivered, the mouth and upper airway are bulb suctioned. In the setting of meconium in the amniotic fluid, the DeLee suction tube is passed down the infant's nares and mouth and vigorous suctioning is performed before delivery of the

Figure 3-11 Near completion of the delivery of the fetal head by the modified Ritgen maneuver. Moderate upward pressure is applied to the fetal chin by the posterior hand covered with a sterile towel while the suboccipital region of the fetal head is held against the symphysis.

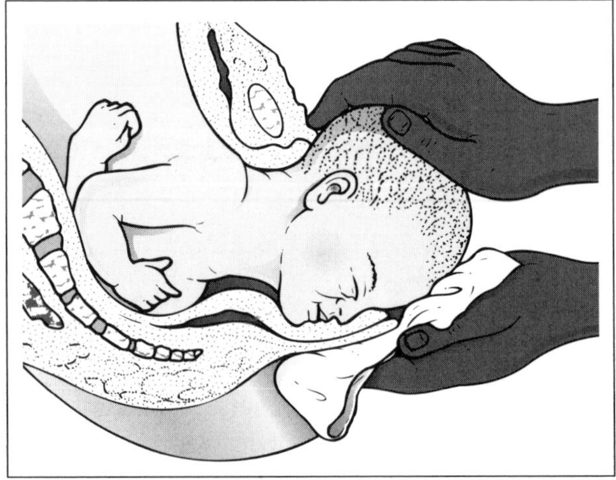

shoulders. After suctioning is completed, the infant's neck is checked for umbilical cord. If a nuccal cord exists, an attempt is made to reduce the cord over the infant's head. If it is too tight, two options exist. If the clinician is extremely confident that delivery will be accomplished shortly, the cord is clamped and cut at this point. If a shoulder dystocia is suspected, an attempt is made to deliver the infant with the nuccal cord intact.

Delivery of the rest of the infant follows first with delivery of the anterior shoulder by exerting direct downward pressure on the infant's head. Once the anterior shoulder is visualized, a direct upward pressure is exerted to deliver the posterior shoulder (Fig. 3-12). After this, exertion of gentle traction will deliver the torso and the rest of the infant. At this point, the cord is clamped and cut and the infant passed off either to the labor nurse and mother or the waiting pediatricians.

Episiotomy An episiotomy is an incision made in the perineum or labia to facilitate delivery. Indications for episiotomy include need to hasten delivery, operative vaginal delivery, and impending shoulder dystocia. A contraindication for episiotomy is assessment that there will be a large perineal laceration. Once the episiotomy is cut, great care should be taken to support the perineum around the episiotomy to avoid extension into the rectal sphincter or rectum itself.

There are two types of episiotomy: median and mediolateral (Fig. 3-13). The median episiotomy uses a vertical midline incision from the posterior forchette and is the most common type used. The mediolateral episiotomy is an oblique incision made from either 5 or 7 o'clock on the vagina. It is used less frequently and reportedly causes more pain and wound infections. However, mediolateral episiotomies are thought to lead to less third- and fourth-degree extensions, particularly in patients with short perineums.

Operative Vaginal Delivery In the setting of prolonged second stage, maternal exhaustion or the need to hasten delivery, an operative vaginal delivery may be indicated. The two possibilities are vacuum-assisted delivery or a forceps delivery. Both are effective methods to facilitate vaginal delivery and have similar indications. The decision of which method to choose is based on knowledge of fetal position and clinician preference and experience.

Forceps Delivery Forceps (Fig. 3-14) have blades that are placed around the infant's head and are shaped with a cephalic curve to accommodate the head. In addition, most have a pelvic curve that conforms to the maternal pelvis. The blade of each forcep is at the end of a shank, which is connected to a handle. The two forceps are connected at the lock, which is between the shank and the handle. Once the forceps are

Figure 3-12 (A) Delivery of the anterior shoulder. (B) Delivery of posterior shoulder.

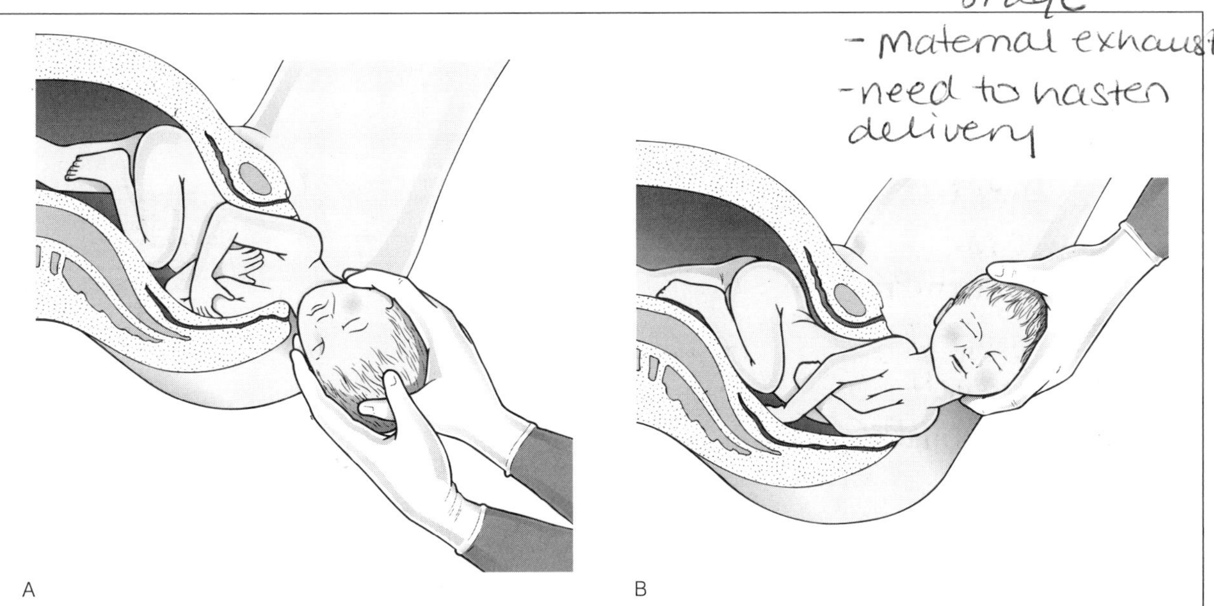

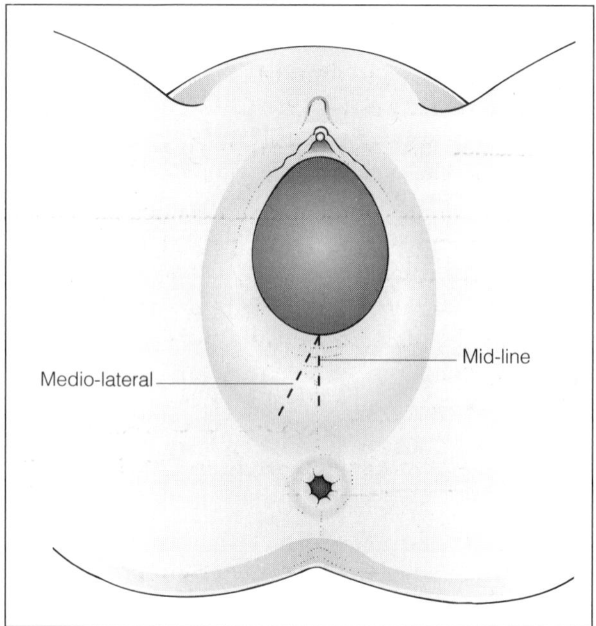

Figure 3-13 Placement of mediolateral and midline episiotomy.

TABLE 3-2

Classification of Forceps Delivery According to Station and Rotation

Type of Procedure	Classification
Outlet forceps	1. Scalp is visible at the introitus without separating the labia 2. Fetal skull has reached pelvic floor 3. Sagittal suture is in anteroposterior diameter or right or left occiput anterior or posterior position 4. Fetal head is at or on perineum 5. Rotation does not exceed 45 degrees
Low forceps	Leading point of fetal skull is at station $\geq \pm 2$ cm, and not on the pelvic floor a. Rotation ≤ 45 degrees (left or right occiput anterior to occiput anterior, or left or right occiput posterior to occiput posterior) b. Rotation >45 degrees
Midforceps	Station above $+2$ cm but head engaged
High	Not included in classification

From Cunningham FG, et al. Williams obstetrics. 19th ed. Norwalk, CT: Appleton & Lange, 1993:557.

placed around the fetal head, the operator pulls on the handles to aid maternal expulsive efforts (Table 3-2).

The conditions necessary for safe application of forceps include full dilation of the cervix, rupture of membranes, head engaged and at least +2 station, absolute knowledge of the position, no evidence of cephalopelvic disproportion, adequate anesthesia, empty bladder, and, most importantly, an experienced operator. Common side effects and complications from forceps application include bruising on the face and head, lacerations to the fetal head at the birth canal, facial nerve palsy, and, rarely, intracranial damage.

Vacuum Extraction The vacuum extractor consists of a vacuum cup that is placed on the fetal scalp and a suction device that is connected to the cup to create the vacuum. Exertion on the cup and consequently on the fetal scalp is made parallel to the axis of

Figure 3-14 Forceps.

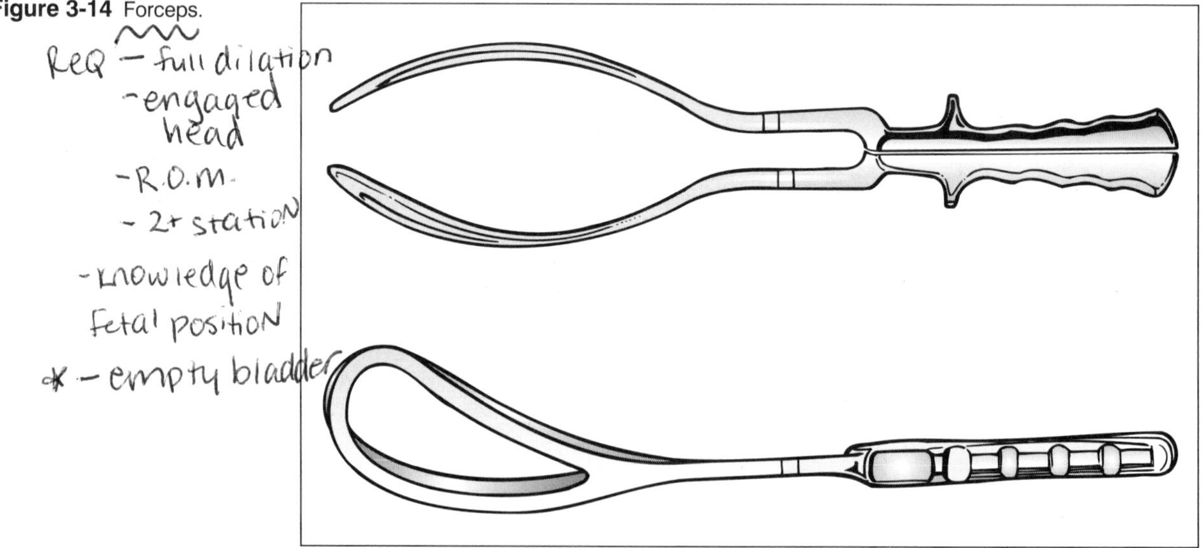

the maternal pelvis concomitant with maternal bearing down efforts and uterine contractions. The most common complications of use of the vacuum are scalp lacerations and cephalohematoma.

Stage 3

Stage 3 begins once the infant has been delivered. It is completed with the delivery of the placenta. Placental separation usually occurs within 5 to 10 minutes of delivery of the infant; however, up to 30 minutes is usually designated within normal limits. With the abrupt decrease in intrauterine cavity size after delivery of the fetus, the placenta is mechanically sheared from the uterine wall with contractions.

The three signs of placental separation include cord lengthening, a gush of blood, and uterine fundal rebound as the placenta is detaching from the uterine wall. Until these signs are noticed, no attempt to deliver the placenta should be made. The placenta is delivered by gentle traction on the cord. It is important not to use too much traction because the cord may tear or uterine inversion may occur.

When the patient begins bearing down for delivery of the placenta, it is imperative that one of the examiner's hands is giving suprapubic pressure to keep the uterus from inverting and prolapsing (Fig. 3-15). When the placenta is evident at the introitus, the delivery should be controlled to avoid both further perineal trauma and tearing of any of the membranes that often trail the placenta at delivery.

Retained Placenta The diagnosis of retained placenta is made when the placenta does not deliver within 30 minutes of the infant. Retained placenta is common in preterm deliveries, particularly previable deliveries. However, it is also a sign of placenta accreta, where the placenta has invaded into or beyond the endometrial stroma. The retained placenta may be removed by manual extraction. A hand is placed in the intrauterine cavity and the fingers used to shear the placenta from the surface of the uterus (Fig. 3-16). If the placenta cannot be completely extracted manually, a curettage is performed to ensure there are no retained POCs.

Laceration Repair Lacerations are repaired after placental delivery. A thorough examination of the perineum, labia, periurethral area, vagina, and cervix is performed to assess lacerations. The most common lacerations are perineal lacerations, which are described by the depth of tissues they involve (Fig. 3-17). A first-degree laceration involves the mucosa or skin. Second-degree lacerations extend into the perineal

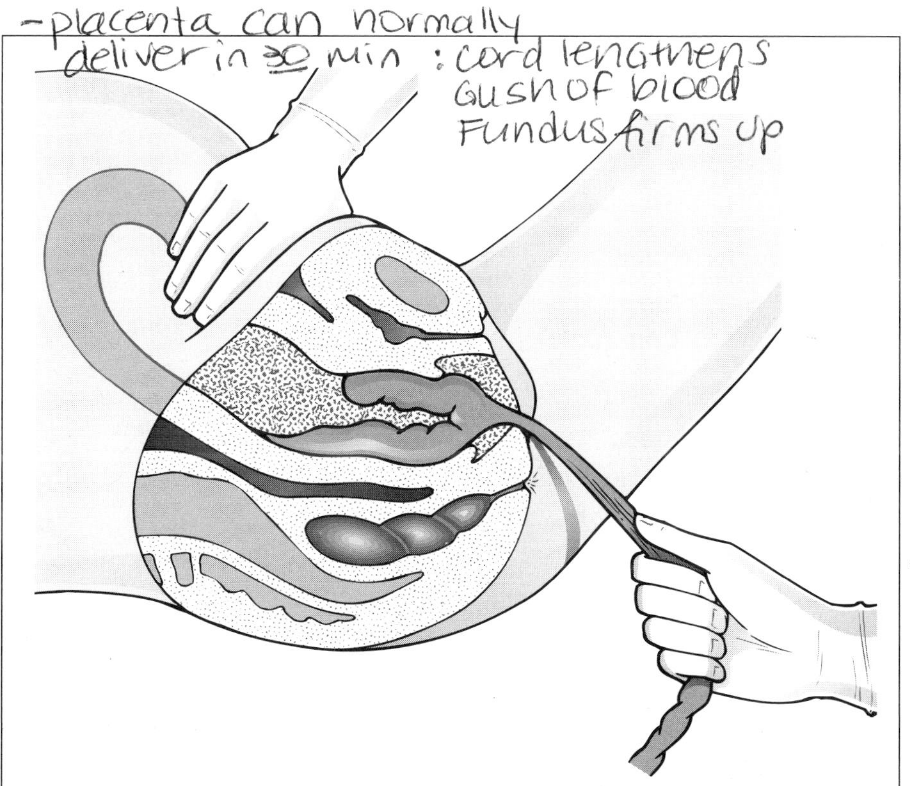

Figure 3-15 Delivery of the placenta with traction on the cord and suprapubic pressure on the internus to prevent uterine inversion.

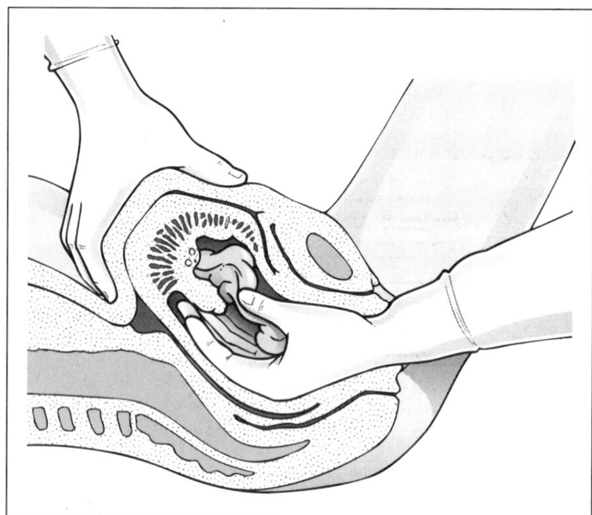

Figure 3-16 Manual removal of placenta. The fingers are alternately abducted, adducted, and advanced until the placenta is completely detached.

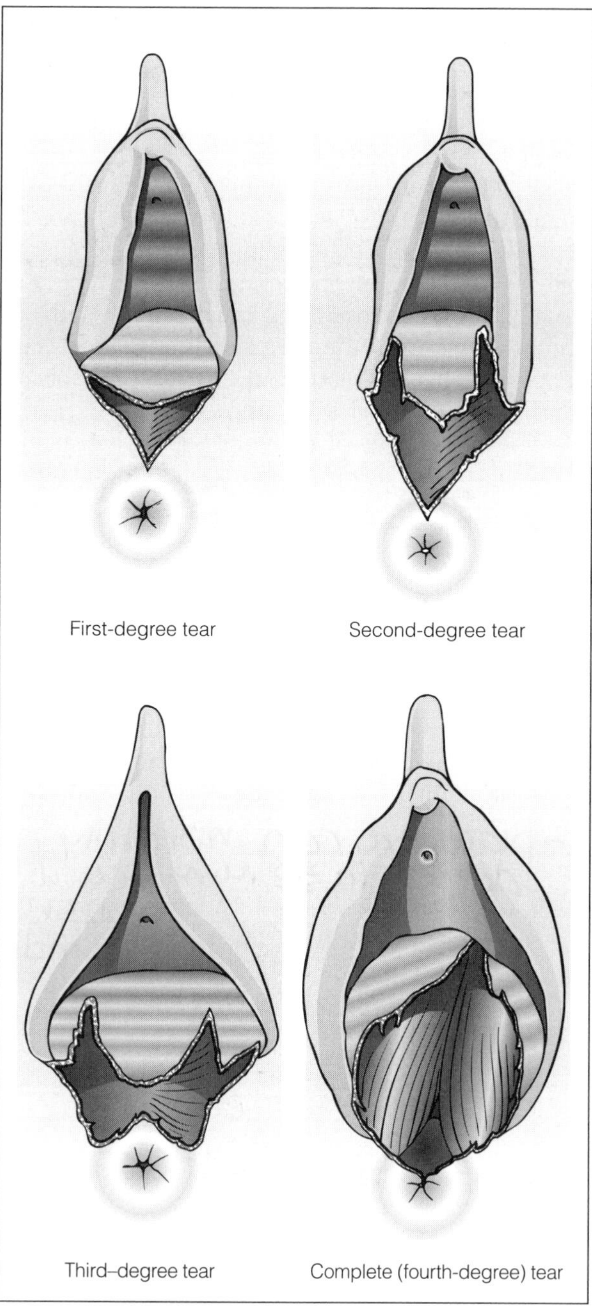

Figure 3-17 Perineal tears.

body but do not involve the anal sphincter. Third-degree lacerations extend into or completely through the anal sphincter, and if the anal mucosa itself is entered it is a fourth-degree tear.

Repair of any superficial lacerations including first-degree perineal tears are usually accomplished with interrupted sutures. The second-degree laceration is repaired in layers. The apex of the laceration, which often lies beyond the hymenal ring, is located and a suture is anchored at the apex. This suture is then run down to the level of the hymenal ring bringing the vaginal tissue together. This suture is then passed beyond the hymenal ring and used to bring the perineal body together. Sometimes a separate suture is used to place a "crown stitch," which brings the perineal body together. Finally, the skin of the perineum is closed with a subcuticular closure (Fig. 3-18).

Third-degree lacerations require repair of the anal sphincter with several interrupted sutures and then the rest of the repair is completed as in a second-degree repair. Fourth-degree repairs are begun with repair of the anal mucosa. Mucosal repair is performed meticulously to prevent fistula formation. Once the rectum is repaired, a fourth-degree laceration is completed as a third-degree repair.

Cesarean Section

Cesarean section has been used effectively throughout this century and is one of the most common operations performed today. Although maternal mortality from cesarean section is low, less than 0.1%, it is still much higher than from vaginal delivery. Furthermore, the morbidity from infections, thrombotic events, wound dehiscence, and increased recovery time is higher than that of vaginal delivery.

The most common indication for primary cesarean section is that of failure to progress in labor. Failure to progress can be caused by problems with any of the three "Ps": powers, pelvis, or passenger. If the pelvis is

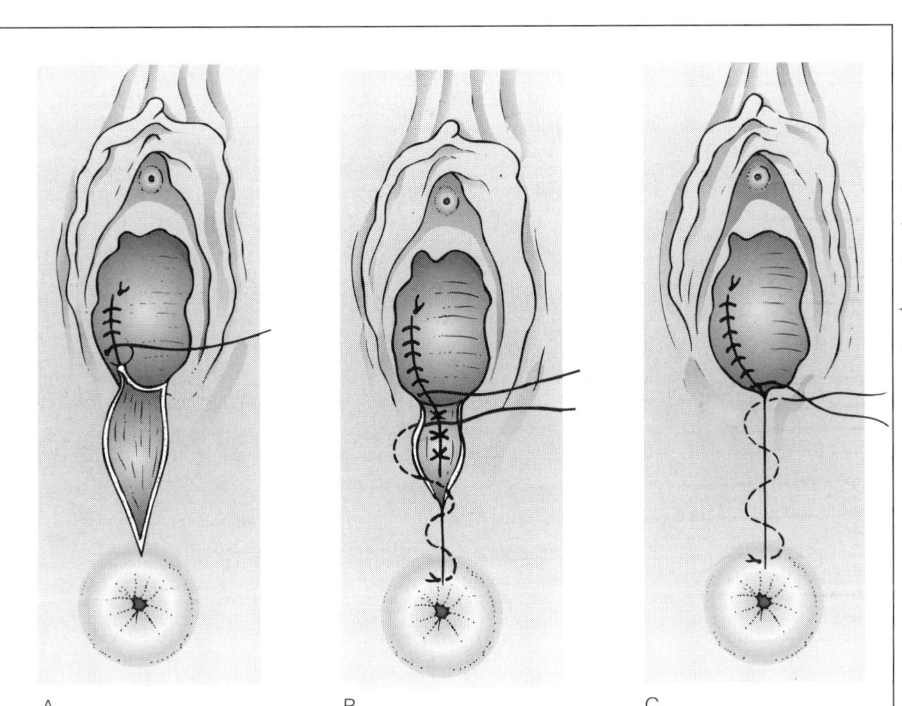

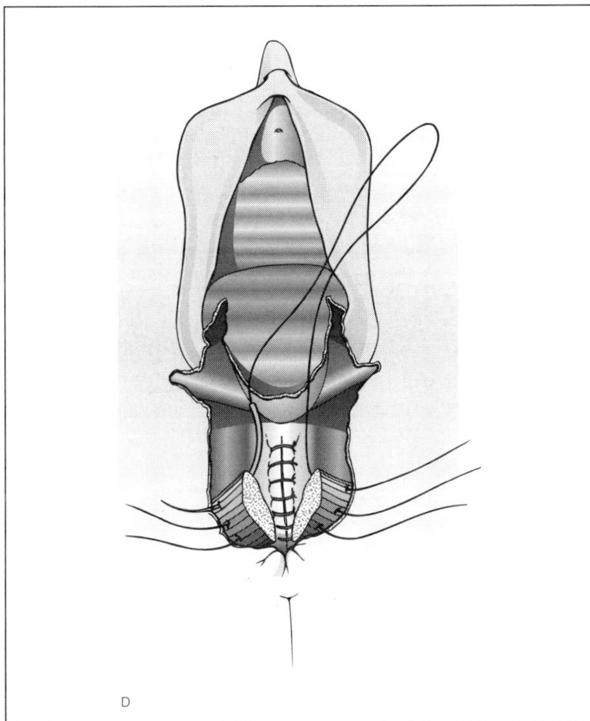

Figure 3-18 (A) Repair of second-degree laceration. (B) Repair of complete perineal tear. The rectal mucosa has been repaired with interrupted, fine chromic catgut sutures. The torn ends of the sphincter ani are next approximated with two or three interrupted chromic catgut sutures. The wound is then repaired, as in a second-degree laceration or an episiotomy.

too small or the fetus too large (depending on the viewpoint taken), the cephalopelvic disproportion (CPD) which results leads to failure to progress. If the uterus simply does not generate enough pressure during contractions, labor can stall and lead to failure to progress. If the labor seems to be stalling, there are a number of measures that can be taken to augment the labor such as pitocin or rupture of membranes.

Other common indications for primary cesarean section (Table 3-3) are breech, shoulder or compound presentation, placenta previa, placental abruption, fetal distress, cord prolapse prolonged second stage, failed operative vaginal delivery, or active herpes lesions. The most common indication for cesarean section is a previous cesarean section.

Vaginal Birth After Cesarean Section

Vaginal birth after cesarean section (VBAC) is commonly attempted with the proper setting. First, the previous hysterotomy needs to be either a Kerr, low horizontal incision, or Kronig, low vertical incision, without any extensions into the cervix or uterine upper segment. The greatest risk in VBAC is that of rupture of the previous uterine scar, which occurs about 1% of the time. Previous classic hysterotomies, or vertical incisions through the thick upper segment of the uterine

TABLE 3-3
Indications for Cesarean Section

Type	Indication
Maternal/fetal	Dystocia
	Cephalopelvic disproportion
	Failed induction of labor
	Abnormal uterine action
Maternal	Maternal diseases
	Eclampsia/severe pre-eclampsia
	Diabetes mellitus
	Cardiac disease
	Cervical cancer
	Previous uterine surgery
	Classic cesarean section
	Previous uterine rupture
	Full-thickness myomectomy
	Obstruction to the birth canal
	Fibroids
	Ovarian tumors
Fetal	Fetal distress
	Cord prolapse
	Fetal malpresentations
	Breech, transverse lie, brow
Placental	Placenta previa
	Abruptio placentae

From Hacker N, Moore JG. Essentials of obstetrics and gynecology. Philadelphia: WB Saunders Company, 1992:309.

corpus, are at a higher risk for uterine rupture in labor and are not allowed to VBAC. Common signs of rupture include abdominal pain, fetal distress, sudden decrease of pressure on an IUPC and a maternal sensation of a "pop" or that something has given away in their abdomen. Thus, the patient needs to be monitored closely in labor and delivered emergently if uterine rupture is suspected.

Key Points

1. Labor is divided into stages: stage 1 until complete cervical dilation, stage 2 until delivery of the infant, and stage 3 until delivery of the placenta.
2. Forceps delivery and vacuum extraction are two forms of operative vaginal delivery.
3. Abdominal delivery is termed cesarean section and is used for delivery of infants who do not deliver vaginally.

▶ OBSTETRIC ANALGESIA AND ANESTHESIA

Natural Childbirth

Much of the pain during labor may actually come from the anticipation of pain and the apprehension that accompanies this event. The idea behind natural childbirth is to educate patients regarding the experiences on labor and delivery to prepare them. In addition, a variety of relaxation techniques, showers, and massage are used to help relax patients. These techniques have been formalized in the Lamaze method, which involves a series of classes for both the patient and a birthing coach that teach both techniques to relax.

Systemic Pharmacologic Intervention

The use of either opiates or sedatives can be useful in the first stage of labor. These medications are useful in relaxing patients and decreasing pain. However, because they cross the placenta, sedating medications should not be used close to the time of expected delivery as they may result in a depressed infant. Other complications of these medications are respiratory depression and increased risk for aspiration.

Pudendal Block

The pudendal nerve travels just posterior to the ischial spine at its juncture with the sacrospinous ligament. With the pudendal block, anesthetic is injected at that site, bilaterally, to give perineal anesthesia. Common use is in the setting of operative vaginal delivery with either forceps or vacuum. It may be combined with local infiltration of the perineum to ensure perineal anesthesia (Fig. 3-19).

Local Anesthesia

In patients without anesthesia who are going to require an episiotomy, local infiltration with an anesthetic is used. Local anesthetic is also used before repair of lacerations.

Epidural and Spinal Anesthesia

Epidurals are commonly performed for patients who wish anesthesia throughout the active phase and delivery of the infant. Many patients have worries about nerve damage and the pain of the epidural itself. An early consult with an anesthesiologist to help answer questions about the epidural can be reassuring. The epidural catheter is then placed in the L3–4 interspace when the patient is requiring analgesia, although usually not until labor is deemed to be in the active phase. Once the catheter is placed, an initial bolus of anesthetic is given and a continuous infusion is started. Again, the epidural does not commonly remove all sensation and can actually be detrimental to the second stage if it does so. However, if the patient requires cesarean delivery, the epidural can be bolused and usually provides adequate anesthesia.

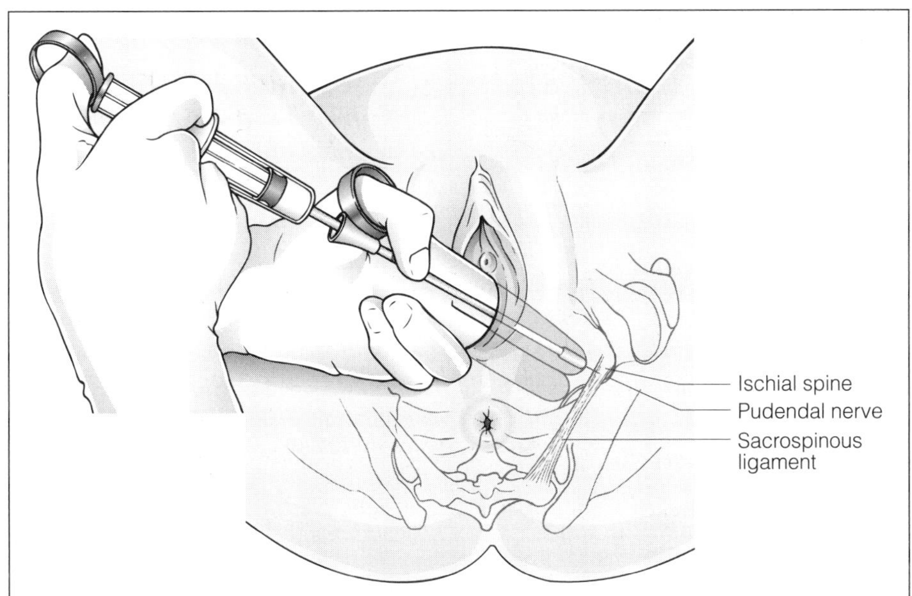

Figure 3-19 Technique for transvaginal pudendal block.

Spinal anesthesia provides anesthesia over a similar region to an epidural; however, it is given in a one-time dose. It is used more commonly for cesarean section than vaginal delivery. A common complication of both forms of anesthesia are maternal hypotension leading to decreased placental perfusion and fetal bradycardia. A more serious complication can be maternal respiratory depression if the anesthetic level goes high enough to affect diaphragmatic innervation. A spinal headache due to the loss of cerebrospinal fluid is a postpartum complication seen in less than 1% of the patients.

General Anesthesia

Although this is rarely used for vaginal delivery, it is used not uncommonly for cesarean section, particularly in the setting of emergent cesarean section. For less urgent cesarean sections, epidural or spinal anesthesia is usually preferred. The two principal concerns of general anesthesia are the risk of maternal aspiration and the risk of hypoxia to mother and fetus during induction. Thus, when choosing the anesthetic for a cesarean section, the urgency of the delivery must be assessed. Common reasons for an emergent cesarean section are abruption, fetal bradycardia, uterine rupture, and hemorrhage from a placenta previa.

Key Points

1. Obstetrical anesthesia allows for more control during the second stage of labor, but can decrease the ability to push.
2. Epidurals are commonly used for labor while spinals are used for cesarean section. Occasionally general anesthesia is used in the emergent setting.

- Opiates/sedatives cross placenta!
- pudendal Block: perineal anesthesia → usually w/ forceps or vacuum
- epidural: @ L-3/4

Spinal: one time dose for section
- maternal hypotension → ↓ placental perfusion + fetal brady.

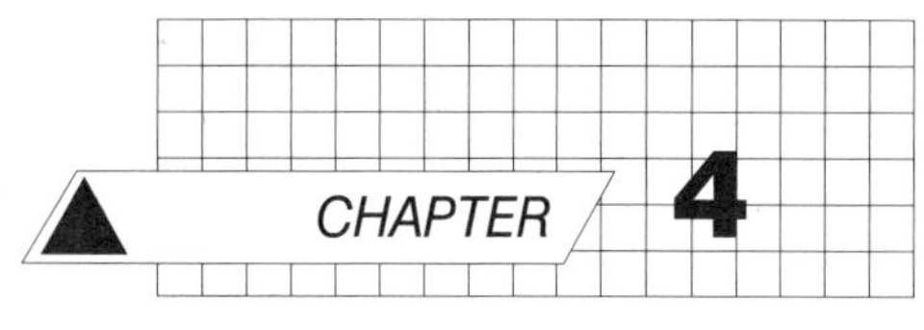

Antepartum Hemorrhage

Hemorrhage is a leading cause of maternal death in the United States and one of the leading causes of perinatal morbidity and mortality. Third trimester vaginal bleeding occurs in 3 to 4% of pregnancies and may be obstetric or nonobstetric (Table 4-1). The major causes of antepartum hemorrhage include placenta previa (20%) and placental abruption (30%).

▶ PLACENTA PREVIA

Pathogenesis

Placenta previa is defined as the abnormal implantation of the placenta over the internal cervical os (Fig. 4-1). **Complete previa** occurs when the placenta completely covers the internal os. **Partial previa** occurs when the placenta covers a portion of the internal os. **Marginal previa** occurs when the edge of the placenta reaches the margin of the os. A low-lying placenta is a placenta that is implanted in the lower uterine segment but does not extend to the internal os.

Bleeding from a placenta previa results from small disruptions in the placental attachment during normal development and thinning of the lower uterine segment during the third trimester. As a result, profuse hemorrhage and shock can occur, leading to significant maternal and fetal mortality and morbidity. Although the maternal and perinatal mortality from placenta previa has dropped rapidly over the past few decades, the perinatal mortality rate is still 10 times that in the general population. Most risk to the fetus comes from **premature delivery,** which is responsible for 60% of perinatal deaths. Other fetal risks associated with placenta previa are shown in Table 4-2.

Placenta previa may also be complicated by an associated **placenta accreta** (placenta previa accreta). Placental accreta is defined as the abnormal invasion of the placenta into the uterine wall. An **accreta** is defined as the superficial invasion of the placenta into the uterine myometrium. An **increta** occurs when the placenta invades the myometrium. A **percreta** occurs when the placenta invades through the myometrium to the uterine serosa.

Placenta accreta causes an inability of the placenta to separate from the uterine wall after delivery of the fetus. This can result in profuse hemorrhage and shock with substantial maternal morbidity and mortality. Two thirds of women with both a placenta previa and an associated accreta require a hysterectomy at the time of delivery (gravid hysterectomy). Table 4-3 summarizes the abnormalities of placentation.

Epidemiology

Placenta previa occurs in 0.5% of pregnancies (1 in 200 births) and accounts for nearly 20% of all antepartum hemorrhages. Placenta previa can also be complicated by an associated placenta accreta (placenta previa accreta) in up to 15% of cases.

Risk Factors

Abnormalities in placentation are the result of events that prevent normal migration of the placenta during normal progressive development of the lower uterine

TABLE 4-1
Differential Diagnosis of Antepartum Bleeding

Obstetric causes	
Placental:	Placenta previa, abruptio placentae, circumvallate placenta
Maternal:	Uterine rupture, clotting disorders
Fetal:	Fetal vessel rupture
Nonobstetric causes	
Cervical:	Severe cervicitis, polyps, benign and malignant neoplasms
Vaginal:	Lacerations, varices, benign and malignant neoplasms
Other:	Congenital bleeding disorder, abdominal or pelvic trauma

Adapted from Hacker N, Moore JG. Essentials of obstetrics and gynecology. Philadelphia: WB Saunders, 1992:155.

TABLE 4-2
Fetal Complications Associated with Placenta Previa

Preterm delivery and its complications
Preterm premature rupture of membranes
Intrauterine growth restriction
Malpresentation
Vasa previa
Congenital abnormalities

Adapted from Hacker N, Moore JG. Essentials of obstetrics and gynecology. Philadelphia: WB Saunders, 1992:155.

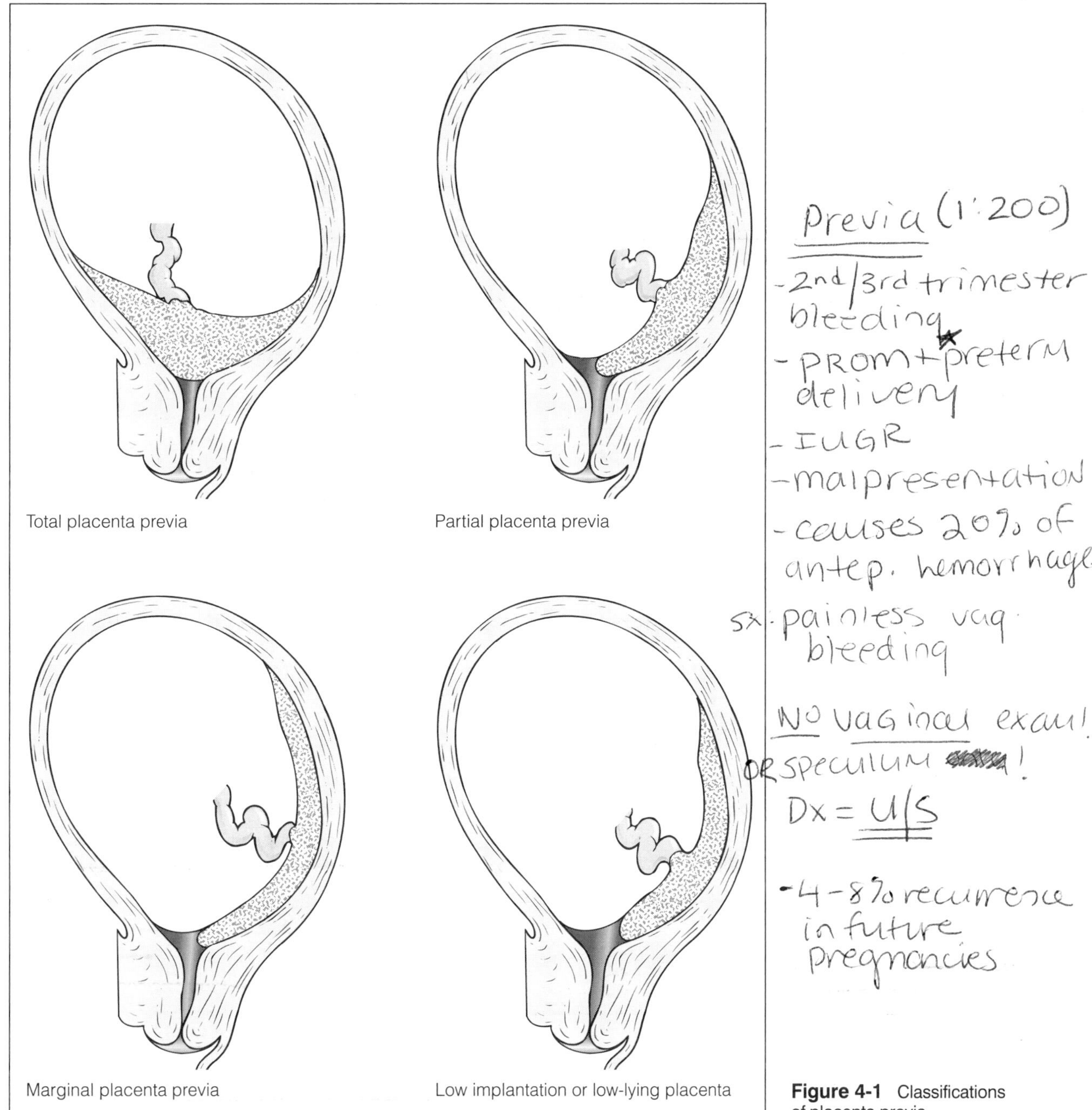

Figure 4-1 Classifications of placenta previa.

segment during pregnancy. **Previous placental implantations and prior uterine scars** are thought to contribute to abnormal placentation in subsequent pregnancies. These factors contribute to the increased rate of placenta previa associated with multiparity, advanced maternal age, and prior cesarean sections. Other factors that predispose to placenta previa include **large placentas** (as seen in multiple gestation pregnancies and erythroblastosis) and **smoking** (affects placental migration). The risk factors for placenta previa are shown in Table 4-4.

Clinical Manifestations

History

Placenta previa classically presents with sudden and profuse **painless vaginal bleeding**. The first episode of

TABLE 4-3
Abnormalities of Placentation

Placenta circumvallata	One in which the membranes double back over the edge of the placenta, forming a dense ring around the periphery of the placenta. Often considered a variant of placental abruption, it is a major cause of second trimester hemorrhage.
Placenta previa	Obstetric complication where the placenta develops over the internal cervical os. Types include complete/total, partial, and marginal.
Placenta accreta	Abnormal adherence of part or all of the placenta to the uterine wall. May be associated with a normally implanted placenta or a placenta previa.
Placenta increta	Placenta accreta where the placenta invades the myometrium. May be associated with a normally implanted placenta or a placenta previa.
Placenta percreta	Placental accreta where the placenta invades through the myometrium to the uterine serosa. May be associated with a normally implanted placenta or a placenta previa.
Vasa previa	Condition where a velamentous cord insertion causes the fetal vessels to pass over the internal cervical os. See also velamentous placenta.
Velamentous placenta	One where the blood vessels insert between the amnion and the chorion away from the margin of the placenta. This leaves the vessels largely unprotected and vulnerable to compression or injury. See also vasa previa.

TABLE 4-4
Predisposing Factors for Placenta Previa

Prior cesarean section
Multiparity
Increasing maternal age
Multiple gestation
Erythroblastosis
Smoking
History of placenta previa

bleeding, the "sentinel" bleed, usually occurs after the 28th week of gestation. During this time, the lower uterine segment develops and thins, causing disruption in the placental attachment and resulting in bleeding. Placenta accretas are usually asymptomatic.

Physical Examination

Vaginal examination is contraindicated in placenta previa because the digital examination can cause further separation of the placenta and trigger catastrophic hemorrhage.

Diagnostic Evaluation

The diagnosis of placenta previa can be made by **ultrasonography** with an accuracy rate of 95%.

Treatment

Unstoppable labor, fetal distress, and life-threatening hemorrhage are indications for immediate cesarean delivery regardless of gestational age. In the case of preterm pregnancy, if the bleeding is not profuse, fetal survival can be enhanced by aggressive expectant management. However, 70% of patients with placenta previa will have a recurrent bleeding episode and will require delivery before 36 weeks gestation.

The following should be done in the case of suspected placenta previa:

1. **Stabilize the patient.** Every patient with vaginal bleeding and a known or suspected previa should be hospitalized, the bleeding controlled, and fetal monitoring started. In an Rh-negative woman, a Kleihauer-Betke test should be performed to determine the extent of any fetomaternal transfusion so that the appropriate amount of RhoGAM can be administered to prevent isoimmunization.
2. **Prepare for future catastrophic hemorrhage.** Expectant management in the stabilized patient includes hospitalization, bedrest, and hematocrit monitoring. Two or more units of blood should be typed, cross-matched, and made available and coagulation studies should be sent. Transfusions should be given to maintain a hematocrit of 30% or greater.
3. **Prepare for premature delivery.** In the preterm pregnancy, beta-methasone may be given to promote fetal lung maturity and tocolysis may be given to assist in prolonging the pregnancy to at least 36 weeks.
4. **Deliver via cesarean section.** In patients who reach 36 weeks gestation without having another bleed, the fetal lung maturity should be checked. If mature indices are obtained, then the patient should be delivered by cesarean section to reduce the risk of repeat hemorrhage.

Follow-Up

Patients with placenta previa have a 4 to 8% risk of having a previa in a subsequent pregnancy.

Key Points

Placenta previa

1. Accounts for 20% of antepartum hemorrhage;
2. Usually presents in the third trimester with painless vaginal bleeding;
3. Is diagnosed by transabdominal ultrasound;
4. Is not diagnosed by vaginal examination; this must be avoided;
5. Patients should be delivered by cesarean section;
6. Has an increased risk of gravid hysterectomy when both placenta previa and placenta accreta are present.

▶ PLACENTAL ABRUPTION

Pathogenesis

Placental abruption (abruptio placentae) is the premature separation of the normally implanted placenta from the uterine wall. It results in hemorrhage between the uterine wall and the placenta. Fifty percent of abruptions occur after the 30th week of gestation, 15% occur during delivery, and 30% are identified only on placental inspection after delivery. Large placental separations may result in premature delivery, uterine tetany, disseminated intravascular coagulation (DIC), and hypovolemic shock. Fetal death from placental abruption occurs in about 1 in 500 deliveries.

The primary cause of placental abruption is unknown although it is associated with a variety of predisposing and precipitating factors (Table 4-5). Of these, maternal hypertension is most commonly associated with placental abruption. Other factors include prior history of placental abruption, external maternal trauma, and rapid decompression of the overdistended uterus.

At the initial point of separation, nonclotted blood courses from the injury site. The enlarging collection of blood may cause further separation of the placenta. In 20% of placental separations, bleeding is confined within the uterine cavity and is referred to as a **concealed hemorrhage** (Fig. 4-2). In the remaining 80% of placental separations, the blood dissects downward toward the cervix, resulting in a **revealed or external hemorrhage**. Because there is an egress for the blood, revealed hemorrhages are less likely than concealed hemorrhages to result in larger retroplacental clots. These clots can cause more complete separation of the placenta and are associated with fetal demise. The result of hemorrhage from torn placental vessels can vary from maternal anemia in mild cases to shock, acute renal failure, and maternal death in severe cases. Twenty percent of patients with placental abruption will develop clinically significant DIC due to the release of thromboplastin into the maternal circulation.

TABLE 4-5

Predisposing and Precipitating Factors for Placental Abruption

- Predisposing factors
  - Hypertension
  - Previous placental separation
  - Advanced maternal age
  - Multiparity
  - Uterine distention
    - Multiple pregnancy
    - Hydramnios
  - Vascular deficiency
    - Diabetes mellitus
    - Collagen vascular disease
  - Cocaine use
  - Cigarette smoking
  - Alcohol use (>14 drinks/wk)
- Precipitating factors
  - Trauma
    - External/internal version
    - Motor vehicle accident
    - Abdominal trauma
  - Placenta circumvallata
  - Sudden uterine volume loss
    - Delivery of first twin
    - Rupture of membranes in hydramnios
  - Preterm premature rupture of membranes
  - Short umbilical cord

Maternal mortality from placental abruption varies from 0.5 to 5%. Most deaths are due to hemorrhage, cardiac failure, or renal failure. **Fetal mortality** occurs in about 35% of all placental abruptions and can be as high as 50 to 80% in cases of severe placental abruption. The cause of demise is due to hypoxia resulting from decreased placental surface area and maternal hemorrhage.

Epidemiology

Placental abruption occurs in about 1 in 120 pregnancies and is responsible for 30% of cases of third trimester bleeding and 15% of perinatal mortality.

Risk Factors

The predisposing and precipitating factors for placental abruption are listed in Table 4-5. The most common factor associated with increased incidence of abruption is hypertension whether it is chronic or a result of pre-eclampsia. In cases of abruption that are severe enough to cause fetal death, 50% are due to hypertension and, of these, half are from chronic hypertension and half are from pre-eclampsia.

Clinical Manifestation

History

The classic presentation of placental abruption is third trimester vaginal bleeding associated with severe abdominal pain. However, about 30% of placental separations are small with few or no symptoms and are identified only after inspection of the placenta at delivery. The signs and symptoms of abruption are shown in Table 4-6.

Figure 4-2 Types of placental separation. Reproduced by permission from DeCherney A, Pernoll M. Current obstetric and gynecologic diagnosis and treatment. Norwalk, CT: Appleton and Lange, 1992:400.

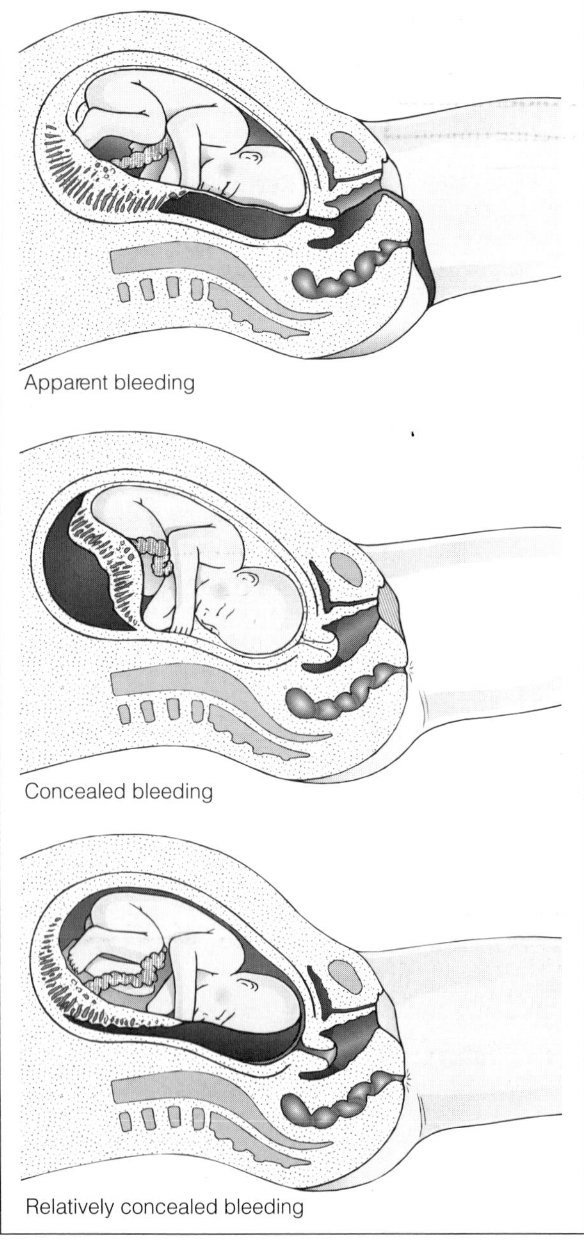

Physical Examination

On physical examination, a patient with placental abruption will have a firm tender uterus and signs of fetal distress due to decreased blood flow.

Diagnostic Evaluation

The diagnosis of placental abruption is primarily a clinical one. Only 2% of abruptions are picked up by **ultrasound** (evidenced by a retroplacental clot). However, because abruption can occur simultaneously with a placenta previa, ultrasonography is routinely performed to rule out previa in cases of suspected abruption. The diagnosis of abruption may be confirmed by inspection of the placenta at delivery. The presence of a retroplacental clot with underlying placental destruction confirms the diagnosis.

Treatment

The potential for rapid deterioration (hemorrhage, DIC, fetal hypoxia) necessitates delivery in some cases of placental abruption. However, most abruptions are small, not catastrophic, and therefore do not necessitate immediate delivery.

The following should be done in the case of suspected placental abruption:

1. **Stabilize the patient.** When placental abruption is known or suspected, the patient should be hospitalized, the bleeding controlled, and fetal monitoring started. In an Rh-negative woman, RhoGAM should be administered to prevent isoimmunization.
2. **Prepare for possibility of future hemorrhage.** Standard antishock measures should be taken, including placement of large-bore intravenous

TABLE 4-6

Presentation of Abruptio Placentae

Symptom	Occurrence (%)
Vaginal bleeding	80
Uterine tenderness/abdominal or back pain	67
Abnormal contractions/increased uterine tone	34
Fetal distress	50
Fetal demise	15

catheters, infusion of lactated Ringer's solution, and preparation of units of crossed-matched blood (whole or packed red blood cells). It is a common mistake to markedly underestimate the volume of blood lost in a placental abruption.

3. **Prepare for premature delivery.** In the preterm pregnancy, beta-methasone may be given to promote fetal lung maturity and tocolysis may be given to assist in prolonging the pregnancy to at least 36 weeks. The patient should remain hospitalized and on bedrest to minimize the likelihood of another hemorrhage.
4. **Deliver if baby is mature or bleeding is life-threatening.** Delivery should be performed in patients with a life-threatening hemorrhage and in patients who reach 36 weeks gestation with verification of fetal lung maturity. Vaginal delivery is preferred as long as bleeding is controlled and there are no signs of fetal distress. Because the uterus is typically hyperactive in patients with an abruption, a rapid labor and delivery should be expected.

Follow-Up

The risk of abruption in future pregnancy is 10% after one abruption and 25% after two abruptions.

Key Points

Placental abruption

1. Accounts for 30% of all third trimester hemorrhages;
2. Has a fetal mortality rate as high as 35%;
3. Usually presents with vaginal bleeding, painful contractions, and a firm tender uterus; 20% of cases present with no bleeding (concealed hemorrhages);
4. Has major risk factors of hypertension (chronic or pregnancy-induced) and previous history of abruption;
5. Can be complicated by hypovolemic shock, DIC, and premature delivery;
6. Patients should be delivered vaginally;
7. Has a high risk of recurrence in subsequent pregnancies.

▶ UTERINE RUPTURE

Pathogenesis

Uterine rupture represents a potential obstetric catastrophe and is a major cause of maternal death. Most complete uterine ruptures occur during the course of labor. Forty percent of all uterine ruptures are associated with a **prior uterine scar** either from cesarean section or other uterine surgery. In the remaining 60% of cases, no prior scarring is present. These ruptures may be related to an **abdominal trauma** (auto accidents, external or internal version procedures), associated with **labor or delivery** (improper oxytocin use, forceps, excessive fundal pressure), or **spontaneously initiated** (placenta percreta, multiple gestation, grand multiparity, invasive mole, choriocarcinoma).

The primary maternal complications from a ruptured uterus include hemorrhage and hypovolemic shock. The overall maternal mortality for uterine rupture is 10 to 15%. The perinatal mortality for uterine rupture ranges from 30 to 50%.

Epidemiology

Uterine rupture is rare, occurring in 0.5% of deliveries.

Risk Factors

Risk factors for uterine rupture are conditions that predispose to a weakened uterine wall, including uterine scars, overdistention, and abnormal placentation (Table 4-7).

Clinical Manifestations

The presentation of uterine rupture is highly variable. Typically, it is characterized by the sudden onset of intense abdominal pain. Vaginal bleeding, if present, may vary from spotting to severe hemorrhage. Fetal distress, abnormal abdominal contouring, cessation of uterine contractions, disappearance of fetal heart tones, and regression of the presenting part are other signs of uterine rupture.

Treatment

Management of uterine rupture requires immediate laparotomy. Classically, **total abdominal hysterectomy is the treatment of choice.** However, in certain cases, it is reasonable to close the site primarily. Future

TABLE 4-7

Risk Factors for Uterine Rupture

Prior uterine scarring
Injudicious use of oxytocin
Grand multiparity
Marked uterine distention
Abnormal fetal lie
Large fetus
External version
Trauma

pregnancy should be discouraged given the high risk for recurrent rupture.

Key Points

Uterine rupture

1. Is a rare obstetric catastrophe;
2. Represents a major cause of maternal death;
3. Has a maternal mortality of 10 to 15% and a fetal mortality of 30 to 50%;
4. Is associated with prior uterine scarring in 40% of cases;
5. Presents with the sudden onset of intense abdominal pain;
6. Usually requires a total abdominal hysterectomy.

▶ FETAL VESSEL RUPTURE

Pathogenesis

Most pregnancies complicated by rupture of a fetal vessel are due to velamentous cord insertion where the blood vessels insert between the amnion and chorion away from the placenta instead of inserting directly into the chorionic plate (see Table 4-3). Because the vessels course unprotected through the membranes before inserting on the placental margin, they are vulnerable to rupture, shearing, or laceration. In addition, these unprotected vessels may cross over the internal cervical os, making them vulnerable to compression by the presenting fetal part or to being torn when the membranes are ruptured. When the vessels cross over the internal cervical os, this is known as vasa previa. Although vasa previa are rare, the perinatal mortality is 50% and increases to 75% if the membranes are also ruptured.

Epidemiology

Only 0.1 to 0.8% of pregnancies are complicated by the rupture of a fetal vessel. The incident rate for vasa previa is 1 in every 5,000 pregnancies.

Risk Factors

The main risk factor for fetal vessel rupture is multiple gestation. Although the rate of velamentous insertion is only 1% in singleton gestations, it increases to 10% for twin gestations and 50% for triplet gestation pregnancies.

Clinical Manifestations

In fortunate cases, the fetal vessels are palpated and recognized through the dilated cervix. More commonly, the presentation of a fetal vessel rupture is vaginal bleeding associated with a sinusoidal variation of the fetal heart rate

Treatment

Given the high risk of fetal exsanguination and death (the vascular volume of the term fetus is less than 250 mL), the treatment for a ruptured fetal vessel is emergency cesarean delivery

Key Points

Fetal vessel rupture

1. Is a rare obstetric complication, usually associated with multiple gestation;
2. Is due primarily to velamentous cord insertion;
3. Is associated with a perinatal mortality of 50%;
4. Can present with vaginal bleeding and a sinusoidal fetal heart rate pattern;
5. Usually requires an emergency cesarean section.

▶ NONOBSTETRIC CAUSES OF ANTEPARTUM HEMORRHAGE

Nonobstetric causes of antepartum hemorrhage are listed in Table 4-1. These conditions usually present with spotting rather than frank bleeding. Typically, there are no uterine contractions or abdominal pain. The diagnosis is usually made by speculum examination, pap smear, cultures, or colposcopy as indicated. Other than advanced maternal neoplasia, which is associated with poor maternal outcome, most nonobstetric causes of antepartum hemorrhage require relatively simple management and have good outcomes. Vaginal lacerations and varices can be located and repaired. Infections may be treated with appropriate agents, and benign neoplasms usually require simple treatment.

Key Points

Nonobstetric causes of antepartum hemorrhage

1. Include cervical and vaginal lacerations, infections, and neoplasms;
2. Typically present with spotting rather than frank bleeding;
3. Generally require simple management and have good outcomes.

CHAPTER 5

Complications of Labor and Delivery

▶ PRETERM LABOR

Labor that occurs before 37 weeks gestation is **preterm labor**. Many patients present with preterm contractions, but only those patients who change their cervix have preterm labor. Preterm labor also is different from **incompetent cervix**, which is silent painless dilatation of the cervix. Both lead to preterm delivery, which is the number one cause of fetal morbidity and mortality in the United States.

Preterm Delivery

Infants born before 37 weeks of gestation are termed premature and have higher rates of morbidity and mortality. Infants are also at risk when they are born weighing less than 2,500 g, termed **low-birth-weight** (LBW) infants. Infants that have not grown appropriately for gestational age are termed **intrauterine growth restricted** (IUGR). Thus, an IUGR baby can be born after 37 weeks but still be LBW. Prematurity puts infants at increased risk of respiratory distress syndrome (RDS) or hyaline membrane disease, intraventricular hemorrhage, sepsis, and necrotizing enterocolitis. The complications and mortality are dramatically affected by gestational age and birthweight. Infants born on the cusp of viability at 24 weeks gestation have a greater than 85% mortality rate, whereas infants born after 36 weeks are quite similar to full-term infants (Fig. 5-1).

Etiology and Risk Factors

Because the defining physiologic mechanism that causes the onset of labor is unknown, the same is true for **preterm labor**. However, there are a variety of risk factors that can be correlated with preterm labor. These include preterm rupture of membranes, chorioamnionitis, multiple gestations, uterine anomalies such as a bicornuate uterus, previous preterm delivery, maternal prepregnancy weight less than 50 kg, placental abruption, maternal disease including pre-eclampsia, infections, intra-abdominal disease or surgery, and low socioeconomic class.

Tocolysis

Tocolysis is the attempt to prevent contractions and the progression of labor. Many tocolytics have been shown only to be effective for an average of 48 hours. The principal benefit from gaining 48 hours in a pregnancy is to allow treatment with steroids. **Betamethasone**, a glucocorticoid, has been shown to reduce the incidence of RDS and other complications from preterm delivery. Thus, before 34 weeks of gestation, the advantage of treating with steroids needs to be weighed against the risk of prolonging the pregnancy. In the setting of preterm rupture of membranes, tocolysis is generally used up to 32 weeks gestation. However, there are many situations in which preterm labor should be allowed to progress. Chorioamnionitis, fetal death, or distress and placental abruption are absolute indications to allow labor to progress and often to hasten delivery. With many other issues such as maternal disease, particularly pre-eclampsia, or in the setting of poor placental perfusion, an assessment of the severity of the situation, the precipitous nature of the complication, the risks from prematurity, and the clinician's prior experience all contribute to the decision of whether or not to tocolyze.

Tocolytics

The goal of tocolytics is to decrease contractions or at least decrease or halt the cervical change resulting from contractions. In the setting of preterm contractions without cervical change, hydration can often decrease the number and strength of the contractions. This works along the principle that a dehydrated patient has increased levels of vasopressin or **antidiuretic hormone** (ADH), the octapeptide synthesized in the hypothalamus along with oxytocin. ADH may cross-react with oxytocin receptors and lead to contractions. Thus, hydration, which decreases the level of ADH, may also decrease the number of contractions. In patients who do not respond to hydration or who are actively changing their cervix, there are a variety of tocolytics that have been used.

Beta-mimetics

Uterine myometrium is composed of smooth muscle fibers. The contraction of these fibers is regulated by myosin light chain kinase, which is activated by calcium ions through their interaction with calmodulin. Thus, by increasing the level of cAMP, the level of free calcium ions decrease, likely by sequestration in sarcoplasmic

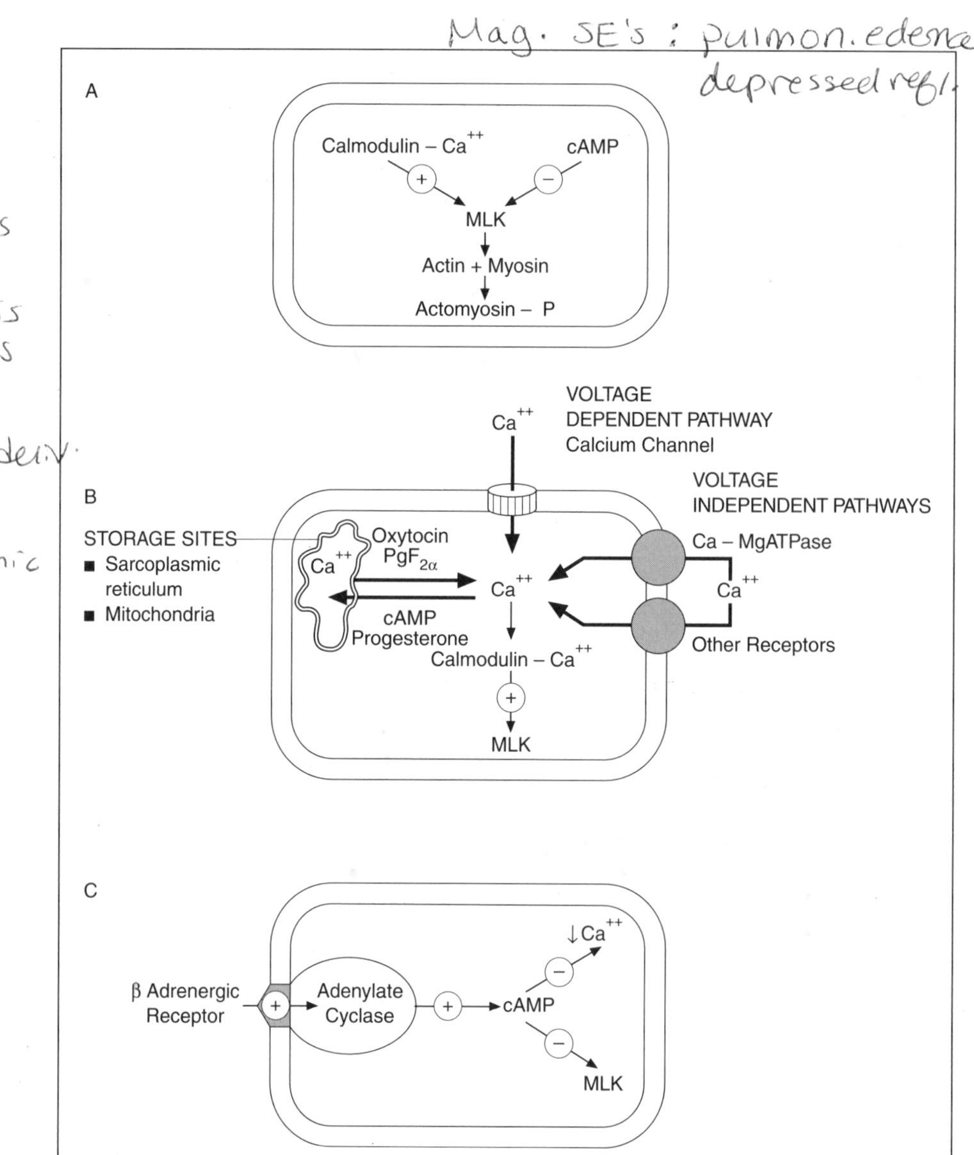

Figure 5-1 Control of myometrial contractility: myosin light-chain kinase (MLK) is the key enzyme.

reticulum, and uterine contractions may be decreased. ATP to cAMP conversion is increased by β-agonists which bind and activate β_2 receptors on myometrial cells.

The two commonly used **beta-mimetics** in the setting of preterm labor are **ritodrine** and **terbutaline**. Although both are certainly effective in halting preterm contractions, in randomized controlled studies where patients were truly in preterm labor, β-agonists gained an average of only 24 to 48 hours further gestation over hydration and bedrest alone. In addition, there are a variety of side effects from use of these drugs, including tachycardia, headaches, and anxiety. More seriously, **pulmonary edema** is a dangerous side effect, and rarely maternal death has been seen.

Magnesium Sulfate

Uterine contractions are likely affected by magnesium because it acts as an antagonist to calcium and acts as a membrane stabilizer. Although magnesium can stop contractions, it has only been shown to effectively forestall true labor an average of 48 hours. Furthermore, it has a variety of side effects. Headaches, fatigue, and depressed reflexes are commonly seen. **Pulmonary edema** has also been demonstrated in women treated with magnesium sulfate; thus, careful monitoring should accompany treatment with this drug.

Calcium Channel Blockers

It is likely that calcium channel blockers decrease the efficacy of calcium in causing uterine contractions and have definitely been shown in vitro to decrease myometrial contractions. In clinical studies, **nifedipine** has been the principal drug studied and seems to have comparable efficacy when compared with ritodrine. Patients experience such side effects as headaches, flushing, and dizziness.

Prostaglandin Inhibitors

Prostaglandins are involved in myometrial contractions and are commonly used to induce labor and to heighten contractions in postpartum patients with uterine atony. Thus, antiprostaglandin agents should theoretically inhibit contractions and possibly halt labor. Indomethacin is the commonly used agent that blocks the enzyme cyclooxygenase and decreases the level of prostaglandins. It has been shown in clinical trials to effectively decrease contractions and forestall labor. However, a variety of complications in the fetus have been demonstrated. These include premature constriction of the ductus arteriosus, pulmonary hypertension, and intraventricular hemorrhage.

Oxytocin Antagonists

Currently, oxytocin antagonists are being studied as a new tocolytic. They have been shown to decrease uterine myometrial contractions, but clinical studies have been small thus far. In theory, they seem to be an obvious choice for an effective tocolytic and should have minimal side effects. Current clinical use has been limited to experimental trials.

▶ PRETERM AND PREMATURE RUPTURE OF MEMBRANES

Rupture of membranes (ROM) occurring before 37 weeks gestation is considered **preterm rupture of the membranes,** whereas rupture of membranes occurring before the onset of labor is termed **premature rupture of the membranes.** If the two occur together it is **preterm premature rupture of the membranes** (PPROM). Anytime rupture of membranes lasts longer than 18 hours before delivery, it is described as **prolonged rupture of membranes.**

Preterm Rupture of Membranes

Spontaneous rupture of the fetal membranes before 37 weeks gestational age is a common cause of preterm labor, preterm delivery, and chorioamnionitis. Without intervention, approximately 50% of patients who have ROM will deliver within 24 hours, and usually 75% will deliver within 48 hours. Commonly, a patient will complain of a gush of fluid per vagina; however, any increased vaginal discharge or complaints of stress incontinence should be evaluated to rule out preterm rupture of membranes.

Diagnosis

The diagnosis is made by obtaining a history of leaking vaginal fluid, performing a speculum examination to look for **pooling** and getting positive **nitrazine** and **fern tests.** If these tests are equivocal, an **ultrasound** can be performed to examine the level of amniotic fluid. If the diagnosis is still unconfirmed, the **amnio/dye test** can be performed with injection of a dye via amniocentesis and observation of whether the dye leaks into the vagina. If there is concern for chorioamnionitis, maternal temperature and white blood count, uterine tenderness, and the fetal heart tracing should all be checked for signs of infection.

Treatment

The management of preterm rupture of membranes varies depending on the gestational age of the pregnancy. The reasoning behind the management of PPROM is that at some gestational age, the risk from prematurity is equal to the risk of infection. That point is somewhere between 32 and 36 weeks; thus, up to this point the risk of prematurity drives intervention, whereas after it the risk of infection motivates delivery. There is debate regarding the point at which the risk of infection is greater; thus, some practitioners would wait until 36 weeks gestational age and others would simply do tests for fetal lung maturity starting at 34 weeks and deliver when mature.

Premature Rupture of the Membranes

The most common concern of **premature rupture of the membranes** is that of chorioamnionitis which increases with the length of ROM. If ROM is expected to last past 18 hours, it is termed **prolonged** rupture of the membranes and treated with antibiotics when in labor. Commonly, if ROM occurs anytime after 36 weeks, labor is induced (or after 34 weeks with documented fetal lung maturity). However, the risks and benefits of this should be discussed with patients before any decision is made.

Key Points

1. Preterm rupture of membranes is ROM before 37 weeks; premature rupture of membranes is ROM that occurs before the onset of labor.

2. Some 75% of patients with PPROM deliver within 48 hours.
3. Once ROM is confirmed, the therapeutic course depends on gestational age and fetal lung maturity.
4. Any patient that shows signs of infection or fetal distress needs to be delivered.

▶ CHORIOAMNIONITIS

Infection of the amniotic fluid surrounding the fetus is termed chorioamnionitis. It is frequently correlated with preterm and prolonged ROM but also occurs without ROM. It is the most common cause of neonatal sepsis, which has a high rate of fetal mortality.

Diagnosis

The common signs of chorioamnionitis are maternal fever, elevated maternal white blood count, uterine tenderness, and fetal tachycardia. Because this problem is of such high concern, other causes of these signs and symptoms should be excluded. Other loci of maternal infection may cause maternal fever and elevated white blood count as well as fetal tachycardia. Fetal tachycardia may be congenital, thus a prior baseline fetal heart rate can be useful. In addition, fetal tachycardia can also be caused by β-agonist tocolytic agents. The maternal white blood cell count is elevated in pregnancy and further elevated with the onset of labor. The white blood cell count is also increased by administration of corticosteroids.

Group B Strep

One commonly suspected organism in causing chorioamnionitis is group B streptococcus. A significant proportion of the population are colonized in the vagina and rectum with this organism, which is correlated with preterm labor, preterm rupture of the membranes, chorioamnionitis, and neonatal sepsis. Neonates with group B strep sepsis have a 25% mortality rate. Among preterm neonates, this figure doubles to over 50%. Thus, antibiotic prophylaxis is recommended in the setting of preterm delivery and prolonged rupture of the membranes even without the diagnosis of frank chorioamnionitis.

Treatment

When chorioamnionitis is suspected, intravenous antibiotics should be started. Commonly, the causative organisms are those that colonize the vagina and rectum; thus, broad-spectrum coverage should be used. In addition to antibiotics, delivery should be hastened with induction, augmentation, or, in the setting of a nonreassuring fetal tracing, by cesarean section.

Key Points

1. Chorioamnionitis is diagnosed by maternal fever, uterine tenderness, elevated maternal white blood count, and fetal tachycardia.
2. Although the infection is often polymicrobial, group B strep colonization has a high correlation with both chorioamnionitis and neonatal sepsis. Treatment involves antibiotics and delivery.

▶ OBSTRUCTION AND MALPOSITION

Although the most common form of delivery is the spontaneous vertex vaginal delivery, there are many other varieties of presentations and deliveries that are not uncommon. Many of the malpresentations lead to cesarean section.

Cephalopelvic Disproportion

One of the most common indications for cesarean section is failure to progress in labor (FTP), most often caused by **cephalopelvic disproportion** (CPD). The three "Ps," pelvis, passenger, and powers, are primarily responsible for a vaginal delivery. If the pelvis is too small, the fetal presenting part is too large or if contractions are inadequate, there will be FTP. Uterine contractions can be measured with IUPCs and augmented with pitocin, but little can be done for the other two factors that make up CPD.

Diagnosis

The maternal pelvis is described as one of four dominant types: gynecoid, android, platypelloid, and anthropoid (Fig. 5-2). Furthermore, many pelves are mixed with different characteristics from more than one of the types of pelves. Common measurements of the pelvis include those of the pelvic inlet, the midpelvis, and the pelvic outlet. The obstetric conjugate, which is the distance between sacral promontory and the midpoint of the symphysis pubis, is the shortest anteroposterior diameter of the pelvic inlet. The anteroposterior diameter of the pelvic outlet, which measures from the tip of the sacrum to the inferior margin of the pubic symphysis, ranges from 9.5 to 11.5 cm. These measurements are performed with both clinical and X-ray pelvimetry, but it is rare to assume CPD based on measurements alone.

The fetal skull is composed of the face, the base, and the vault. The face and base are composed of fused bones, which do not change during labor; however, the bones of the vault are not fused and can undergo molding to conform to the maternal pelvis. The vault is composed of five bones: two frontal, two parietal, and one occipital. The spaces between the bones are known as sutures, and the two spots where the sutures intersect are the **anterior** and **posterior fontanelles**. How the fetal head presents to the maternal pelvis is important in accomplishing a vaginal delivery. There is great variation in the diameter of the skull at various levels and with various inclinations. When the fetal skull is properly flexed, the suboccipitobregmatic diameter presenting to the pelvis averages 9.5 cm in a term infant. When the sagittal suture is not located midline in the pelvis (**asynclitism**), the diameter of the skull being accommodated is effectively increased.

Treatment

If cephalopelvic disproportion is suspected, it is still often worthwhile to attempt a trial of labor. In the setting of fetal macrosomia, induction of labor may be chosen before the opportunity for vaginal delivery passes. This practice leads to a similar or greater cesarean section rate for failed induction rather than CPD.

Breech Presentation

Breech presentation, or buttocks first, is present in 3 to 4% of all singleton deliveries. Factors associated with breech presentation include previous breech delivery, uterine anomalies, polyhydramnios, oligohydramnios, multiple gestations, hydrocephalus, and anencephalus. Persistent breech presentation is also associated with placenta previa and fetal anomalies. Complications of a vaginal breech delivery include prolapsed cord and entrapment of the aftercoming head. Thus, breech presentations are often delivered via cesarean section.

Types of Breech

There are three categories of the breech presentation (Fig. 5-3): **frank, complete**, and **incomplete** or **footling**. The frank breech has flexed hips and extended knees and thus the feet are near the fetal head. The complete breech has flexed hips, but one or both knees are flexed as well with at least one foot near the breech. The incomplete or footling breech has one or both of the hips not flexed so that the foot or knee lies below the breech in the birth canal.

Diagnosis

The breech presentation may be diagnosed in a variety of fashions. With abdominal examination using the Leopold maneuvers, the fetal head can be palpated near the fundus while the breech is palpated in the pelvis. With vaginal examination, the breech can be palpated, the common landmarks being the gluteal cleft and the anus or, in the setting of an incomplete

Figure 5-2 Characteristics of four types of pelves.

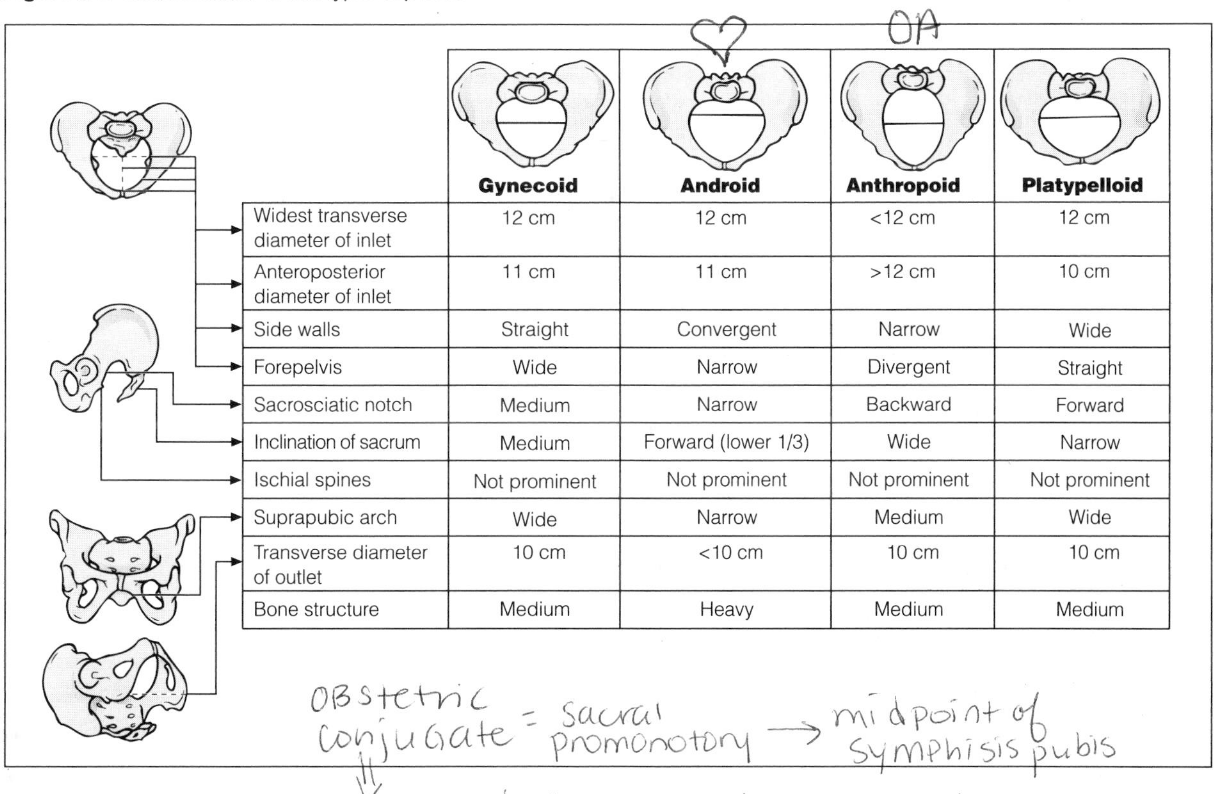

	Gynecoid	Android	Anthropoid	Platypelloid
Widest transverse diameter of inlet	12 cm	12 cm	<12 cm	12 cm
Anteroposterior diameter of inlet	11 cm	11 cm	>12 cm	10 cm
Side walls	Straight	Convergent	Narrow	Wide
Forepelvis	Wide	Narrow	Divergent	Straight
Sacrosciatic notch	Medium	Narrow	Backward	Forward
Inclination of sacrum	Medium	Forward (lower 1/3)	Wide	Narrow
Ischial spines	Not prominent	Not prominent	Not prominent	Not prominent
Suprapubic arch	Wide	Narrow	Medium	Wide
Transverse diameter of outlet	10 cm	<10 cm	10 cm	10 cm
Bone structure	Medium	Heavy	Medium	Medium

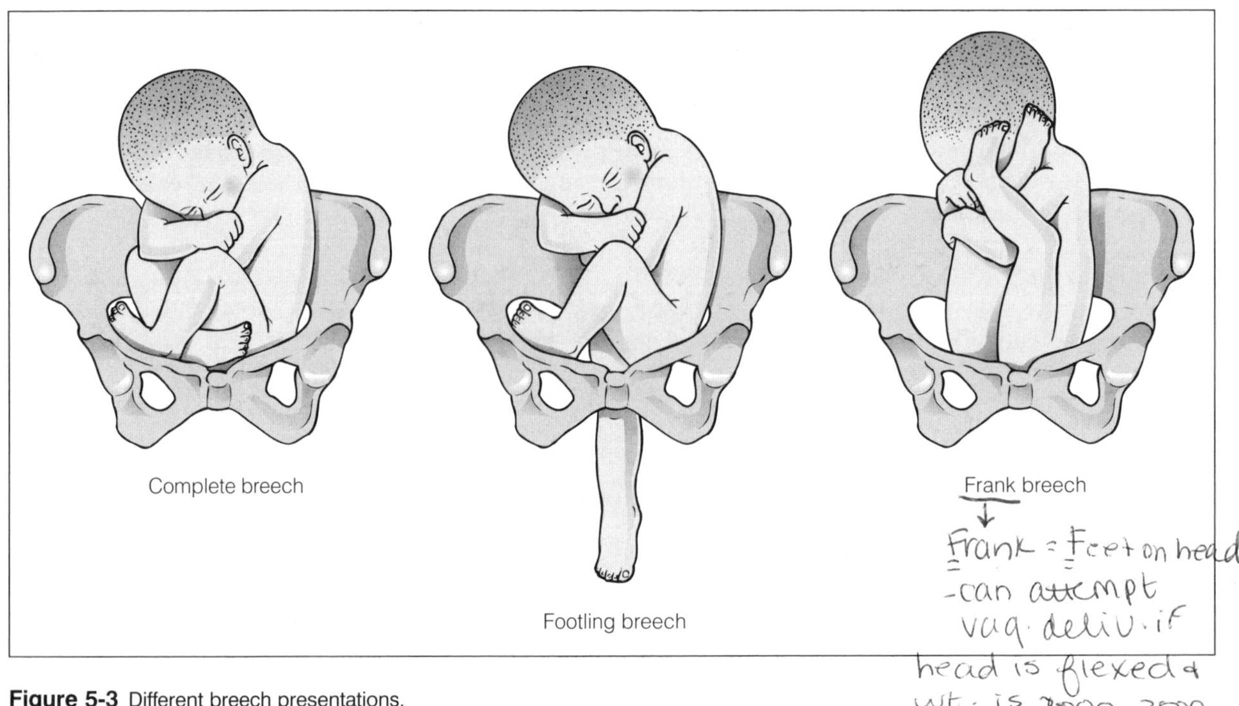

Figure 5-3 Different breech presentations.

breech, the fetal lower extremity. Often diagnosis is made or confirmed with ultrasound. On ultrasound, it is easy to confirm breech and then to determine the type of breech.

Treatment

In most settings, cesarean section is recommended for breech presentation. However, there are two other variations: external version of the breech and trial of breech vaginal delivery. External version consists of manipulation of the breech infant into a vertex presentation. It is rarely performed before 37 weeks gestational age because of the likelihood of spontaneous version before this point. Version also carries the risk of preterm labor, vabruption, or rupture of membranes.

Trial of breech vaginal delivery can be attempted in the proper setting. There must be a favorable pelvis, a flexed head, estimated fetal weight between 2,000 and 3,500 g, and frank breech presentation. Contraindications including nulliparity, complete or incomplete breech presentation, and estimated fetal weight greater than 3,500 g should be presented to the patient along with recommendation for cesarean section. However, if a patient insists on attempted vaginal delivery, careful monitoring of the fetus and progress of labor is imperative.

Key Points

1. There are three types of breech: frank, complete, and incomplete or footling.
2. Breech presentations are usually delivered via cesarean section, but in the proper setting, trial of vaginal delivery may be pursued.

Malpresentation of Vertex

Even in the setting of a vertex presentation, there can be malpresentation. The face, brow, persistent occiput posterior (OP), or a compound presentation with a fetal upper extremity can complicate the vertex presentation. In addition, the shoulder can present in the setting of a transverse lie.

Face

The diagnosis of face presentation (Fig. 5-4) can be made with vaginal examination and palpation of the nose, mouth, eyes, or chin (mentum). If the fetus is mentum anterior, vaginal delivery will often ensue. However with a mentum posterior or transverse, the fetus must rotate to mentum anterior for the fetus to deliver vaginally. Of note, many anencephalic fetuses have a face presentation.

Brow

Brow presentation (Fig. 5-5) occurs when the portion of the fetal skull just above the orbital ridge presents. With the brow presenting, a larger diameter must pass

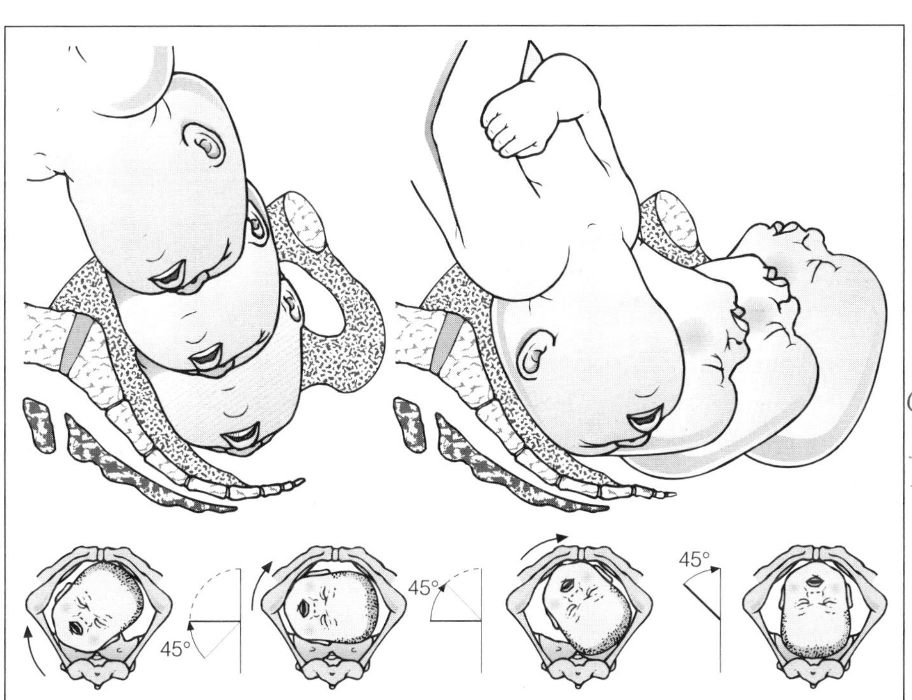

Figure 5-4 (A) Mechanisms of labor for right mentoposterior position with subsequent rotation of mentum anterior and delivery. (B) Face presentation. Well engaged in the mentolateral position.

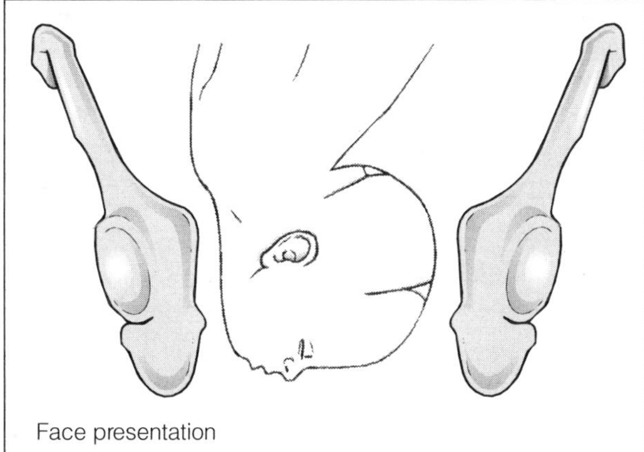

Figure 5-4 (continued)

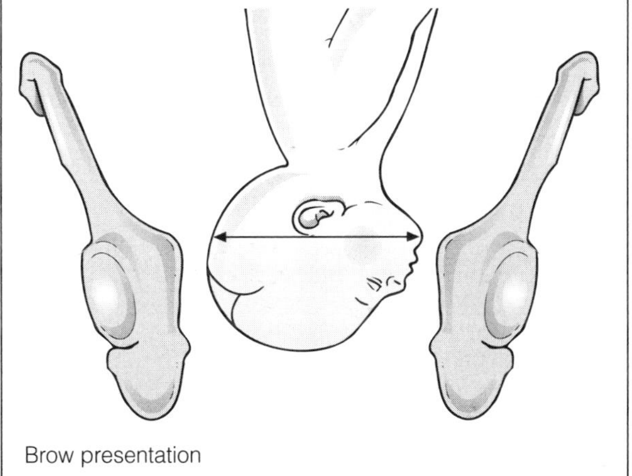

Figure 5-5 Brow presentation with mentovertex diameter presenting.

through the pelvis. Thus, unless the fetal head is particularly small or the pelvis is particularly large, the brow presentation must convert to occiput or face to deliver.

Shoulder

If the fetus is in a transverse lie, often the shoulder is presenting to the pelvic inlet. Diagnosis of this malpresentation can be made with abdominal or vaginal examination and ultrasound confirmation. Unless there is spontaneous conversion to vertex, shoulder presentations will be delivered via cesarean section because of the increased risk of cord prolapse, increased risk for uterine rupture, and the difficulty of vaginal delivery.

Compound Presentation

A fetal extremity presenting alongside the vertex or breech is considered a compound presentation (Fig. 5-6). This occurs in less than 1 in 1,000 pregnancies. It is increased with prematurity, multiple gestations, polyhydramnios, and CPD. A common complication of

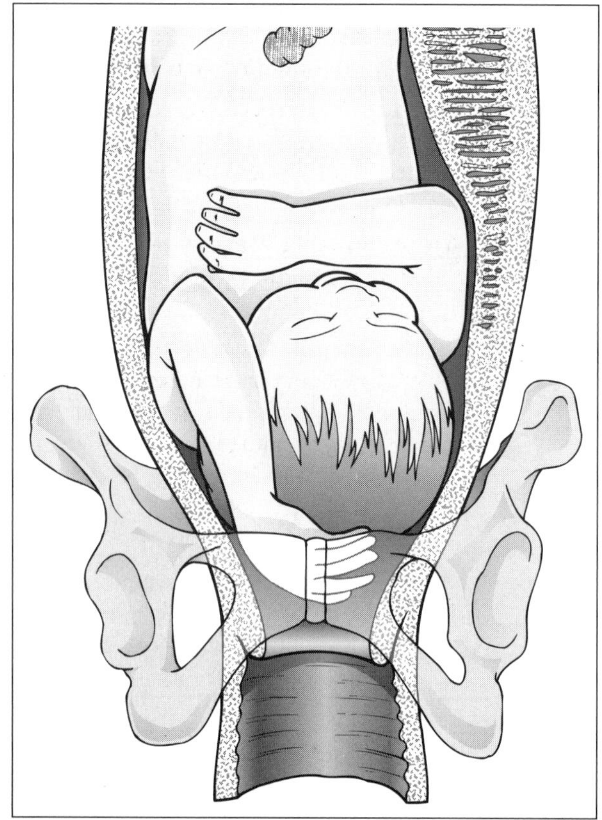

Figure 5-6 Compound presentation. The left hand is lying in front of the vertex. With further labor the hand and arm may retract from the birth canal and the head may then descend normally.

compound presentation is umbilical cord prolapse. The diagnosis is often made with vaginal examination when the fetal extremity is palpated alongside the presenting part. At this point it should be determined whether the prolapsed fetal part is a hand or foot. Ultrasound may be used as well to determine the type of extremity presenting.

Treatment

Often times, if an upper extremity is presenting alongside the vertex, the part may be gently reduced; however, prolapse of a lower extremity in vertex presentation is much less likely to deliver vaginally. Compound presentation of a lower extremity with a breech is considered a **footling** or **incomplete breech** presentation and should be taken to cesarean section. In all cases of compound presentation, umbilical cord prolapse should be suspected and careful monitoring with continuous fetal heart tracings and frequent vaginal examinations should ensue.

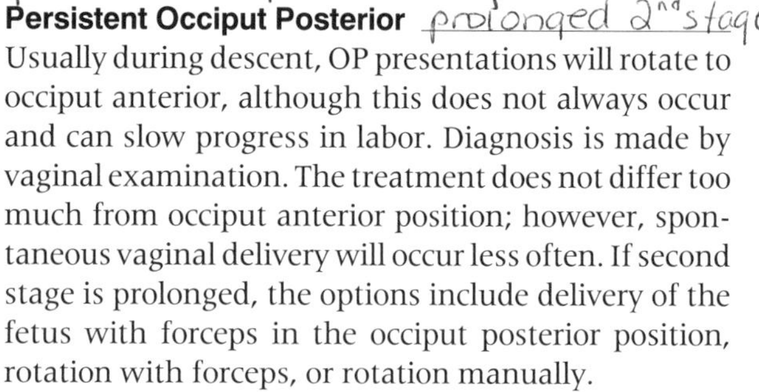

Persistent Occiput Posterior

Usually during descent, OP presentations will rotate to occiput anterior, although this does not always occur and can slow progress in labor. Diagnosis is made by vaginal examination. The treatment does not differ too much from occiput anterior position; however, spontaneous vaginal delivery will occur less often. If second stage is prolonged, the options include delivery of the fetus with forceps in the occiput posterior position, rotation with forceps, or rotation manually.

Key Points

1. There are a variety of vertex malpresentations including **face**, **brow**, **compound**, and **persistent OP**.
2. These presentations will often deliver vaginally but need closer monitoring and sometimes require different maneuvers.

Shoulder Dystocia

Once the head of the fetus is delivered, difficulty in delivering the shoulders, particularly because of impaction of the anterior shoulder behind the pubic symphysis, is termed **shoulder dystocia**. Risk factors for shoulder dystocia include fetal macrosomia, gestational diabetes, previous shoulder dystocia, obese patients, postdates pregnancy, and prolonged second stage of labor. There is increased morbidity and mortality associated with shoulder dystocia. Fetal complications include fractures of the humerus and clavicle, brachial plexus nerve injuries (Erb's palsy), hypoxia, and death.

Diagnosis

The actual diagnosis of a shoulder dystocia is made when routine obstetric maneuvers fail to deliver the infant. However, because of the antepartum risk factors, some shoulder dystocias may be predicted and prevented or at least prepared for. In diabetic patients with EFW > 4,200 g, cesarean section is the recommended mode of delivery. In patients with gestational diabetes or macrosomia, an induction may be attempted before the fetus becomes larger than 4,000 g. Preparation for a shoulder dystocia includes placing the patient in the dorsal lithotomy position, having adequate anesthesia, cutting a generous episiotomy, and having several experienced clinicians present at birth.

Treatment

There are a series of maneuvers to deliver an infant with a shoulder dystocia:

▲ **Suprapubic pressure:** This is to dislodge the anterior shoulder from behind the pubic symphysis (Fig. 5-7).

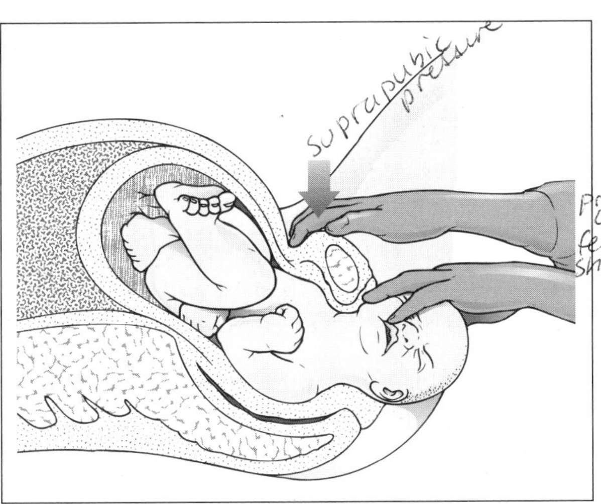

Figure 5-7 Moderate suprapubic pressure is often the only additional maneuver necessary to disimpact the anterior fetal shoulder.

- **McRoberts maneuver:** Sharp flexion of the maternal hips that decreases the inclination of the pelvis and can free the anterior shoulder (Fig. 5-8).
- **Rubin maneuver:** Pressure on an accessible shoulder to push it toward the anterior chest wall of the fetus to decrease the bisacromial diameter and free the impacted shoulder (Fig. 5-9).
- **Woods corkscrew maneuver:** Pressure behind the posterior shoulder to rotate the infant and dislodge the anterior shoulder.
- **Delivery of the posterior shoulder:** By sweeping the posterior shoulder across the chest and delivering the arm, the bisacromial diameter can then be rotated to an oblique diameter of the pelvis and the anterior shoulder is freed.

If these maneuvers are unsuccessful, they may be performed again. If the infant is still undelivered, there are several other maneuvers that can be performed. Cutting or fracturing the clavicle or cutting the pubic symphysis will often release the infant. If none of these

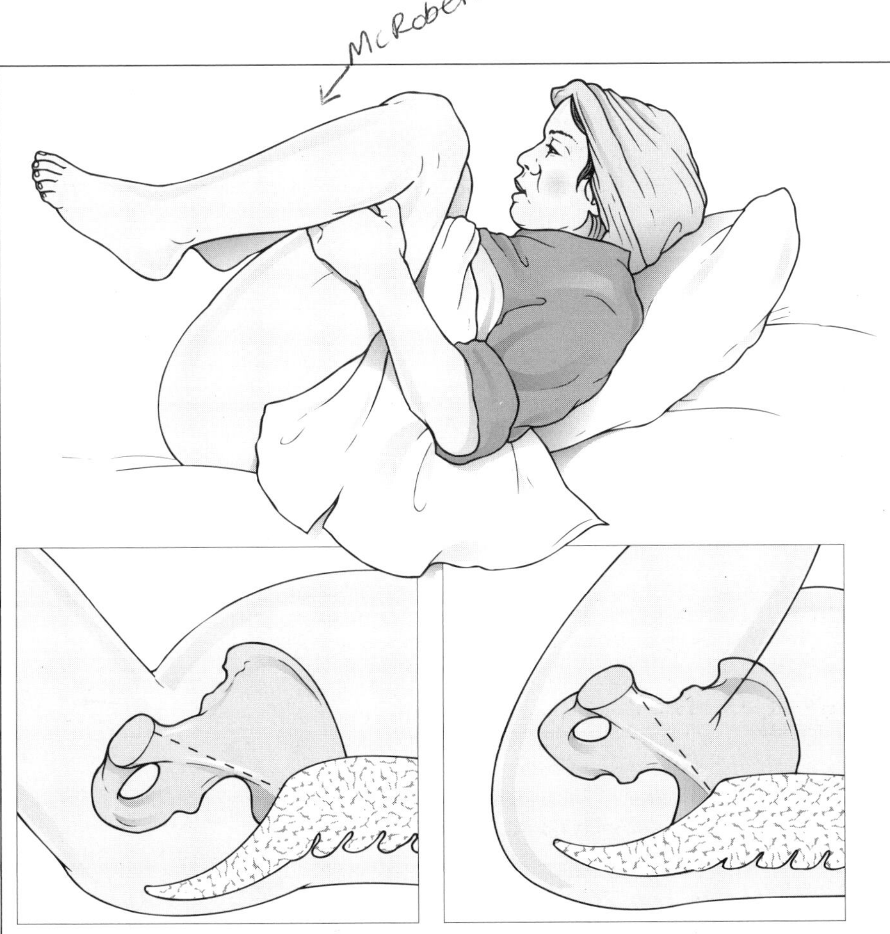

Figure 5-8 Sharp ventral rotation of both maternal hips (McRoberts maneuver) brings the pelvic inlet and outlet into a more vertical alignment, facilitating delivery of the fetal shoulders.

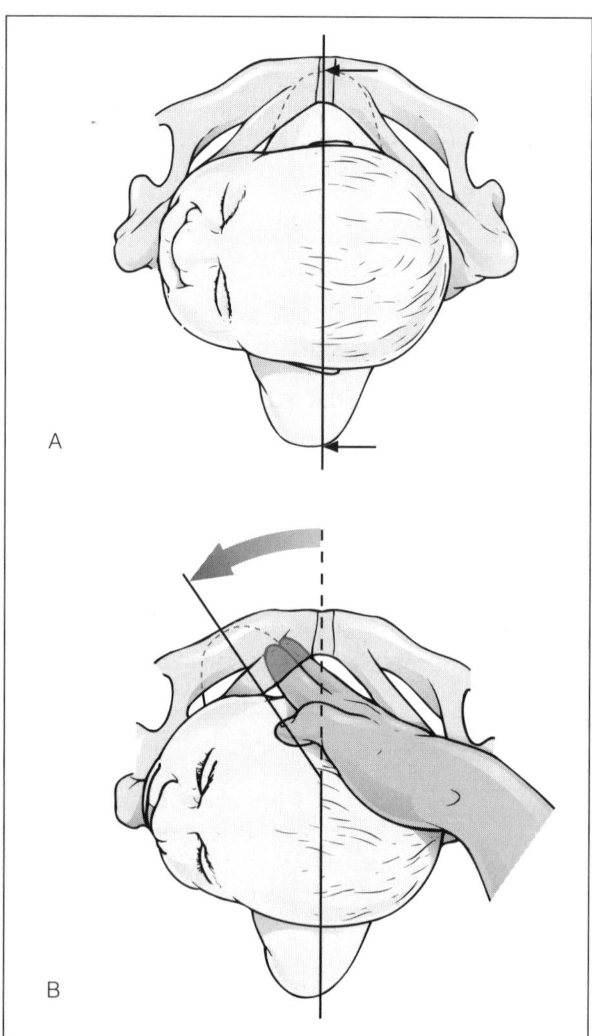

Figure 5-9 Rubin (second) maneuver. (A) The shoulder-to-shoulder diameter is shown as the distance between the two small arrows. (B) The most easily accessible fetal shoulder (the anterior is shown here) is pushed toward the anterior chest wall of the fetus. Most often, this results in abduction of both shoulders, reducing the shoulder-to-shoulder diameter and freeing the impacted anterior shoulder.

maneuvers is successful, the **Zavanelli** maneuver involves placing the infant's head back into the pelvis and performing cesarean delivery.

Key Points

1. Shoulder dystocias can result in fetal fractures, nerve damage, and hypoxia.
2. Risk factors for shoulder dystocia include fetal macrosomia, diabetes, previous dystocia, maternal obesity, postdate deliveries, and prolonged second stage of labor.
3. The maneuvers to reduce a shoulder dystocia include suprapubic pressure, McRoberts maneuver, Wood's corkscrew, delivery of posterior shoulder, fracture or cutting the clavicle or pubic symphysis, and the Zavanelli maneuver.

CHAPTER 6

Fetal Complications of Pregnancy

▶ DISORDERS OF FETAL GROWTH

Fetuses less than the 10th percentile for growth are termed **small for gestational age** (SGA). Those greater than the 90th percentile are termed **large for gestational age** (LGA). SGA fetuses are further described as either symmetric or asymmetric. Symmetric implies that the fetus is proportionately small. Asymmetric implies that there are organs of the fetus that are disproportionately smaller. Classically, an asymmetric infant will have wasting of the torso and extremities while preserving the brain. Thus, the skull will be at a greater percentile than the rest of the body. Before making the diagnosis of either SGA or LGA, it is imperative that accurate dating of the pregnancy is ascertained.

Small for Gestational Age

SGA infants are associated with higher rates of mortality and morbidity for their **gestational age**. However, they do better than infants with the same weight delivered at earlier gestational ages. An SGA baby born at 34 weeks that weighs the same as a 28-week infant will have lower morbidity and mortality rates. The causes of SGA infants can be divided into those that lead to decreased growth potential and those that lead to **intrauterine growth restriction** (IUGR) (Table 6-1). These two categories can be correlated with symmetric and asymmetric growth respectively.

Decreased Growth Potential

Congenital abnormalities cause approximately 10 to 15% of SGA infants. Trisomy 21 (Down's syndrome), trisomy 18 (Edward's syndrome), and trisomy 13 (Patau's syndrome) all lead to SGA babies. Turner's syndrome (45,XO) leads to a decrease in birth weight. Infants with osteogenesis imperfecta, achondroplasia, neural tube defects, anencephaly, and a variety of autosomal recessive syndromes may all be SGA.

Intrauterine infections of all varieties, particularly **cytomegalovirus** and **rubella**, lead to SGA infants. They are probably the cause of 10 to 15% of all SGA babies. Exposure to **teratogens** and other drugs during pregnancy can also lead to decreased potential for growth. The two most common are alcohol and cigarettes, which both lead to SGA infants. It should be noted that up to 10% of SGA fetuses are constitutionally small based purely on parental stature.

Intrauterine Fetal Growth Restriction

Growth restriction results in asymmetric growth, usually sparing the fetal brain. This results from decreased nutrition and oxygen being transmitted across the placenta. Maternal factors include baseline hypertension, anemia, chronic renal disease, and severe malnutrition. Furthermore, severe diabetes with extensive vascular disease may lead to IUGR infants.

Placental factors leading to diminished placental blood flow leads to IUGR. These factors include placenta previa and placental infarction. Multiple gestations often lead to lower birth weights both because of earlier delivery as well as SGA infants.

Diagnosis

Infants are at an increased risk to be SGA in mothers with a previous SGA baby or with any of the above etiologies. These fetuses should be followed carefully for intrauterine growth. Fundal height is measured at each prenatal visit. Oligohydramnios and small infants lead to fundal heights less than expected. Any patient with a fundal height 3 cm less than expected should receive an ultrasound for fetal growth.

If SGA is suspected, the accuracy of the patient's dating should be verified. Any infant at risk for IUGR or being SGA is followed with serial ultrasound scans for growth. A fetus with decreased growth potential will usually start small and stay small, whereas one with IUGR will fall off the growth curve.

Treatment

For patients with a history of SGA infants, the underlying etiology should be explored. If nutrition, alcohol, cigarettes, or other drugs were issues in the prior pregnancy, they should be dealt with at each prenatal visit. Patients with a history of placental insufficiency, preeclampsia, collagen vascular disorders, or vascular disease are placed on a baby aspirin per day.

For SGA fetuses who have consistently been small throughout the pregnancy, there is no indication to expedite delivery. For SGA fetuses near term that have fallen off the growth curve, the risk of prematurity is

TABLE 6-1

Risk Factors for SGA Infants

Decreased growth potential
Genetic and chromosomal abnormalities
Intrauterine infections
Teratogenic exposure
Substance abuse
Radiation exposure
Small maternal stature
Pregnancy at high altitudes
Female fetus
Intrauterine growth restriction
Maternal factors including hypertension, anemia, chronic renal disease, malnutrition, and severe diabetes
Placental factors including placenta previa, chronic abruption, placental infarction, multiple gestations

likely less than the risk of the intrauterine environment. This is assessed with fetal testing such as a nonstress test (NST), oxytocin challenge test (OCT), or biophysical profile (BPP). If fetal testing is nonreassuring, these patients should be delivered. For SGA fetuses remote from term, the decision of whether to deliver must weigh how the infant will do in a neonatal intensive care unit versus how it will be maintained in the intrauterine environment. For those left undelivered, frequent antenatal testing with NSTs, OCTs, and BPPs; weekly ultrasounds for fetal growth; and possibly admission to the hospital may be indicated.

Key Points

1. Infants less than the 10th percentile are small for gestational age or SGA.
2. Small infants can have symmetric or asymmetric growth.
3. Common causes of decreased growth potential include congenital abnormalities, drugs, infections, radiation, and small maternal stature.
4. IUGR infants are commonly born to women with systemic diseases leading to poor placental blood flow.

Large for Gestational Age and Fetal Macrosomia

An LGA fetus is defined as those with an **estimated fetal weight** greater than the 90th percentile. However, LGA is less important than the diagnosis of **fetal macrosomia**. Although definitions of macrosomia vary, the American College of Obstetricians and Gynecologists use a birth weight **greater than 4,500 g**. A birth weight of greater than 4,000 g is also used by many clinicians and researchers to define macrosomia. Macrosomic infants have a higher risk of shoulder dystocia and birth trauma with resultant brachial plexus injuries with vaginal deliveries. Other neonatal risks include low apgar scores, hypoglycemia, polycythemia, hypocalcemia, and jaundice. LGA infants are at a higher risk for childhood leukemia, Wilm's tumor, and osteosarcoma.

Mothers with LGA macrosomic infants are at increased risk for cesarean section, perineal trauma, and post-partum hemorrhage. There is a higher rate of cesarean section for macrosomic infants both due to failure to progress in labor and electively because of suspected increased risk for shoulder dystocia.

Etiology

The most classically associated risk factor for fetal macrosomia is **maternal diabetes**. There is not a clear-cut picture between the different varieties of diabetes including type I, type II, or gestational or whether insulin is required in terms of differences as being more or less predictive of macrosomia. **Maternal obesity**, weight greater than 90 kg, is correlated with an increased risk for fetal macrosomia. This correlation is seemingly independent of maternal stature and gestational diabetes.

Any woman who has previously delivered an LGA infant is at increased risk in ensuing pregnancies for fetal macrosomia. **Postterm** pregnancies have an increased rate of macrosomic infants. **Multiparity** and **advanced maternal age** are risk factors (Table 6-2) but mostly secondary to the increased prevalence of diabetes and obesity.

Diagnosis

Upon routine prenatal care, patients with macrosomic infants will often be a size greater than dates on measurement of the fundal height. By late third trimester, Leopold's examination of the infant will seem large. As with SGA fetuses, dating should be verified. Any

TABLE 6-2

Risk Factors for Macrosomic Infants

Diabetes
Maternal obesity
Postterm pregnancy
Previous LGA or macrosomic infant
Maternal stature
Multiparity
Advanced maternal age
Male infant
Beckwith-Wiedemann syndrome (pancreatic islet-cell hyperplasia)

patient with diabetes or a previous LGA infant merits estimated fetal weights by ultrasound every week to 2 weeks late in pregnancy. Patients that are size greater than dates are also referred to ultrasound. Ultrasound uses the biparietal diameter, femur length, and abdominal circumference to estimate the fetal weight. These estimates are usually accurate to within 10 to 15%.

Treatment

The management of LGA and macrosomic infants includes prevention, surveillance, and induction of labor before the attainment of macrosomia. Patients with diabetes need tight control of their blood glucose during pregnancy. Well-controlled sugars are thought to decrease the incidence of macrosomic infants in this population, although this has not been confirmed by large randomized studies.

Obese patients can be counseled to lose weight before conception. Once pregnant, these patients are advised to gain less weight than the average patient and should be referred to a nutritionist for assistance in maintaining adequate nutrition with some control of caloric intake.

Because of the risk for birth trauma and failure to progress in labor secondary to cephalopelvic disproportion, LGA pregnancies are often induced before the fetus can attain macrosomic status. The risks for this course of action is increased rate of cesarean section for failed induction and prematurity in a poorly dated pregnancy. Vaginal delivery of the suspected macrosomic infant involves preparing for a shoulder dystocia. Furthermore, it is not prudent to use forceps or vacuum in this setting, which can lead to a shoulder dystocia.

Key Points

1. LGA is a fetus or infant greater than the 90th percentile. Both 4,000 and 4,500 g have been used as the threshold for fetal macrosomia.
2. LGA and macrosomic infants are at greater risk for birth trauma, hypoglycemia, jaundice, lower apgar scores, and tumors of childhood.
3. Increased size is seen in the fetus with maternal diabetes, maternal obesity, increased maternal height, postterm pregnancies, multiparity, advanced maternal age, and male sex.

▶ DISORDERS OF AMNIOTIC FLUID

The amniotic fluid reaches its maximum volume of about 800 mL at about 28 weeks. This volume is maintained until close to term when it begins to fall to about 500 mL at 40 weeks. The balance of fluid is maintained by production by the fetal kidneys and lungs and resorption by fetal swallowing and the interface between the membranes and the placenta. A disturbance in any of these functions may lead to a pathologic change in amniotic fluid volume.

With the use of ultrasound in pregnancy as an antepartum diagnostic tool, the amniotic fluid in addition to the fetus can be evaluated. The classic measure of amniotic fluid is the amniotic fluid index (AFI). The AFI is calculated by dividing the maternal abdomen into quadrants and finding the largest vertical pocket of fluid in each quadrant. The vertical measurements of each pocket in centimeters are summed. An AFI of less than 5 is considered oligohydramnios. If it is greater than 20 it is diagnostic of polyhydramnios.

Oligohydramnios

Oligohydramnios in the absence of rupture of membranes is associated with a 40-fold increase in perinatal mortality. It is also associated with congenital anomalies particularly of the genitourinary system and growth restriction. In labor, nonreactive nonstress tests, fetal heart rate decelerations, meconium, and cesarean section for nonreassuring fetal testing are all increased with an AFI of less than 5.

Etiology

The cause of oligohydramnios can be thought of as either decreased production or increased withdrawal. Amniotic fluid is produced by the fetal kidneys and lungs. It can be resorbed by the placenta, swallowed by the fetus, or leaked out into the vagina. Chronic uteralplacental insufficiency (UPI) can lead to oligohydramnios because the fetus likely does not have the nutrients or blood volume to maintain adequate glomerular filtration rate. UPI is commonly associated with growth restricted infants.

Congenital abnormalities of the genitourinary tract can lead to decreased urine production. These malformations include renal agenesis (Potter's syndrome), polycystic kidney disease, or obstruction of the genitourinary system. The most common cause of oligohydramnios is rupture of membranes. Even without a history of leaking fluid, the patient should be examined to rule out this possibility.

Diagnosis

Diagnosis of oligohydramnios is made by ultrasound. Patients screened for amniotic fluid volume include those measuring size less than dates, with a history of ruptured membranes, with suspicion for IUGR pregnancy, and that have a postterm pregnancy.

Treatment

The management of oligohydramnios is entirely dependent on the underlying etiology. In pregnancies that are IUGR, a host of other data need consideration, including the rest of the BPP, cord Doppler flow, gestational age, and the cause of the IUGR. A postdate pregnancy with oligohydramnios should be induced. In the setting of an infant with congenital abnormalities, the patient should be referred to genetic counseling. A plan should be made for delivery in coordination with the pediatricians.

Patients with rupture of membranes at term are induced if not already in labor. If there is meconium or in the setting of frequent decelerations, an amnio infusion may be performed to increase the AFI. Amnio infusion is performed to dilute any meconium present in the amniotic fluid and to theoretically decrease the number of decelerations. Preterm premature rupture of membranes is discussed in Chapter 5.

Key Points

1. Oligohydramnios is defined as an AFI of less than 5.
2. Oligohydramnios can be caused by decreased placental perfusion, decreased production by the fetus, and rupture of membranes.
3. Pregnancies at term complicated by oligohydramnios should be delivered.

Polyhydramnios

Polyhydramnios, an AFI greater than 20, is present in 2 to 3% of pregnancies. Fetal structural and chromosomal abnormalities are more common in the setting of polyhydramnios. It is associated with such malformations as neural tube defects, obstruction of the fetal alimentary canal, and hydrops.

Etiology

Polyhydramnios is not as ominous a sign as is oligohydramnios. It is correlated with an increase in congenital anomalies. It is also more common in pregnancies complicated by diabetes, hydrops, and multiple gestation. In an obstruction of the gastrointestinal tract, the infant is unable to swallow the amniotic fluid, leading to polyhydramnios. Multiple gestations can lead to transfusion syndromes with polyhydramnios around one fetus and oligohydramnios around the other.

Diagnosis

Polyhydramnios is diagnosed by ultrasound of patients being scanned for size greater than dates, routine screening of diabetic or multiple gestation pregnancies, or is an unsuspected finding on an ultrasound performed for other reasons. An AFI of greater than 20 is diagnostic of polyhydramnios.

Treatment

As in oligohydramnios, the particular setting of polyhydramnios dictates the management of the pregnancy. Patients with polyhydramnios are at risk for malpresentation and should be carefully evaluated in labor. There is an increased risk of cord prolapse with polyhydramnios; thus, rupture of membranes should be performed in a controlled setting if possible or only if the head is truly engaged in the pelvis. Upon spontaneous rupture of membranes, a sterile vaginal examination should be performed to verify presentation and rule out cord prolapse.

Key Points

1. Polyhydramnios is diagnosed by an AFI greater than 20 on ultrasound.
2. Polyhydramnios is associated with diabetes, multiple gestations, hydrops, and congenital abnormalities.
3. Obstetric management of polyhydramnios should include careful verification of presentation and observation for cord prolapse.

▶ OTHER FETAL COMPLICATIONS

Rh Incompatibility

If a woman is Rh negative and her fetus is Rh positive, there is a possibility that she may be sensitized to the Rh antigen and develop antibodies. These antibodies cross the placenta and cause hemolysis of fetal red blood cells. The incidence of Rh negativity varies among race (Table 6-3). Commonly, most individuals only become sensitized during pregnancy and blood transfusion. In the United States, the incidence of sensitization is decreasing from both causes.

If the antibodies do cross and cause hemolysis, the infant can have disastrous complications. The anemia

TABLE 6-3
Prevalence of Rh Negativity by Race

Race	Percent Rh Negative
Caucasian	15
African-American	8
African	4
Native American	1
Asian	$\ll 1$

caused by hemolysis leads to increased extramedullary production of fetal red cells. Erythroblastosis fetalis, or fetal hydrops, a syndrome with a hyperdynamic state, heart failure, diffuse edema, ascites, and pericardial effusion, is the result of serious anemia. The bilirubin, which is a breakdown product of red blood cells, is cleared by the placenta before birth but in the neonate can lead to jaundice and neurotoxic effects.

The Unsensitized Rh-Negative Patient

If a patient is Rh negative but has a negative antibody screen, the goal of the pregnancy is to keep her from becoming sensitized. Any time during the pregnancy that there is a possibility that a patient may be sensitized, such as amniocentesis, miscarriage, vaginal bleeding, abruption, and delivery, she should be given RhoGAM, an anti-D immunoglobulin (Rh IgG). Antibody screen is performed at the initial visit. RhoGAM is given at 28 weeks. Postpartum RhoGAM is given if the neonate is Rh positive.

A standard dose of RhoGAM, 0.3 mg of Rh IgG, will eradicate 15 mL of fetal red blood cells (30 mL of fetal blood with a hematocrit of 50). This dose is adequate for a routine pregnancy. However, in the setting of placental abruption or any antepartum bleeding, a Kleihauer-Behtke test for amount of fetal red blood cells in the maternal circulation can be sent. If the amount of bleeding is more than can be eliminated by the single RhoGAM dose, further Rh IgG can be given.

The Sensitized Rh Negative Patient

If on initial visit the antibody screen for Rh comes back positive, the titer is checked as well. Antibody titers greater than 1:8 are worrisome. If paternity is not in question, blood type can be performed on the father of the baby to determine whether the fetus is at risk. However, because approximately 5% of all pregnancies have unknown or incorrect paternity, the safest course is to treat all pregnancies as if erythroblastosis is a risk.

Frequent fetal surveys are performed to examine the fetus for ascites and pericardial effusion. Amniocentesis is begun at 16 to 20 weeks. Fetal cells from the amniocentesis can be analyzed for Rh status. The amniotic fluid is analyzed by a spectrophotometer, which measures the light absorbance by bilirubin resulting as a breakdown product of hemolysis. These absorbance measurements are plotted on the Liley curve (Fig. 6-1), which predicts the severity of disease. The curve is broken up into three regions.

Zone 1 is suggestive of a mildly affected fetus, and amniocentesis can be performed approximately every 2 to 3 weeks. Zone 2 is suggestive of a moderately affected fetus, and amniocentesis should be repeated every 1 to 2 weeks. The severely affected fetus will fall into zone 3. Amniocentesis is repeated weekly. Percutaneous umbilical blood sampling (PUBS) may be performed to obtain a fetal hematocrit. If the hematocrit is low, the PUBS needle can be used for transfusion. Before PUBS, intraperitoneal transfusion had been performed.

Other Causes of Immune Hydrops

There are a variety of other red blood cell antigens including the **ABO** blood type, antigens **CDE** in which D is the Rh antigen, **Kell**, **Duffy**, **Lewis**, and many others. Some also carry the risk for causing fetal hydrops (e.g., Kell and Duffy), whereas others may lead to a mild hemolysis but not severe immune hydrops (e.g., ABO, Lewis). With the advent of treatment with RhoGAM, the incidence of Rh isoimmunization has decreased and the other causes of immune related fetal hydrops are leading to an increased percentage of the cases. Sensitized patients are managed similarly to Rh-negative patients with antibody titers, amniocentesis, PUBS, and transfusions.

Figure 6-1 Liley graph used to depict severity of fetal hemolysis with red cell isoimmunization.

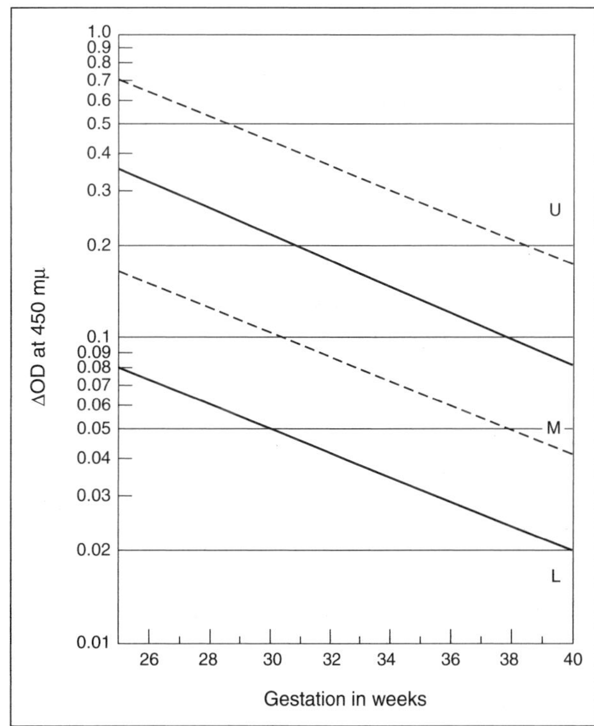

Key Points

1. Rh-sensitized women with Rh-positive infants have antibodies that cross the placenta, leading to hemolysis and anemia in the infant. If the anemia is low enough, a hyperdynamic state develops with edema, ascites, and heart failure.
2. Rh-negative patients who are not sensitized should be treated with antepartum RhoGAM to prevent sensitization. Postpartum, they should receive another shot of RhoGAM if the fetus is Rh positive.
3. Patients undergoing miscarriage, abruption, amniocentesis, ectopic pregnancy, and vaginal bleeding who are Rh negative are given RhoGAM.
4. Rh-negative patients who are sensitized are followed closely with serial ultrasounds and amniocentesis. The amniocentesis is done to measure the amount of bilirubin in the fluid, which is indicative of the amount of hemolysis.

Fetal Demise

Intrauterine fetal death (IUFD) is a rare but disastrous occurrence. It can be seen with a variety of medical and obstetric complications of pregnancy, including abruption, congenital abnormalities, and postterm pregnancy. Most commonly, there is no explanation for a fetal demise. A retained IUFD greater than 3 to 4 weeks can lead to hypofibrinogenemia secondary to the release of thromboplastic substances from the decomposing fetus. In some cases, full-blown disseminated intravascular coagulation (DIC) can result.

Diagnosis

Early in pregnancy, before 20 weeks, the diagnosis of fetal death (missed abortion) is suspected by lack of uterine growth or cessation of symptoms of pregnancy. Diagnosis is confirmed with serially falling human chorionic gonadotropin (hCGs) and ultrasound documentation. After 20 weeks' gestation, fetal death is suspected with absence of fetal movement noted by the mother and absence of uterine growth. Diagnosis can be confirmed by ultrasound.

Treatment

Because of the risk of DIC with retained IUFD, the best treatment is delivery. Early gestations can be terminated by dilatation and evacuation. After 20 weeks, the pregnancy must be terminated by induction of labor.

Key Points

1. IUFD is more common with disorders of the placenta.
2. The cause of IUFD is usually unknown but is often attributed to cord accidents.
3. Retained IUFD can lead to DIC; thus, delivery upon diagnosis is indicated.

Postterm Pregnancy

A postterm pregnancy is defined as one that goes beyond 42 weeks gestational age or greater than 294 days past the last menstrual period (LMP). It is estimated that 3 to 10% of all pregnancies will go postterm. It is an important obstetric issue because of the increased risk of macrosomic infants, oligohydramnios, meconium aspiration, intrauterine fetal death, and dysmaturity syndrome. There is also greater risk to the mother because of a greater rate of cesarean sections (approximately doubled) and delivery of larger infants.

Etiology

The most common reason for the diagnosis of postterm pregnancy is inaccurate dating; thus, accurate dating is imperative early in pregnancy. Because the physiologic basis for the onset of labor is poorly understood, the mechanisms for preterm or postterm labor are also not understood. There are a few rare conditions of the fetus associated with postterm pregnancy. These include anencephaly, fetal adrenal hypoplasia, and absent fetal pituitary. All are notable for diminished levels of circulating estrogens.

Diagnosis

Again, it should be stressed that the diagnosis is made by accurate dating. Because ultrasound can be off by as much as 3 weeks near term, this cannot be used to confirm dating. Accurate dating is made by a firm LMP consistent with a bimanual examination in the first trimester or a first trimester ultrasound. Dating by a second trimester ultrasound or unsure LMP is more suspect.

Treatment

The approach to the postterm pregnancy is varied but generally involves more frequent visits, increased fetal testing, and plans for eventual induction. A typical plan for following a postterm pregnancy is listed below.

Pregnancies that go past 40 weeks should usually receive a nonstress test (NST) in the 41st week. Induction is indicated with nonreassuring fetal testing. During the 42nd week, the patient should be seen twice and receive a biophysical profile (BPP) at one of the visits and NST at the other. Induction is indicated with nonreassuring fetal testing or electively with an inducible cervix (Bishop score >6). After 42 weeks, often the patient is induced regardless of cervical examination.

Key Points

1. Postterm pregnancy is defined as greater than 42 weeks gestational age.
2. Postterm pregnancies are at increased risk for fetal demise, macrosomia, meconium aspiration, and oligohydramnios.
3. Increased fetal surveillance and induction are the most common management options for postterm pregnancies.

Multiple Gestations

If a fertilized ovum divides into two separate ova, monozygotic, or "identical," twins result. If ovulation produces two ova and both are fertilized, dizygotic twins result. Without assisted fertility, the rate of twinning is approximately 1 in 80 pregnancies, with 30% of those monozygotic. The rate of naturally occurring triplets is approximately 1 in 7,000 to 8,000 pregnancies. However, with ovulation enhancing drugs and in vitro fertilization, the incidence of dizygotic multiple gestations is increasing.

Complications of Multiple Gestation

Multiple gestations result in an increase in a variety of obstetric complications including preterm labor, placenta previa, cord prolapse, postpartum hemorrhage, and pre-eclampsia. The fetuses are at increased risk for preterm delivery, congenital abnormalities, being small for gestational age, and malpresentation. The average gestational age for twins is between 36 and 37 weeks; for triplets it is 33 to 34 weeks. Monozygotic twins with a monochorionic placenta can develop **twin-twin transfusion syndrome**. Vascular communication between the twins can result in one fetus with hypervolemia, cardiomegaly, glomerulotubal hypertrophy, edema, and ascites and the other with hypovolemia, growth restriction, and oligohydramnios.

Pathogenesis

Monozygotic twinning results from division of the fertilized ovum or cells in the embryonic disk. If separation occurs before the differentiation of the trophoblast, two chorions and two amnions result. After trophoblast differentiation and before amnion formation (days 5 to 10), separation leads to a single placenta, one chorion, and two amnions. Division after amnion formation leads to a single placenta, one chorion, and one amnion and occasionally conjoined or "Siamese" twins. There are no risk factors for monozygotic twins and it does not follow any inheritable pattern.

Dizygotic twins primarily result from fertilization of two ova by two sperm. There are a variety of risk factors associated with dizygotic twinning. Dizygotic twins tend to run in families and are more common in people of African descent. Around the world the rate of dizygotic twins ranges from 1 in 1,000 in Japan to 1 in 20 in several tribes in Nigeria. The rate of all multiple gestations has increased sharply since the onset of medical treatment of infertility. Clomid, a fertility-enhancing drug, increases the rate of dizygotic twinning to 8%.

Diagnosis

Multiple gestations are usually diagnosed by ultrasound. It is suspected with rapid uterine growth, excessive maternal weight gain, or palpation of more than two fetal large parts (vertex and breech). The level of hCG, human placental lactogen (hPL), and maternal serum alpha-fetoprotein (MSAFP) are all elevated for gestational age. Rarely, diagnosis will be made after delivery of the firtst fetus with palpation of the aftercoming fetus(es).

Treatment

Because of the increased risk for complications, multiple gestation pregnancies are managed as high-risk pregnancies. Aside from the management of the complications, the principal issue in multiple gestations is mode of delivery.

Delivery of Twins

There are four possibilities for twin presentation, both vertex (40%), both breech, vertex then breech (40%), and breech then vertex. When deciding mode of delivery, all breech presenting twins (20%) are considered together.

Vertex/vertex twins may be delivered vaginally with a cesarean section for fetal distress. Vertex/nonvertex twins may be delivered vaginally if the twins are concordant or the presenting twin is larger. The twins should be between 2,000 and 3,500 g by classic criteria, although current data suggest that delivery is safe above 1,500 g. Either version to vertex of the second twin or breech extraction is used for delivery of the second twin. Nonvertex presenting twins are delivered via cesarean section.

Delivery of Triplets

Most triplet gestations (>90%) are delivered via cesarean section. Rarely, triplets will be concordant, with vertex presenting, all greater than 1,500 to 2,000 g and a vaginal delivery can be attempted. Multiple gestations beyond triplets are all delivered via cesarean section if possible.

Key Points

1. Monozygotic twins carry the same genetic material, whereas dizygotic twins are from separate ova and sperm and are only as related as siblings.
2. Multiple gestations are at increased risk for preterm labor and delivery, placenta previa, postpartum hemorrhage, pre-eclampsia, cord prolapse, malpresentation, and congenital abnormalities.
3. There is a genetic predisposition for dizygotic twinning, whereas the rate of monozygotic twinning is the same throughout all races and families.
4. Vaginal delivery of vertex/vertex presenting twins is preferred, vertex/nonvertex twins is possible with the right circumstances, and nonvertex/nonvertex twins are delivered by cesarean section.

Congenital
TB = 50% mortality

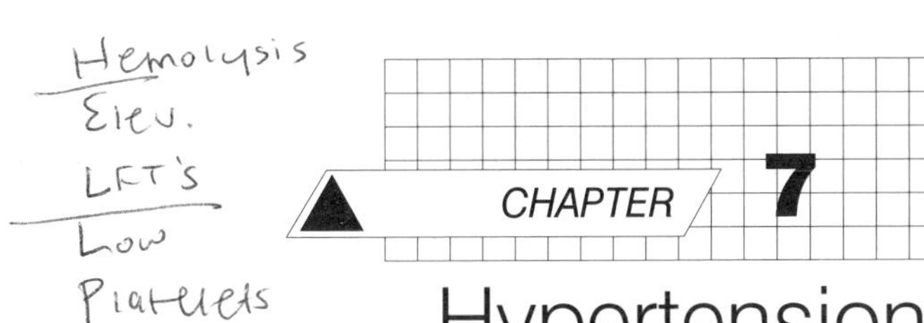

Hypertension in Pregnancy

In the obstetric patient, hypertension is defined as a blood pressure of at least 140/90 mm Hg. Hypertension may be present before pregnancy, as with chronic hypertension, or may be induced by pregnancy as with pre-eclampsia and eclampsia. The American College of Obstetricians and Gynecologist's recommended classification of the hypertensive states of pregnancy are shown in Table 7-1. Complications from these disorders are consistently among the three most common causes of maternal death in all developed countries.

▶ PRE-ECLAMPSIA

Pathogenesis

Pre-eclampsia is the presence of edema, hypertension, and proteinuria in the pregnant woman. It occurs primarily in, but is not limited to, nulliparous women in their third trimester. Although no definite cause for pre-eclampsia has been determined, it is well accepted that the underlying pathophysiology involves **a generalized arteriolar constriction** (vasospasm) and intravascular depletion that can produce symptoms related to ischemia, necrosis, and hemorrhage of organs.

As shown in Table 7-2, major fetal complications of pre-eclampsia are due to prematurity. Also, the generalized vasocontriction of pre-eclampsia can result in a decreased blood flow to the placenta. This may manifest itself as acute uteroplacental insufficiency, resulting in abruption or fetal distress. The uteroplacental insufficiency may also be chronic in nature and result in a fetus with poor uterine growth (intrauterine growth restriction).

Maternal complications associated with pre-eclampsia (Table 7-3) are related to the generalized arteriolar vasoconstriction that has an impact on the brain (seizure and stroke), kidneys (oliguria and renal failure), liver (edema and subcapsular hematoma), and small blood vessels (thrombocytopenia and disseminated intravascular coagulation [DIC]). Pre-eclampsia results in both an increased rate of premature delivery and cesarean section. About 10% of patients with severe pre-eclampsia develop HELLP syndrome.

HELLP syndrome is a subcategory of pre-eclampsia in which the patient presents with hemolytic anemia, elevated liver enzymes, and low platelets. Hypertension may be minimal in these patients. Although HELLP syndrome is uncommon, patients can have a rapidly accelerating downhill course, resulting in poor maternal and fetal outcomes. Despite careful management, HELLP syndrome still has a high rate of stillbirth (10 to 15%) and neonatal death (20 to 25%).

Epidemiology

Pre-eclampsia occurs in 5 to 6% of all live births and can develop any time after the 20th week of gestation but is most commonly seen in the third trimester near term. When hypertension is seen in the early second trimester (14 to 20 weeks), a hydatidiform mole or previously undiagnosed chronic hypertension should be considered.

Unlike other pre-eclamptic patients, the patient with HELLP is more likely to be multiparous, 25 years of age or older, and at less than 36 weeks gestation at the time of presentation. Although 80% of patients develop HELLP after being diagnosed with pre-eclampsia (30% with mild pre-eclampsia and 50% with severe

TABLE 7-1

Hypertensive States of Pregnancy

- ▲ Pre-eclampsia and eclampsia (hypertension specific to pregnancy)
- ▲ Chronic hypertension (regardless of origin)
- ▲ Chronic hypertension with superimposed pre-eclampsia
- ▲ Transient hypertension

TABLE 7-2

Fetal Complications of Pre-eclampsia

Complications related to prematurity (if early delivery is necessary)

Acute uteroplacental insufficiency
- Placental infarct abruption
- Intrapartum fetal distress
- Stillbirth (in severe cases)

Chronic uteroplacental insufficiency
- Asymmetric and symmetric small-for-gestational age fetuses
- Intrauterine growth restriction

Oligohydramnios

TABLE 7-3
Maternal Complications of Pre-eclampsia

Medical manifestations
- Seizure
- Cerebral hemorrhage
- DIC and thrombocytopenia
- Renal failure
- Hepatic rupture or failure
- Pulmonary edema

Obstetrical complications
- Uteroplacental insufficiency
- Placental abruption
- Increased premature deliveries
- Increased cesarean section deliveries

TABLE 7-4
Major Risk Factors for Pre-eclampsia

Nulliparity
Maternal age (<20 or >35 years)
Black race
Chronic hypertension
Multiple gestation
Family history of pre-eclampsia (first-degree female relative)

pre-eclampsia), 20% of patients with HELLP have no previous history of hypertension before their diagnosis.

Risk Factors

The major risk factors for pre-eclampsia include nulliparity, maternal age less than 20 or greater than 35, multiple gestation, and underlying chronic hypertension (Table 7-4).

Clinical Manifestations

Mild Pre-eclampsia

As shown in Table 7-5, mild pre-eclampsia is classically defined as a third trimester blood pressure greater than 140 systolic or 90 diastolic on two occasions at least 6 hours apart (or a 30 mm Hg rise in systolic or 15 mm Hg rise in diastolic pressure above previous levels) accompanied by proteinuria greater than 300 mg/24 hours and nondependent edema (face and/or hands). It has been determined that edema is not essential to the diagnosis of pre-eclampsia, but the occurrence of hypertension and proteinuria is diagnostic. Proteinuria is generally the last sign to develop.

Severe Pre-eclampsia

Criteria for severe pre-eclampsia (see Table 7-5) include blood pressure greater than 160 systolic or 110 mm Hg diastolic on two occasions at least 6 hours apart accompanied by proteinuria greater than 5 g/24 hours (or 3 to 4+ protein on dipstick). A woman with mild pre-eclampsia by blood pressure and proteinuria parameters would be classified as having severe pre-eclampsia if she also developed certain associated conditions. These include altered consciousness, headache or visual changes, epigastric or right upper quadrant pain, significantly impaired liver function (>2 times normal), oliguria (<400 mL in 24 hours), pulmonary edema or cyanosis, and significant thrombocytopenia (<100,000/mm^3). Many clinical manifestations associated with pre-eclampsia are explained on the basis of vasospasm, leading to necrosis and hemorrhage of organs.

HELLP Syndrome

The disorder is characterized by rapidly deteriorating liver function and thrombocytopenia. In addition, a

TABLE 7-5
Criteria for Classification of Pre-eclampsia and Eclampsia

Disorder	Blood Pressure (mm Hg)	Proteinuria	Edema	Other Signs/Symptoms
Pre-eclampsia				
Mild	140/90–160/110 or ≥30 incr SBP ≥15 incr DBP	<5 g/24 hr or 1–2 plus dipstick	Hands and/or face	
Severe	>160/110	>5 g/24 hr or 3–4 plus dipstick	Hands and/or face	Any mild pre-eclamptic with oliguria (<400 mL/24 hr), pulmonary edema, RUQ Pain, headache/scomata, altered LFTs, or thrombocytopenia is classified with severe pre-eclampsia
Eclampsia				Any pre-eclamptic with seizures not due to other causes is classified with eclampsia

* Blood pressure taken at rest on two occasions at least 6 hours apart.

number of patients will develop DIC. The criteria for diagnosis and relevant laboratory tests are shown in Table 7-6. Liver capsule distention produces epigastric pain, often with progressive nausea and vomiting, and can lead to hepatic rupture.

Treatment

Mild Pre-eclampsia

Because delivery is the ultimate treatment for pre-eclampsia, induction of labor is the treatment of choice for pregnancies at term, unstable preterm pregnancies, or pregnancies where there is evidence of fetal lung maturity. In these cases, vaginal delivery may be attempted with the assistance of prostaglandins, pitocin, or amniotomy as needed. Cesarean delivery need only be performed for obstetric indications. For preterm patients who are stabilized, bedrest and expectant management may be used. Once the patient reaches term, shows evidence of fetal lung maturity, or worsening pre-eclampsia, delivery is advised.

All pre-eclamptic patients should be started on magnesium sulfate therapy for seizure prophylaxis (4- to 6-g load and 2 g/h) during labor and delivery and it should be continued until 12 to 24 hours after delivery.

Severe Pre-eclampsia

The goals of treatment in severe pre-eclampsia are to prevent eclampsia, control maternal blood pressure, and deliver the fetus. Patients with severe pre-eclampsia should be stabilized using magnesium sulfate for seizure prophylaxis and hydralazine (a direct arteriolar dilator) for blood pressure control. Once the patient is stabilized, delivery should ensue immediately. In general, conservative therapy is discouraged for patients with severe pre-eclampsia. In fact, some providers recommend that if the pregnancy has progressed beyond 28 weeks and a tertiary nursery is available, then delivery is the treatment of choice even in the stable patient with severe pre-eclampsia.

TABLE 7-6

Criteria for the Diagnosis of HELLP Syndrome

*H*emolytic anemia
- Schistocytes on peripheral blood smear
- Elevated total bilirubin
- Elevated lactate dehydrogenase

*E*levated *L*iver enzymes
- Elevated aspartate amino-transferase
- Elevated lactate dehydrogenase

*L*ow *P*latelets
- Thrombocytopenia

HELLP Syndrome

Delivery is the definitive treatment for HELLP syndrome.

Follow-Up

Women who develop pre-eclampsia during their first pregnancy will have a 25 to 33% recurrence rate in subsequent pregnancies. In patients with both chronic hypertension and pre-eclampsia, the risk of recurrence is 70%. Low doses of aspirin during subsequent pregnancies has been found to decrease the risk of recurrence.

Key Points

Pre-eclampsia

1. Is the presence of hypertension (>140/90 mm Hg), proteinuria (>300 mg/day), and significant non-dependent edema after 20 weeks gestation;
2. Has an incidence of 5 to 6% of all live births and occurs most commonly in nulliparous women in their third trimester;
3. Is characterized by a generalized multiorgan vasospasm that can lead to seizure, stroke, renal failure, liver damage, DIC, or fetal demise;
4. Has risk factors including nulliparity, multiple gestation, and chronic hypertension;
5. Is ultimately treated with vaginal delivery using magnesium sulfate and hydralazine as indicated.

▶ ECLAMPSIA

Eclampsia is the occurrence of grand mal seizures in the pre-eclamptic patient not attributed to other causes (see Table 7-5). Although patients with severe pre-eclampsia are at greater risk to develop seizures, 25% of women with eclampsia were originally found to have only mild pre-eclampsia before the onset of seizures. Of note, eclampsia may also occur without proteinuria. Complications of eclampsia include cerebral hemorrhage, aspiration pneumonia, hypoxic encephalopathy, and thromboembolic events.

Clinical Manifestations

Seizures in the eclamptic patient are tonic-clonic in nature and may or may not present with an aura. These seizures may develop before labor (25%), during labor (50%), or after delivery (25%). Most postpartum seizures occur within the first 48 hours after delivery but occasionally will occur as late as 7 to 10 days after delivery.

Treatment

Treatment strategy for eclamptic patients includes seizure management, blood pressure control, and prophylaxis against further convulsions. Hypertension management can usually be achieved using hydralazine to lower the blood pressure. For seizure control and prophylaxis, eclamptic patients are treated with magnesium sulfate ($MgSO_4$) to decrease hyperreflexia and prevent further seizures by raising the seizure threshold. This should not be confused with the use of $MgSO_4$ as a tocolytic in cases of premature labor.

In eclampsia, $MgSO_4$ therapy is initiated at the time of diagnosis and continued for 12 to 24 hours after delivery. The goal of magnesium sulfate therapy is to reach a therapeutic level while avoiding toxicity through careful clinical monitoring (Table 7-7). In the case of overdose, 10 mL 10% calcium chloride or calcium gluconate should be rapidly administered intravenously.

Once the eclamptic patient is stabilized and convulsions have been controlled, only then should delivery be initiated. In the case of eclampsia, the best way to treat the fetus is to stabilize the mother. Cesarean delivery should be reserved for obstetric indications.

Key Points

Eclampsia

1. Is the occurrence of grand mal seizures in the pre-eclamptic patient that cannot be attributed to other causes;
2. Presents with seizures occurring before labor (25% of patients), during labor (50%), or after delivery (25%);
3. Is treated with seizure management and prophylaxis with magnesium sulfate, hypertension management with hydralazine, and vaginal delivery only after the patient has been stabilized.

TABLE 7-7

Clinical Response to Serum Magnesium Sulfate Concentrations

Serum Concentration $MgSO_4$ (mg/mL)	Clinical Response
4.8–8.4	Therapeutic seizure prophylaxis
8	Central nervous system depression
10	Loss of deep tendon reflexes
15	Respiratory depression/paralysis
17	Coma
20–25	Cardiac arrest

▶ CHRONIC HYPERTENSION

Pathogenesis

Chronic hypertension is defined as hypertension present before conception, before 20 weeks gestation, or persisting more than 6 weeks postpartum. Approximately one third of patients with chronic hypertension in pregnancy will develop superimposed pre-eclampsia. Because of poor vascular development, the fetus may suffer from intrauterine growth restriction (IUGR) and the woman is at increased risk for superimposed pre-eclampsia, premature delivery, and abruptio placentae.

Treatment

Treatment of mild chronic hypertension is controversial; however, mothers with controlled blood pressures tend to have fewer problems. In general, women with chronic hypertension are continued on their medications throughout pregnancy. Methyldopa (a central alpha-adrenergic agonist) is the only antihypertensive agent whose long-term maternal and fetal safety has been assessed, although more severe hypertension may require hydralazine, beta blockers, labetalol, or calcium channel blockers. Low doses of aspirin have been found to decrease the risk of pre-eclampsia.

Key Points

Chronic hypertension

1. Is defined as hypertension occurring before conception, before 20 weeks gestation, or persisting more than 6 weeks postpartum;
2. Can lead to superimposed pre-eclampsia in 30% of patients;
3. Is generally treated with continuation of antihypertensives, especially Methyldopa, throughout pregnancy.

▶ CHRONIC HYPERTENSION WITH SUPERIMPOSED PRE-ECLAMPSIA

Chronic hypertension with superimposed pre-eclampsia is defined as worsening hypertension (increases of 30 mm Hg systolic or 15 mm Hg diastolic above the patient's average values) or worsening proteinuria in the latter half of pregnancy. Approximately one third of patients with chronic hypertension will develop superimposed pre-eclampsia. Eighty percent of these patients have a hypertensive disorder of renal origin that is aggravated by the pregnancy. When pre-eclampsia occurs in women with chronic hypertension, the prognosis is worse for the mother and fetus than with either condition alone. These patients have an increased risk of complications, including abruptio placentae, DIC, and acute tubular necrosis. Fetal risk of prematurity is 20 to 30% and the risk of IUGR is 10 to 15%.

Key Points

Chronic hypertension with superimposed pre-eclampsia

1. Is worsening hypertension or proteinuria in the chronic hypertensive patient;
2. Develops during pregancy in one third of chronic hypertensive patients;
3. Is associated with a worse prognosis than either chronic hypertension or pre-eclampsia alone.

▶ TRANSIENT HYPERTENSION

Transient hypertension describes the new onset of hypertension that develops between midpregnancy and the first 48 hours after delivery. It is also known as late or gestational hypertension. It is distinguished from the other hypertensive disorders of pregnancy in that it occurs without other signs of pre-eclampsia (i.e., proteinuria remains less than 300 mg/L) and there is no pre-existing history of hypertension. It is particularly difficult to distinguish transient hypertension from pre-eclampsia. Therefore, the diagnosis should be made only in retrospect, when the pregnancy is completed without the development of proteinuria.

Key Points

Transient hypertension

1. Is hypertension occurring for the first time in the second half of pregnancy, during labor, or within 48 hours of delivery without significant proteinuria (<300 mg/L);
2. Is also known as late or gestational hypertension.

CHAPTER 8

Diabetes During Pregnancy

▶ PATHOGENESIS

Diabetes during pregnancy encompasses a range of disease entities including gestational diabetes and overt diabetes mellitus (Table 8-1). True gestational diabetes mellitus (GDM) is an impairment in carbohydrate metabolism that first manifests itself during pregnancy. This category may include a small number of previously undiagnosed type I and type II diabetic women, although the incidence is quite small.

Diabetes during pregnancy can have devastating impacts on both mother (Table 8-2) and fetus (Table 8-3). Diabetic women are four times more likely to develop pre-eclampsia or eclampsia than nondiabetic women and twice as likely to have a spontaneous abortion. Similarly, the rates of infection, hydramnios, postpartum hemorrhage, and cesarean section are all increased for diabetic mothers. In the long term, GDM is also associated with impaired insulin tolerance and the manifestation of diabetes later in life.

Control of maternal glucose levels in overtly diabetic women is an important factor in determining fetal outcome. In the absence of prepregnancy and prenatal care, the rate of perinatal mortality in the setting of diabetes can be as high as 40%. However, with adequate care the rate can be reduced to only 3 to 5%. Major fetal effects include a fivefold increase in perinatal death and a two- to threefold increase in the rate of congenital malformations. Early in pregnancy, the fetus is at risk of congenital malformations and poor fetal growth. Late in pregnancy, the fetus is at risk for fetal growth abnormalities and sudden intrauterine fetal death. Ironically, although macrosomia is a major risk in diabetic pregnancies, the macrosomic infant is more likely to have delayed organ development.

▶ EPIDEMIOLOGY

The incidence of GDM ranges from 1 to 12% of pregnant women depending on the population, whereas that of overt diabetes is less than 1% of women of childbearing age.

▶ RISK FACTORS

The risk for diabetes during pregnancy includes age 25 years or older, obesity, family history, previous infant weighing more than 4,000 g, previous stillborn infant, previous congenitally deformed infant, previous polyhydramnios, and history of recurrent abortions.

▶ DIAGNOSTIC EVALUATION

The best time to screen for diabetes during pregnancy is at the end of the second trimester between 24 and

TABLE 8-1

White Classification for Diabetes During Pregnancy

Classification	Description
Gestational diabetes	Diabetes discovered for the first time during pregnancy
Class A	Diet controlled; any age or onset
Class B	Onset: age 20 or older Duration: less than 10 years
Class C	Onset: age 10–19 years Duration: 10–19 years
Class D	Onset: before age 10 years Duration: greater than 20 years
Class R	Proliferative retinopathy or vitreous hemorrhage
Class F	Diabetic nephropathy
Class RF	Retinopathy and nephropathy
Class H	Arteriosclerotic heart disease, clinically evident
Class T	Prior renal transplantation

TABLE 8-2

Maternal Complications of Diabetes During Pregnancy

Obstetric complications
- Polyhydramnios
- Pre-eclampsia

Diabetic emergencies
- Hypoglycemia
- Ketoacidosis
- Diabetic coma

Vascular and end organ involvement
- Cardiac
- Renal
- Ophthalmic
- Peripheral vascular

Neurologic
- Peripheral neuropathy
- Gastrointestinal disturbance

TABLE 8-3

Fetal Complications of Diabetes Mellitus

Macrosomia with traumatic delivery
Delayed organ maturity
  Pulmonary
  Hepatic
  Neurologic
  Pituitary-thyroid axis
Congenital abnormalities
  Cardiovascular
  Neural tube defect
  Caudal regression syndrome
Intrauterine growth restriction
  Intrauterine death
  Abnormal fetal heart rate patterns
  Small-for-date babies

28 weeks gestation. Patients with one or more risk factors for developing gestational diabetes should be screened at their first prenatal visit and during each subsequent trimester.

There are a variety of proposed methods of screening for diabetes during pregnancy (Table 8-4). The most common screening test consists of giving a 50-g glucose load and then measuring the plasma glucose 1 hour later. If the 1-hour glucose level is greater than 140 mg/dL, then the test is positive and glucose tolerance testing is necessary.

Women with a positive screening test need a 3-hour oral glucose tolerance test (OGTT) to evaluate their carbohydrate metabolism (Table 8-5). The OGTT involves the administration of 100 mg of oral glucose given after an 8-hour overnight fast preceded by a 3-day special carbohydrate diet. Glucose levels are measured immediately before glucose administration and again at 1, 2, and 3 hours after the dose. If two or more values are elevated, including the fasting glucose, then a diagnosis of gestational diabetes is made.

Once the diagnosis of diabetes mellitus is made, the **White classification** system is used to determine the patient's diabetes type. This classification is important because it is prognostic for perinatal survival. Although the overall perinatal mortality in the setting of diabetes is less than 5% in the United States, the outcome in any given case is associated with the severity of illness. For example, White class A patients have a perinatal survival of over 95% compared with survival rates of only 50 to 65% for diabetic patients with hypertension, proteinuria, and nephropathy. Along with the White classification, other **"prognostically bad signs"** include hypertension, pyelonephritis, ketoacidosis, and poor compliance.

TABLE 8-4

Glucose Screening Tests During Pregnancy

Test	Normal Glucose Level (mg/dL)
Fasting	< 100
1 hr after a 50-g glucose load	< 140
2 hr after a 100-g glucose load	< 165

TABLE 8-5

Three-Hour Glucose Tolerance Test: Venous and Plasma Criteria for GDM

Timing of Glucose Measurement	Normal Whole Venous Blood Glucose (mg/dL)	Normal Plasma Glucose
Fasting	90	105
1 hr	165	190
2 hr	145	165
3 hr	125	145

▶ TREATMENT

The goals of managing the diabetic patient include thorough patient education, control of maternal glucose, and proper fetal growth and development. To achieve these goals, tight glucose control should be maintained throughout the pregnancy and just before conception. Studies now show that stricter control of serum glucose levels during pregnancy can decrease the rate of maternal and neonatal complications. To achieve euglycemia, diet, insulin, and exercise must each be regulated. Patient education and close maternal and fetal monitoring are major components of successful therapy.

An American Diabetic Association (ADA) diet of at least 1,800 calories per day is recommended for all patients with diabetes during pregnancy. Both the timing and content of meals is important; therefore, a meal plan based on intake of 30 to 35 kcal/kg of ideal body weight is suggested.

Oral hypoglycemic agents are generally not used in pregnancy because they cross the placental barrier and are potentially teratogenic. Insulin has a molecular weight of 6,000 and therefore does not cross the placenta. Women with GDM can usually achieve euglycemia with management of diet without the use of insulin. Women with White classes A through H require insulin for the management of their plasma glucose.

TABLE 8-6

Glucose Monitoring and Insulin Dosing During Pregnancy

Insulin Type and Dose Time	Time Impact Seen	Target Glucose Level (mg/dL)
Evening NPH	Fasting	75–100
Morning regular	Pre-lunch	120–140
Morning NPH	Pre-dinner	120–140
Evening regular	Pre-evening snack	120–140

TABLE 8-7

Instructions for Adjusting Insulin Dosage

1. Establish a fasting glucose level between 75 and 100 mg/dL.
2. Only adjust one dosing level at a time.
3. Do not change any dosage by more than two to three units per day.
4. Wait 24 hr between dosage changes to evaluate the response.

Table 8-6 demonstrates the relationship between the time of insulin dose, the time of glucose testing, and the target blood glucose levels. When adjusting a patient's dosing schedule, one needs to consider other factors that may alter insulin requirements, including diet, exercise, stress, and infection. When insulin changes become necessary, there are a few simple rules that aid in the process (Table 8-7).

Because the level of physical activity affects the plasma glucose level, a consistent level of physical activity is suggested. Keep in mind that a hospitalized patient who achieves euglycemia in the context of relatively low activity may encounter bouts of hypoglycemia when at home on the same insulin regime because her physical activity level increases thus lowering the need for insulin.

In the patient with overt diabetes mellitus, renal, cardiac, and ophthalmic functioning is monitored along with monthly glycosylated hemoglobin levels ($Hgb\ A_{1C}$) that correlate with long-term (6 to 8 weeks) glucose control.

In the patient with insulin-requiring GDM, antenatal testing usually begins between 30 and 32 weeks gestation to evaluate the growth and well being of the fetus. Earlier testing is recommended if polyhydramnios, hypertension, or macrosomia is detected. Fetal assessment includes serial ultrasound examination at least every 4 to 6 weeks after the 30th week to look for fetal anomalies, macrosomia, intrauterine growth restriction, and polyhydramnios. Testing typically also consists of daily kick counts, non-stress tests, or biophysical profiles.

In general, in the well-controlled diabetic with no complications, induction of labor and vaginal delivery are undertaken at 38 to 40 weeks gestation given the increased risk of fetal death after 40 weeks. Delivery before the 38th week of gestation may be necessary in the setting of acidosis, hypertension, worsening diabetic state, or fetal compromise. In the case of elective delivery, verification of **fetal lung maturity** is essential given that even mild GDM can delay lung maturity. Cesarean delivery is used if the expected fetal weight is greater than 4,500 g or if other obstetric indications are present.

The laboring woman requires an increased amount of insulin due to the stress levels imposed on the body during this period. If levels exceed 100 to 120 mg/dL, a continuous infusion of insulin with dextrose can be used to achieve euglycemia during labor. Insulin is to be discontinued after delivery of the placenta.

After delivery, the maternal insulin requirements drop significantly because of the removal of the placenta, which contains many insulin antagonists. Patients with gestational diabetes do not usually need insulin in the postpartum period. They are, however, given an oral glucose tolerance test at 6 weeks postpartum. At discharge, insulin-dependent diabetes mellitus patients are started on two thirds of their *prepregnancy* insulin dose and adjustments are made as needed.

▶ FOLLOW-UP

Among patients who develop GDM during pregnancy, 50% will experience GDM in subsequent pregnancies and 25 to 35% will go on to develop overt diabetes within 5 years. The infants of patients with GDM have an increased incidence of childhood obesity and type II diabetes during early adulthood and later in life.

▶ KEY POINTS

1. Gestational diabetes occurs in 1 to 12% of pregnant women, whereas overt diabetes mellitus affects less than 1% of women of childbearing age.
2. All pregnant women should be screened for diabetes between 24 and 28 weeks gestation. A positive screening test should be followed with an oral glucose tolerance test.
3. Maternal complications of diabetes during pregnancy include hyperglycemia, hypoglycemia, urinary tract infection, hypertension, hydramnios, and retinopathy.

4. Fetal complications of diabetes during pregnancy include spontaneous abortion, macrosomia, congenital anomalies, neonatal hypoglycemia, respiratory difficulties, and perinatal death.
5. Pregnancy management should include frequent health care visits, thorough patient education, ADA diet, glucose monitoring, fetal monitoring, and insulin as indicated.
6. Patients should generally be induced between 38 and 40 weeks with verification of fetal lung maturity. Intrapartum insulin and dextrose are used to maintain tight control during delivery. Cesarean section is recommended for fetal weight over 4,500 g.

most common Deffect = in pt w/diab: Cardiac (VSD)

most classic = caudal regression syndrome (sacral agenesis)

- 50% pts will have GDM in subsequent preg.

CHAPTER 9

Other Medical Complications of Pregnancy

In the previous two chapters, two important medical complications of pregnancy were discussed: hypertensive states and diabetes in pregnancy. In this chapter a variety of the other common medical complications of pregnancy are discussed. Pregnancy impacts every physiologic system in the body as well as many disease states. When considering disease management in pregnancy, the possible teratogenic effects of any treatment or imaging modality must be kept in mind.

▶ INFECTIOUS DISEASES IN PREGNANCY

Urinary Tract Infections

The rate of urinary tract infections (UTIs) is increased in pregnancy. Multiple studies show that asymptomatic bacteriuria with greater than 100,000 colonies on culture occurs in roughly 5% of all pregnancies. Although this is similar to the nonpregnant population, it can lead to episodes of cystitis and pyelonephritis at higher rates than in nonpregnant women. Asymptomatic bacteriuria will proceed to UTI, cystitis, or pyelonephritis in 25% of the patients. Of the cases of pyelonephritis, 15% will be complicated by bacteremia, sepsis, or adult respiratory distress syndrome (ARDS). In sickle cell patients, the rate of asymptomatic bacteriuria doubles to 10% of patients.

Pathogenesis

There are a number of factors in pregnancy that can lead to cystitis and pyelonephritis. During pregnancy, the smooth muscle dilatory effects of estrogen and progesterone as well as the mechanical compressive effects of the uterus decrease bladder tone and cause uteral dilation. Both cystitis and vesicoureteral reflux are increased, leading to more ascending infections.

Diagnosis

UTIs are diagnosed with clinical signs and symptoms of dysuria, urinary frequency, and urinary urgency in conjunction with a positive urine culture. The urinalysis and sediment have elevated white blood cells and bacteria. Cystitis is diagnosed with suprapubic tenderness upon palpation and complaints of lower abdominal pain in the setting of a UTI. Pyelonephritis presents with costovertebral angle tenderness along with fever and an elevated white blood count.

Treatment

Escherichia coli accounts for greater than 70% of all UTIs. The remainder are usually due to enterococcus, proteus, coagulase negative staphylococcus, and group B streptococcus. Because most UTIs are caused by *E. coli*, initial treatment of asymptomatic bacteriuria is usually with amoxicillin, macrodantin, or Bactrim. Symptomatic UTIs and cystitis are also treated in this fashion with adjustment of medication based on culture sensitivity results.

Because of the serious sequelae, pyelonephritis in pregnancy is treated with intravenous (IV) antibiotics until the patient is afebrile for 48 hours. Currently, the possibility of treating these patients with a single dose of IV antibiotics and continuing with oral antibiotics or treating with oral antibiotics alone is being investigated.

Key Points

1. Five percent of pregnant women will have asymptomatic bacteria and are at increased risk for cystitis and pyelonephritis.
2. Once diagnosed, pyelonephritis is treated with IV antibiotics.

Bacterial Vaginosis

Recent studies demonstrated that bacterial vaginosis increases the risk for preterm delivery and low-birth-weight infants. Common symptoms are a malodorous discharge or vaginal irritation. Diagnosis can be made by performing the "whiff" test with vaginal discharge (see Chapter 14), examination of slides for clue cells, or upon culture of the cervix or vagina. Common organisms include *Gardnerella vaginalis*, Bacteroides, and *Mycoplasma hominis*. Metronidazole (Flagyl) is the treatment of choice but is not currently recommended in the first trimester.

Group B Streptococcus

Group B streptococcus is responsible for UTIs, chorioamnionitis, and endomyometritis during pregnancy. It is also a major pathogen in neonatal sepsis due to vertical transmission, which has severe implications. Although sepsis occurs in only 2 to 3 per 1,000 live births, the mortality rate with group B streptococcal sepsis ranges from 25 to 50%. Various studies demonstrated a wide range of colonization in pregnant women from 10 to 35%. To protect infants from group B streptococcus infections, women with known group B strep status are treated with **IV penicillin G** when in labor. Furthermore, women with an unknown group B strep status who are delivering before 37 weeks gestation or have rupture of membranes greater than 18 hours are also treated with penicillin G until delivery.

Herpes Simplex Virus

Herpes simplex virus (HSV) is a DNA virus that has two types, HSV-1 and HSV-2. Genital herpes infections are primarily caused by HSV-2; however, there are extragenital HSV-2 infections as well as genital HSV-1 infections. Patients with a history of herpes should have a careful examination of the labia, vagina, and cervix for lesions when presenting in labor because of the risk for vertical transmission during delivery. If lesions are seen, cesarean section is the optimal mode of delivery.

Primary herpes infections in pregnancy can also be transmitted across the placenta. A primary infection can be differentiated from a secondary by checking antibody titers. A previously infected person will have circulating IgG antibodies. A primary infection transmitted late in the third trimester, particularly close to delivery, is much more dangerous because of the lack of maternal antibodies transmitted to the fetus.

HSV can cause severe infections in the neonate. Herpetic lesions may occur on the skin and mouth of approximately 50% of infected infants. These infections can be diagnosed by viral cultures of the oropharynx and eyes or herpetic lesions, if present. The infection can progress to a viral sepsis and herpes encephalitis, which can lead to neurologic devastation and death. Infected infants are treated as soon as infection is suspected with IV acyclovir.

Varicella Zoster Virus

Varicella zoster virus (**VZV**) causes chickenpox. Because it is primarily a disease of childhood, more than 90% of adults are immune to VZV infection. The infection in adults tends to be more serious than in children with a higher rate of varicella pneumonia. Routine varicella titers are not drawn in pregnancy. However, any patient who is not certain whether they have had chickenpox should avoid contact with the disease and be tested immediately if they are exposed.

Vertical transmission occurs transplacentally. In the first trimester, there is an increased risk of spontaneous abortion. It is thought that VZV may pose some teratogenic threat. Infections near term may lead to a postnatal infection that may range from a benign course like chickenpox or a fulminant disseminated infection, leading to death. Other infants may show no signs of infection at birth; however, they will develop shingles at some point later in childhood.

Varicella zoster immune globulin (VZIG) may prevent transmission of the disease. Thus, any patient without a history of chickenpox with an exposure in pregnancy should receive VZIG within 72 hours of exposure. Infants of mothers who develop varicella disease within 5 days before delivery or 2 to 3 days after should receive VZIG.

Cytomegalovirus

Cytomegalovirus (**CMV**) infections of mothers usually causes either a subclinical or mild viral illness. Only rarely will it lead to hepatitis or a mononucleosis like syndrome; thus, maternal infections are rarely diagnosed. CMV causes in utero infections in approximately 1% of all newborns; however, probably less than 10% of these will result in a clinically recognized illness.

Infants that are symptomatic will develop cytomegalic inclusion disease manifested by a diffuse collection of findings including hepatomegaly, splenomegaly, thrombocytopenia, jaundice, cerebral calcifications, chorioretinitis, and an interstitial pneumonitis. Affected infants have a high mortality rate (30%) and may develop mental retardation, sensorineural hearing loss, and neuromuscular disorders. Less than 10% of these infants will have no sequelae of the disease.

Currently, there is no treatment or prophylaxis for the disease. Antiviral medications have been tried, currently without success. A vaccine for the prevention of disease in the mother is being investigated as well.

Rubella Virus

Rubella infection in adults leads to a mild illness with a maculopapular rash, arthritis, arthralgias, and a diffuse lymphadenopathy that lasts 2 to 4 days. The infection can be transmitted to the fetus and cause congenital rubella infection, which may lead to **congenital rubella syndrome** (CRS). The maternal-fetal transmission rate is highest during the first trimester as are the rates of congenital abnormalities. However, transmission may occur at anytime during pregnancy.

The congenital abnormalities associated with CRS include deafness, heart abnormalities, cataracts, and mental retardation. However, with rubella infection during organogenesis, it is likely that any organ system may be affected. There are a variety of latent sequelae that include the delayed onset of diabetes, thyroid disease, deafness, ocular disease, and growth hormone deficiency. The diagnosis of rubella infections relies on serologies. IgM titers will result from primary and reinfection with rubella. Because IgM does not cross the placenta, titers in the infant are indicative of infection. IgG titers that are elevated over time support the diagnosis of CRI in an infant as well.

Currently, there is no treatment for rubella once acquired. However, the institution of rubella immunization has decreased the number of CRS cases to less than 20 per year. In pregnancy, the rubella titer is checked during the first trimester. Because of theoretic risk of transmission of the live virus in the vaccine, patients do not receive the measles, mumps, and rubella vaccine until postpartum. Women who are known to have low or nonexistent titers should be advised to avoid anyone with possible rubella infections.

Human Immunodeficiency Virus

Approximately 25% of infants born to human immunodeficiency virus (HIV)-infected mothers will become infected with HIV. Increased transmission can be seen with higher viral burden or advanced disease in the mother, rupture of the membranes, and events during labor and delivery that increase neonatal exposure to maternal blood. Transmission is believed to occur late in pregnancy or during labor and delivery. Although it has been suggested that cesarean section delivery can lower transmission rates, this theory has not been confirmed by clinical trials. Current evidence does suggest, however, that zidovudine or AZT administration during the antepartum (after the first trimester), intrapartum, and neonatal period can reduce the risk of maternal-fetal HIV transmission by two thirds in women with mildly symptomatic HIV disease. These findings underline the importance of offering HIV screening to all expectant mothers.

Neisseria gonorrhoeae

Gonococcal infections are transmitted during passage of the neonate through the birth canal. The infection in neonates can be of the eye, oropharynx, external ear, and anorectal mucosa. These infections can become disseminated causing arthritis and meningitis.

Because there are antibiotic therapies for *N. gonorrhoeae*, it should be screened for in early pregnancy and eradicated. In high-risk populations, third-trimester screening is common. The diagnosis is made via culture or by DNA probe. Treatment can be with ceftriaxone or penicillin and probenecid. Because they often accompany one another, patients should be treated with azithromycin or erythromycin for presumed chlamydial infection as well.

Chlamydia trachomatis

Chlamydial infections in the newborn can lead to serious sequelae. In infected patients with vaginal deliveries, 40% of their infants will develop conjunctivitis and greater than 10% will develop chlamydial pneumonia. The infection is transmitted during delivery from the genital tract to the infant.

Because asymptomatic infection is common, all patients should be screened during pregnancy and treated if positive. Because tetracycline and doxycycline are not advised in pregnancy, the treatment of choice is erythromycin or azithromycin. Usually patients positive for chlamydia are treated for gonococcus as well, because the two infections tend to be transmitted together.

Hepatitis B

Viral hepatitis caused by the hepatitis B DNA virus can be acquired from sexual contact, exposure to blood products, and transplacentally. The clinical manifestations of the disease range from mild hepatic dysfunction to fulminant liver failure and death. It can be diagnosed using a variety of antibody and antigenic markers.

During the prenatal period, all patients are screened for hepatitis B surface antigen (HBsAg). Those with HBsAg are likely to have chronic disease and are at risk for transmission to their fetus. If patients are exposed during pregnancy, they can be given HepB immunoglobulin, which may be protective. Neonates of mothers who are HBsAg positive should be given HepB immunoglobulin at birth, 3 months, and 6 months. All infants are routinely being immunized with the hepatitis B vaccine.

Syphilis

Syphilis is caused by infection with the spirochete *Treponema pallidum* and is usually transmitted via sexual contact or transplacentally to the fetus. Because there must be spirochetemia for vertical transmission to occur, pregnant women with latent syphilis may not transmit the disease, whereas those with primary or secondary syphilis are quite likely to do so. Despite prenatal screening and easily available treatment, there are still several hundred cases of congenital syphilis annually in the United States.

Syphilis in pregnancy resulting in vertical transmission may present with a late abortion, a stillborn infant, or a congenitally infected infant. Congenital syphilis presents as a systemic illness with hepatomegaly, splenomegaly, hemolysis, lymphadenopathy, and jaundice. Diagnosis can be made by identification of IgM antitreponemal antibodies, which do not cross the placenta, whereas a noninfected fetus of an infected mother will have maternal IgG antibodies that do cross the placenta. Treatment is with penicillin as discussed in Chapter 14.

Toxoplasmosis

Toxoplasma gondii is a common protozoan parasite that can be found in humans and domestic animals. The infections in immunocompetent hosts are often subclinical. Occasionally, a patient will get fevers, malaise, lymphadenopathy, and a rash similar to most viral infections. Pregnant women who are infected can transmit the disease transplacentally to their fetus. Transmission is more common when the disease is acquired in the third trimester, although neonatal manifestations are usually mild or subclinical. Infections acquired in the first trimester are transmitted less commonly; however, the infection has much more serious consequences in the fetus. Severe congenital infection can involve fevers, seizures, chorioretinitis, hydro- or microcephaly, hepatosplenomegaly, and jaundice. Thus, the differential diagnosis for this infection includes nearly all other commonly acquired intrauterine infections. Diagnosis of toxoplasmosis in the neonate can be made with detection of IgM antibodies, but lack of the antibodies does not necessarily rule out infection.

Because women with previous *Toxoplasma* exposure are likely to be protected from further infections, it is a reasonable policy to screen all patients in the antepartum period for the disease to determine whether they are at risk for infection. As the disease is transmitted commonly to and from cats, patients are advised to avoid cats in pregnancy. Toxoplasmosis in pregnancy can be diagnosed maternally with IgM and IgG titers. If diagnosis is made or suspected early in pregnancy, verification of fetal infection can be made by obtaining fetal blood via **percutaneous umbilical blood sampling**. Diagnosis may influence the decision of whether to terminate a pregnancy in the first two trimesters. The disease can be treated with pyrimethamine and a sulfonamide after 14 weeks gestation or spiramycin. Spiramycin is preferable in pregnant women because no teratogenic effects are known.

Key Points

1. It is important to differentiate between infections that are transmitted transplacentally and ones that are acquired from the birth canal.
2. Infections during the first trimester during organogenesis are more likely to cause congenital abnormalities and spontaneous abortions.
3. Congenital infections can lead to serious infections of the neonatal period often with disastrous long-term sequelae, including mental retardation, blindness, and deafness.
4. Because IgM does not cross the placenta, IgM in the mother's circulation implies an acute infection. IgG implies that there has been a previous infection.

▶ HYPEREMESIS GRAVIDARUM

Nausea and vomiting in pregnancy, or "morning sickness" is common; seen in 88% of pregnancies, it usually resolves by the 16th week of pregnancy. A variety of etiologies have been proposed for these symptoms in pregnancy. Elevated levels of human chorionic gonadotropin, thyroid hormone, or the intrinsic hormones of the gut have all been hypothesized. There seems to be a disordered motility of the upper gastrointestinal tract that contributes to the problem. Despite the nausea and vomiting, often patients will be able to maintain adequate nutrition. However, occasionally patients will become dehydrated and have electrolyte abnormalities. When this occurs, hyperemesis gravidarum is the diagnosis given.

Treatment and Prognosis

For patients with true hyperemesis gravidarum, their symptoms may persist into the third trimester and rarely until term. The goal of therapy is to maintain adequate nutrition. Upon presentation with dehydration, patients should be rehydrated and electrolyte abnormalities should be normalized. A hypochloremic alkalosis from extensive vomiting will often be seen, so normal saline with 5% dextrose is commonly used. The nausea and vomiting itself may respond to antiemetics. Compazine, Phenergan, Tigan, and Reglan are commonly used. Antiemetics should ge given IV, intramuscularly, or as suppositories because oral medications will often lead to further emesis.

Long-term management of hyperemesis includes maintaining hydration, adequate nutrition, and symptomatic relief from the nausea and vomiting. Many patients will respond to antiemetics and IV hydration. Once they are rehydrated, they will be able to use the antiemetic to control their nausea so that they are able to maintain oral intake. However, a small percentage of patients will require feeding tubes or even parenteral nutrition for the course of the pregnancy. As long as hydration and adequate nutrition are maintained, pregnancy outcomes are usually good.

Key Points

1. Nausea and vomiting in pregnancy is common; however, patients with hyperemesis gravidarum will not be able to maintain hydration and nutrition.
2. Acute management is with IV hydration, electrolyte repletion, and antiemetics.
3. Chronic treatment is with antiemetics and occasionally tube feeds or parenteral nutrition.

▶ COAGULATION DISORDERS

Pregnancy is generally considered a "hypercoaguable" state. The pathogenesis of this state has not been elucidated, but there are several hypotheses as to the etiology that include increased coagulation factors, endothelial damage, and venous stasis. Interestingly, the risk for superficial vein thrombosis (SVT), deep vein thrombosis (DVT), and pulmonary embolus (PE) is increased postpartum. These coagulation problems present difficulty in treatment during pregnancy (Table 9-1), and pulmonary embolus is one of the leading causes of maternal mortality.

Pathogenesis

A single cause of the hypercoagulability of pregnancy has not been found, but there are several possible mechanisms hypothesized. The first is that there is an intrinsic increase in coagulability of the serum itself. In pregnancy, the production of clotting factors is increased and levels of all the clotting factors except XI and XIII are noted. Also noted in pregnancy is that the turnover time for fibrinogen is decreased and that there are increased levels of fibrinopeptide A, which is cleaved from fibrinogen to make fibrin. Furthermore, there are increased levels of circulating fibrin monomer complexes. These levels increase further at the time of delivery and immediately postpartum. Finally, it has been hypothesized that the placenta synthesizes a factor that decreases fibrinolysis, but there is minimal evidence for this.

TABLE 9-1

Thrombotic Events in Pregnancy

	Antepartum	Postpartum
Superficial vein thromboses	20 per 10,000	110 per 10,000
Deep vein thromboses	5 per 10,000	10 per 10,000
Pulmonary embolus	4 per 10,000	13 per 10,000

Another proposed source for the hypercoagulability is increased exposure to subendothelial collagen secondary to increased endothelial damage during pregnancy, although a mechanism has not been proposed. It has also been hypothesized that endothelial damage in the venous system during parturition increases the amount of thrombogenesis. This seems feasible, particularly as the pathogenesis behind ovarian vein thrombosis, but it does not entirely account for the hypercoagulability before parturition.

Venous stasis also may account for some of the increase in venous thromboses during and after pregnancy. There are two principal causes for venous stasis in pregnancy. The first is decreased venous tone during pregnancy, which may be related to the smooth muscle reactant properties of this high estrogen and progesterone state. Second, the uterus, as it enlarges, compresses the inferior vena cava, the iliac, and pelvic veins. This compression, in particular, likely contributes to the increase in pelvic vein thromboses.

Superficial Vein Thrombosis

Although this is a painful complication of hypercoagulability, it is thought to be unlikely to lead to emboli. The diagnosis is usually obvious with a palpable, usually visible, venous cord that is quite tender with local erythema and edema. Because of the low risk of emboli from SVT, it is not routinely treated. However, the patient should be given the signs and symptoms of DVTs and PEs as they may be at an increased risk for either.

Deep Vein Thrombosis

Diagnosis of DVT is often made clinically with confirmation by Doppler studies or venography. The usual patient will present with lower extremity pain and swelling, usually unilateral. On examination they will often have edema, local erythema, tenderness, venous distention, and a palpable cord underlying the region of pain and tenderness. When clinical suspicion is high, the patient is usually sent for lower extremity noninvasive studies with the Doppler ultrasound for confirmation of a venous obstruction. Rarely, venography, the gold standard, will be used.

Treatment of DVT during pregnancy involves the use of heparin. Initially, the treatment is with IV heparin, which often is continued with subcutaneous heparin throughout the remainder of the pregnancy and postpartum. Currently, the use of low molecular heparin in pregnancy is being studied and may have some use. Coumadin therapy is contraindicated in pregnancy secondary to evidence of fetal abnormalities caused by coumadin. When given in the first trimester, it causes warfarin embryopathy, which involves nasal hypoplasia and skeletal abnormalities. In addition, it seems to cause diffuse central nervous system abnormalities and optic atrophy when given anytime in pregnancy.

Pulmonary Embolus

Pulmonary embolus results when emboli from DVTs travel to the right heart and then lodge in the pulmonary arterial system, leading to **pulmonary hypertension, hypoxia,** and, depending on the extent of the emboli, **right-sided heart failure and death.** Clinical suspicion of pulmonary embolus is raised whenever a patient presents with acute onset of **shortness of breath,** simultaneous onset of **pleuritic chest pain, hemoptysis,** and concordant signs of DVT.

The diagnosis of PE usually involves the clinical picture correlated with a variety of diagnostic tests. A **chest radiograph,** or chest X-ray, may be entirely normal; however, two common signs seen are the abrupt termination of a vessel as it is traced distally and an area of radiolucency in the area of the lung beyond the PE. An **electrocardiogram** may also be entirely normal; however, it occasionally shows signs of right heart strain with right axis deviation, nonspecific ST-T changes, and peaked T-waves. A **ventilation/perfusion scan** is a radionuclide scan that first examines the perfusion of the lungs by detecting a radioisotope in the pulmonary circulation (Fig. 9-1). An entirely normal perfusion scan rules out PE. However, if there is a defect in perfusion, a ventilation scan is performed by having the patient inhale a radioisotope and detecting the ventilation. Mismatched defects in the ventilation and perfusion scans are indicative of PE. A **pulmonary angiography** is the gold standard for diagnosis of PE. The pulmonary artery is catheterized and a radiopaque dye is injected. Diagnosis is made if there are intraluminal filling defects or if sharp vessel cutoffs are seen (Fig. 9-2).

Treatment of mild PE is similar to treatment of DVT with IV heparin and eventually subcutaneous heparin therapy. In the postpartum period, coumadin can be used as well. Massive PE leading to an unstable hypoxic patient is often treated with streptokinase for thrombolysis in addition to supportive measures. Patients are treated for a minimum of 6 months.

Key Points

1. Pregnancy is a hypercoagulable state with increased clotting factors, endothelial damage, and venous stasis.
2. Pulmonary embolus is the leading cause of maternal death.
3. DVT and PE may be treated with heparin. Thrombolysis may be necessary for the unstable patient.

▶ SUBSTANCE ABUSE IN PREGNANCY

Substance abuse in pregnancy contributes to both the maternal and fetal morbidity and mortality both antepartum and postpartum. The most commonly used substances are alcohol and cigarettes, both of which contribute to poor outcomes of pregnancy. The two most common illicit drugs used in pregnancy are cocaine and opiates. These each have their associated problems for the infant. Finally, even when infants are born with minimal effects of the intrapartum insult, substance abuse is an indicator for other social problems that may contribute to a poor environment for child rearing.

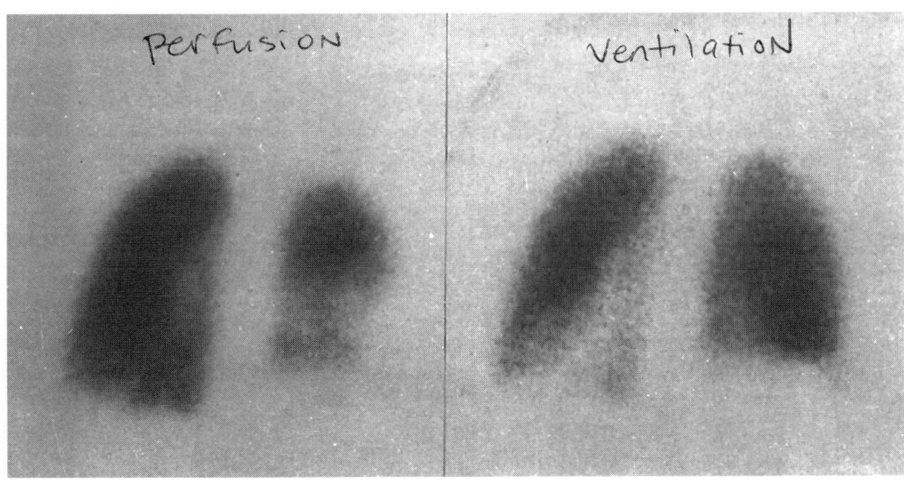

Figure 9-1 In these posterior views, the perfusion lung scan (left) reveals segmental defects, which are not "matched" in the normal ventilation scan (right). This is consistent with a high probability of pulmonary embolism.

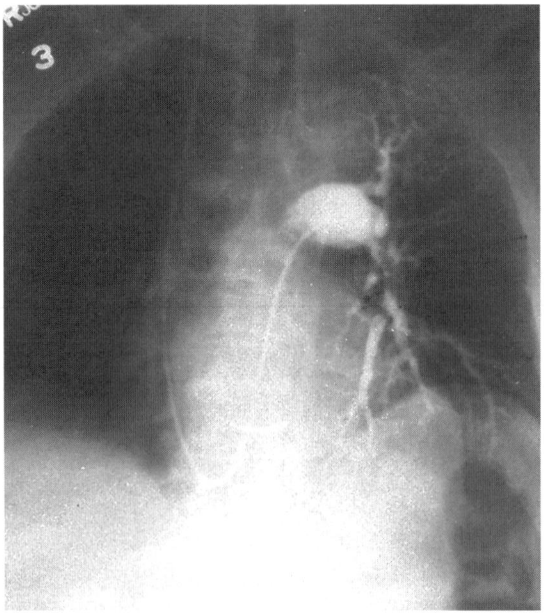

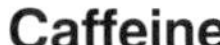

Figure 9-2 Arteriogram of the left pulmonary artery shows filling defects and an unperfused segment of lung as shown by the absence of contrast dye.

Alcohol

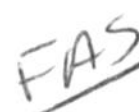

A constellation of abnormalities in the infants born to women who abuse alcohol during pregnancy have been included in the diagnosis of fetal alcohol syndrome (FAS). The syndrome tends to occur with increased severity in patients who drank "heavier" (two to five drinks per day) in pregnancy. FAS, which includes growth retardation, central nervous system effects, and abnormal facies, is estimated to occur in approximately 1 in every 2,000 live births. However, there may be many other milder cases that are not recognized. Diagnosis is made by a history of alcohol abuse in the mother combined with the constellation of infant abnormalities. There are other teratogenic effects of alcohol that include almost every organ system; in particular, cardiac defects are associated with alcohol abuse.

Treatment

Several studies have shown that aggressive counselling programs for expectant mothers has led to a significant decrease in alcohol intake in greater than 50% of the participants. For patients who are at risk for alcohol withdrawal, barbiturates are often used for withdrawal symptoms because of the potential teratogenicity of benzodiazepines. Because alcoholics are at higher risk for nutritional deficiencies, special care should be taken to ensure adequate nutrition during pregnancy.

Caffeine

Caffeine is found in coffee (30 to 170 mg/cup), tea (10 to 100 mg/cup), and caffeinated soft drinks (30 to 60 mg/12 oz). It is the most commonly used drug in pregnancy, with almost 80% of all pregnant women being exposed in the first trimester. Studies on rats showed teratogenicity at high levels of caffeine exposure. There does appear to be an increased risk of first and second trimester miscarriages with consumption of greater than150 mg/day of caffeine. Patients should be advised of this risk and to cut down caffeine consumption during pregnancy to less than 150 mg/day.

Cigarettes

Cigarette smoking in pregnancy has been correlated with increased risk of spontaneous abortions, preterm births, abruptio placenta, and decreased birth weight. Furthermore, infants exposed to cigarette smoking in the womb are at an increased risk for sudden infant death syndrome and respiratory illnesses of childhood. A dose-response effect has been noted for many of these outcomes. In the Ontario Perinatal Mortality Study, smokers were divided into less than 1 pack per day (PPD) and more than 1 PPD. An increased risk of fetal death of 20% was found in those pregnancies in the less than 1 PPD and of 35% in the greater than 1 PPD group.

Treatment

Because of the demonstrated dose-response effect of smoking, patients should be counseled as to the increased risks for their infant and advised at the very minimum to decrease cigarette use, although there is no demonstrated safe amount of smoking. Furthermore, primary care physicians caring for women of child-bearing age should begin this counseling before pregnancy.

Cocaine

The use of cocaine in pregnancy is correlated with abruptio placenta, growth-restricted infants, and an increased risk for preterm labor and delivery. There has been a reported delivery of an infant with a massive cerebral infarction born to a woman who took a large dose of cocaine within 72 hours before delivery. The physiologic effects of cocaine, which cause vasoconstriction and hypertension, are consistent with this event, as well as the increased risk for abruption. Increasing amounts of evidence show that children who were exposed to cocaine in utero are at increased risk for central nervous system problems including developmental delay.

Treatment

Patients who admit to cocaine use should be advised of its risks to themselves and their infant. Social services should be involved during the prenatal care, and patients who continue to abuse the drug should be encouraged to enter a detoxification center to quit.

Opiates

The two most common opiates used in pregnancy are heroin and methadone. There are no known teratogenic effects of opiates. In fact, there is likely to be more danger to fetuses from heroin withdrawal syndrome, including miscarriage, preterm delivery, and fetal death, than from chronic opiates use. Thus, patients using heroin in pregnancy should be enrolled in methadone programs rather than advised to quit outright. Once infants are delivered, they will need careful monitoring and slow withdrawal from their narcotic addiction using tincture of opium. Once patients have delivered, an aggressive effort should be made to taper their methadone.

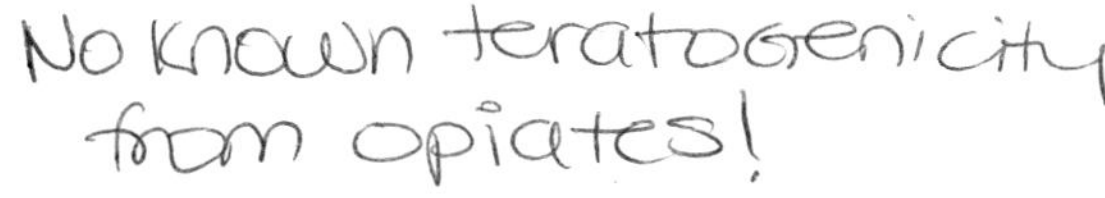

Key Points

1. Heavy alcohol abuse is correlated with FAS, which includes a constellation of growth restriction, central nervous system effects, and abnormal facies. Alcohol has been also correlated with other teratogenic effects, particularly cardiac defects.
2. Caffeine use greater than 150 mg/day has been correlated with increase risk of spontaneous abortions.
3. Cigarette use during pregnancy has been correlated with growth restriction, abruptions, preterm delivery, and fetal death. Strong encouragement should be given to patients to decrease use during pregnancy.
4. Cocaine has been correlated with abruptio placenta and central nervous system effects in children, and patients should be advised to quit outright.
5. Narcotic abusers should be enrolled in methadone programs because the acute withdrawal effects of narcotics are more dangerous than chronic use.

CHAPTER 10

Postpartum Care and Complications

▶ ROUTINE POSTPARTUM CARE

Vaginal Deliveries

Routine care issues in patients after vaginal delivery include pain control and perineal care. Usually, the pain can be reduced with nonsteroidal anti-inflammatory drugs (NSAIDs) or acetaminophen. Low-dose narcotics are occasionally required to get a patient comfortable, particularly at the hour of sleep. For patients with vaginal deliveries that involved either episiotomies or lacerations, perineal care is particularly important. Ice packs around the clock can be quite beneficial for both pain and edema in the perineum and labia. When inspecting the perineum of a patient postpartum, it is important to ensure that the perineal repair is intact and that no hematomas have developed. It is also important to assess the patient for hemorrhoids, which are common in pregnancy and postpartum, particularly after a long second stage. These should resolve, but patients benefit from over-the-counter hemorrhoidal medications, stool softeners, and ice packs.

Cesarean Section

Wound care and pain management are key issues in postcesarean section care. Local wound care and observation for signs of wound infection or separation are part of the routine care. Pain is usually managed with narcotics, which can contribute to a postoperative ileus. Thus, patients on narcotics should also be on stool softeners and occasionally laxatives. NSAIDs should be used concomitantly for the cramping pain caused by uterine involution.

Breast Care

All postpartum patients need breast care regardless of whether they are nursing. Patients will usually have milk "let down," and the onset of lactation approximately 24 to 72 hours postpartum. When this occurs, the breasts usually get uniformly warmer, firmer, and tender. Patients often complain of pain or warmth in the breasts and may experience a low-grade fever. For patients not breastfeeding, ice packs, a tight bra, analgesics, and anti-inflammatories are all useful. Patients that are breastfeeding get some relief from the breastfeeding itself, although this act can lead to its own difficulties, such as tenderness and erosions around the nipple.

Postpartum Contraception

Contraception is an important issue to address while patients are still in the hospital. Condoms are particularly good because of the prophylaxis against sexually transmitted infections. The other barrier methods of the diaphragm and cervical cap should be avoided until 6 weeks postpartum when the cervix has returned to its normal shape and size. Intrauterine devices (IUDs) may be inserted postpartum; however, they have a higher rate of extrusion in the immediate postpartum period because of the dilated cervix.

For patients that are not breastfeeding, oral contraceptive pills (OCPs), norplant, and Depo-provera are all options. OCPs have been shown to decrease the amount of milk produced by breastfeeding mothers. Depo-provera may decrease milk production as well, but it is unlikely to be clinically significant. For patients that are dedicated to breastfeeding and interested in hormonal forms of birth control, Depo-provera is the better choice.

Key Points

1. Abstinence is the best form of contraception; a close second is tubal ligation. However, most patients use neither and need a contraceptive plan.
2. Condoms with a spermicidal foam or gel can be used by anyone postpartum.
3. Diaphragms and cervical caps need to be refitted at 6 weeks.
4. IUDs, norplant, and Depo-provera can be given postpartum.
5. OCPs can be used in nonbreastfeeding patients but may cause decreased lactation in breastfeeding mothers.

▶ POSTPARTUM COMPLICATIONS

The primary medical complications that arise postpartum usually occur 1 to 2 weeks after delivery (Table 10-1). Probably the most common and important are

TABLE 10-1

Complications of Vaginal and Cesarean Deliveries

	Vaginal Delivery	Cesarean Section
Common complications	Postpartum hemorrhage Vaginal hematoma Cervical laceration Retained POCs	Postpartum hemorrhage Surgical blood loss Wound infection Endomyometritis
Rare complications	Endomyometritis Episiotomy infections Episiotomy breakdown	Wound dehiscence

postpartum hemorrhage, endomyometritis, and mastitis. Postpartum depression can also occur and may begin within the first week after delivery.

Postpartum Hemorrhage

Postpartum hemorrhage is defined as blood loss exceeding 500 mL in a vaginal delivery and greater than 1,000 mL in a cesarean section. If the hemorrhage occurs before the first 24 hours, it is deemed early postpartum hemorrhage; after that it is late or delayed postpartum hemorrhage. Common causes of bleeding postpartum include uterine atony, retained products of conception (POCs), placenta accreta, cervical lacerations, and vaginal lacerations (Tables 10-2 and 10-3). While investigating the cause for the hemorrhage, the patient is simultaneously started on fluid resuscitation, and preparations are made to give blood transfusions. If patients become hypovolemic and hypotensive, a rare outcome is Sheehan's syndrome, or pituitary infarction. These patients present either with the absence of milk let down secondary to the absence of prolactin or failure to restart menstruation secondary to the absence of gonadotropins.

Vaginal Lacerations

Vaginal lacerations with uncontrolled bleeding should be the first thing ruled out in the initial postpartum period. Initially after a delivery, one examines the perineum, labia, periurethral area, and deeper aspects of the vagina for lacerations. These should be repaired at that time. However, deep sulcal tears or vaginal lacerations behind the cervix may be quite difficult to visualize without careful retraction. Adequate anesthesia, an experienced obstetrician, and assistance in retracting are all necessary to perform an adequate exploration. These lacerations can be repaired with absorbable sutures.

TABLE 10-2

Conditions that Predispose to or Worsen Obstetrical Hemorrhage

- Abnormal placentation
  - Placental previa
  - Abruption placentae
  - Placenta accreta
  - Ectopic pregnancy
  - Hydatidiform mole
- Trauma during labor and delivery
  - Episiotomy
  - Complicated vaginal delivery
  - Low- or midforceps delivery
  - Cesarean section or hysterectomy
  - Uterine rupture
- Small maternal blood volume
  - Small woman
  - Pregnancy hypervolemia constricted
    - Severe pre-clampsia
    - Eclampsia
- Uterine atony
  - Overdistended uterus
    - Large fetus
    - Multiple fetuses
    - Hydramnios
  - Anesthesia or analgesia
  - Exhausted myometrium
    - Rapid labor
    - Prolonged labor
    - Oxytocin or prostaglandin stimulation
    - Chorioamnionitis
- Coagulation defects—intensify other causes
  - Placental abruption
  - Prolonged retention of dead fetus
  - Amnionic fluid embolism
  - Severe intravascular hemolysis
  - Massive transfusions
  - Severe pre-eclampsia and eclampsia
  - Congenital coagulopathies
  - Anticoagulant treatment

Adapted from Cunningham FG et al. Williams Obstetrics. 19th ed. Norwalk, CT: Appleton & Lange, 1993:820.

TABLE 10-3

Etiology of Postpartum Hemorrhage in Vaginal and Cesarean Deliveries

Vaginal Delivery	Cesarean Section
Vaginal lacerations	Uterine atony
Cervical lacerations	Surgical blood loss
Uterine atony	Placenta accreta
Placenta accreta	Uterine rupture
Vaginal hematoma	
Retained POCs	
Uterine inversion	
Uterine rupture	

Cervical Lacerations

Cervical lacerations can be seen in any delivery where the cervix has dilated. Commonly they are a result of rapid dilation of the cervix during the first stage of labor or if a patient has begun second stage without complete dilation of the cervix. If a patient is bleeding at the level of the cervix or above, a careful exploration of the cervix should be performed.

The patient should have adequate anesthesia, either epidural, spinal, or pudendal block. The walls of the vagina should be retracted so the cervix can be well visualized. When the anterior lip of the cervix is seen, it can be grasped with a ring forcep. Then, another ring forcep can be used to grasp beyond the first and in this fashion the cervix should be "walked" around its entirety so that no lacerations, particularly on the posterior aspect, are missed. If any lacerations are seen they can be repaired with either interrupted or running absorbable sutures.

Uterine Atony

Patients are at a higher risk for uterine atony if they are multiparous, particularly a grand multip (more than five deliveries) or if they have a history of atony with any previous pregnancies. Uterine abnormalities or fibroids may also interfere with uterine contractions and lead to atony and increased bleeding. The diagnosis of atony is made by palpation of the uterus and finding it soft rather than firm. Atony is often treated by pitocin IV, which is often given prophylactically to most postpartum patients. While pitocin is being administered, strong uterine massage should be performed to assist the uterus to contract down. If atony continues, the next step is Methergen (methylergonovine). If the uterus is still atonic, the next step is to give Prostin ($PGF_{2\alpha}$). The prostaglandin is thought to be more effective if given directly into the uterine musculature, either transabdominally or transcervically.

Retained POCs

Careful inspection of the placenta should always be performed. However, with vaginal delivery, it can often be difficult to determine whether a small piece of the placenta has been left behind in the uterus. Oftentimes, these retained fetal membranes or placenta pass in the lochia. However, they occasionally lead to endomyometritis and postpartum hemorrhage. These complications usually present several days after delivery. If the suspicion is high for retained POCs, the uterus should be explored either manually if the cervix has not contracted down or by **dilatation and curettage** (D&C). Once it has been ascertained that there are no POCs via exploration, if hemorrhage continues, either accreta or atony should be suspected.

Accreta

Placenta accreta, increta, and percreta are discussed briefly in Chapter 4 with antepartum hemorrhage. These conditions are the result of placental tissue invading into or beyond the uterine myometrium leading to incomplete separation of the placenta postpartum and postpartum hemorrhage. Accreta presents with bleeding unresponsive to contractile agents such as pitocin, ergonovines, and prostaglandins and to uterine massage. If these fail to stop the bleeding, accreta is suspected and the patient is brought to the operating room for surgical management.

To stop the hemorrhage due to accreta, the first step is usually bilateral O'Leary sutures to tie off the uterine artery. The second step is unilateral ligation of the hypogastric, or internal iliac, artery. If these fail to provide hemostasis, often the patient requires a gravid hysterectomy.

Uterine Rupture

Uterine rupture is estimated to occur in 1 of every 2,000 deliveries. It is an intrapartum complication but may present with bleeding postpartum. It is rare for rupture to occur in a nulliparous patient. Risk factors include previous uterine surgery, breech extraction, obstructed labor, and high parity. Symptoms usually include abdominal pain and a "popping" sensation intra-abdominally. Treatment involves laparotomy and repair of the ruptured uterus. If hemorrhage cannot be controlled, hysterectomy may be indicated.

Uterine Inversion

Uterine inversion may occur in 1 of 2,500 deliveries. Risk factors include fundal implantation of the placenta, uterine atony, accreta, and excessive traction on the cord during third stage. Diagnosis is made by witnessing the fundus of the uterus attached to the placenta upon placental delivery. The first step in treatment is to attempt to manually reinvert the uterus. Uterine relaxants such as nitroglycerin may be given to aid reinversion. If this is unsuccessful, laparotomy is required to reinvert the uterus with an abdominal approach (Fig. 10-1).

Key Points

1. Postpartum hemorrhage is an obstetric emergency.
2. The causes include uterine atony, uterine rupture, uterine inversion, retained POCs, placenta accreta, and cervical or vaginal lacerations.
3. Treatment may require use of blood products including fresh frozen plasma and cryoprecipitate in patients who develop disseminated intravascular coagulation (DIC).

Endomyometritis

Endomyometritis is a polymicrobial infection of the uterine lining that often invades into the underlying wall. It is most commonly seen after cesarean sections

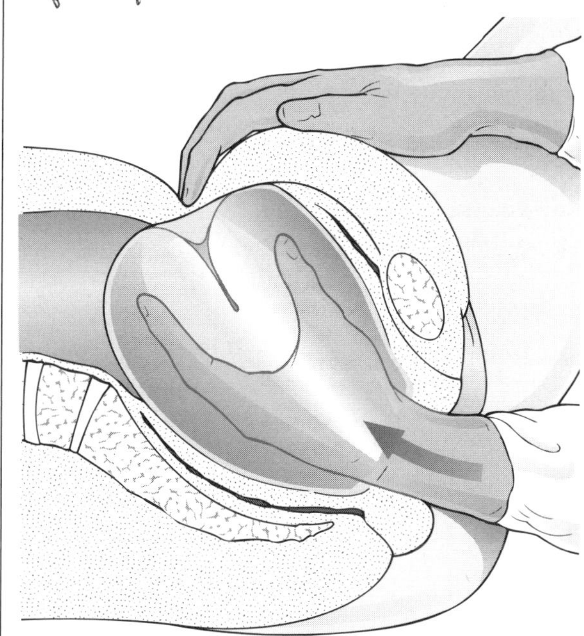

Figure 10-1 Manual replacement of an inverted uterus.

but can be seen in vaginal deliveries as well, particularly if manual removal of the placenta was required.

Diagnosis is made in the setting of fever, elevated white blood count, and uterine tenderness, with a higher suspicion after cesarean sections. It commonly occurs 5 to 10 days after delivery but should still be suspected when all other sources of infection have been ruled out for several weeks after delivery. Because retained POCs can be the etiology of infection, often an ultrasound is obtained to examine the intrauterine contents.

Treatment of endomyometritis is usually with broad-spectrum intravenous antibiotics, or "triple" antibiotics. If retained POCs are suspected, a D&C is performed. Because the postpartum uterus is at greater risk for perforation, great care should be taken during dilation and a blunt rather than sharp curette should be used. Antibiotics are continued until the patient is afebrile for 48 hours, uterine pain and tenderness is absent, and the white blood count normalizes.

Key Points

1. Endomyometritis is more common in patients with cesarean section than vaginal delivery, although patients with manual removal of the placenta are also at increased risk.
2. Diagnosis is clinical with fever, elevated white blood cell count, and uterine tenderness.
3. Treatment is with broad-spectrum antibiotics and D&C for retained POCs.

Mastitis

Mastitis is a regional infection of the breast, commonly caused by the patient's skin flora or the oral flora of breastfeeding infants. The organisms enter an erosion or cracked nipple and proliferate, leading to infection. Lactating women will often have warm, diffusely tender, and firm breasts, particularly at the time of engorgement or milk let down. This should be differentiated from focal tenderness, erythema, and differences in temperature from one region of the breast to another. Classically, a patient with mastitis is able to differentiate between lactation and infection because of the focality and the change in symptoms. The diagnosis can be made with physical examination, a fever, and an elevated white blood count.

Mastitis can be treated with oral antibiotics; commonly dicloxacillin is used. Patients should also continue to breastfeed, which prevents intraductal accumulation of infected material. Patients who are not breastfeeding should breast pump in the acute phase of the infection. Patients who are unresponsive to oral antibiotics are admitted for intravenous antibiotics until they remain afebrile for 48 hours.

Key Points

1. Mastitis is more common in breastfeeding women.
2. It is differentiated from engorgement by focal tenderness, erythema, and edema.
3. Treatment is with oral antibiotics and breast pumping or feeding.

Postpartum Depression

Many patients have the postpartum "blues" with mood swings and changes in appetite and sleep if not frank postpartum depression. The pathophysiology of depression is poorly understood, but particularly in postpartum patients, the rapid changes in estrogen, progesterone, and prolactin may be involved. The incidence of postpartum blues is greater than 50% in the postpartum patient, whereas postpartum depression complicates greater than 5% of pregnancies.

Diagnosis

Most patients have normal changes in appetite, energy level, and sleep patterns in the initial postpartum period that do not necessarily indicate procession to frank depression. However, patients who experience low energy level, anorexia, insomnia, hypersomnolence, and extreme sadness and other depressive symptoms for greater than a few weeks may have postpartum depression. These patients often have feelings of being entirely incapable of caring for their infants. Occasionally, depressed patients have suicidal ideation; this is a much clearer marker for depression and merits close observation.

Therapy and Prognosis

In patients with transient postpartum depression, usually the symptoms pass on their own with support and encouragement. However, these patients can occasionally progress to a more severe postpartum depression or psychosis. In these situations, the caregiver needs to determine whether the patient is having suicidal or homicidal ideation. A social worker and professional counselor should be involved as should the immediate family and any other individuals who are close to the patient and provide support. Most patients improve without psychopharmacology, but if the depression, and particularly the suicidal ideation, does not resolve, antidepressant medications are indicated. Most patients without a history of depression or other mental illness improve, usually to their prepregnancy state.

Key Points

1. Changes in appetite, sleep patterns, and energy level are common in the first few weeks postpartum.
2. Postpartum depression is common and probably underdiagnosed.
3. In most patients, the depressive symptoms resolve on their own, but occasionally antidepressants are required.

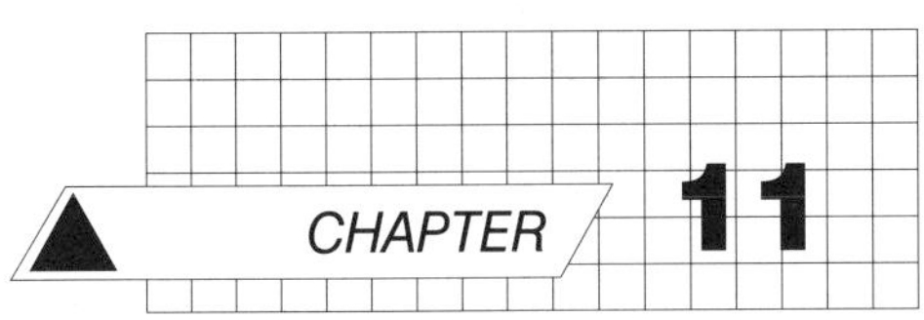

Benign Disorders of the Lower Genital Tract

▶ BENIGN LESIONS OF THE VULVA AND VAGINA

Many benign lesions and conditions of the vulva and vagina are infectious in nature and are covered in Chapter 14. However, noninfections lesions, including vulvar dystrophies, cysts, and benign tumors, are also found.

▶ CONGENITAL ANOMALIES

A variety of congenital defects occur in the external genitalia and vagina. Included are labial fusion, imperforate hymen, vaginal septum, and vaginal agenesis.

Labial Fusion

Labial fusion is associated with excess androgens. The etiology may be exogenous androgens or from an enzymatic error leading to increased androgen production. The most common form of enzymatic deficiency is 21-hydroxylase deficiency (Chapter 19) leading to congenital adrenal hyperplasia. This may be phenotypically demonstrated in the neonate with ambiguous genitalia. The neonates often present with adrenal crisis and loss of salt. This autosomal recessive trait occurs in roughly 1 in 40,000 to 50,000 pregnancies.

Treatment of this defect is to give cortisol, which is not being produced by the adrenal cortex. The exogenous cortisol then negatively feeds back on the pituitary to decrease the release of adrenal corticotrophic hormone (ACTH), thus inhibiting the stimulation of the adrenal gland that is shunting all steroid precursors into androgens. The labial fusion and other ambiguous genitalia may require reconstructive surgery.

Imperforate Hymen

The hymen is at the junction between the sinovaginal bulbs and the urogenital sinus. If it is not perforated during the organogenesis of the reproductive tract, it will be left as an obstruction to the outflow tract of the reproductive system. It is usually diagnosed at puberty with primary amenorrhea and the occurrence of menstrual cramps. On physical examination there may be hematocolpos, which is a buildup of blood behind the hymen. Before puberty, there may be hydrocolpos or mucoculpos, which are buildup of secretions behind the hymen. Treatment of imperforate hymen is with surgical correction.

Vaginal Septum

The vagina is formed as the Müllerian system from above joins the sinovaginal bulb at the mullerian tubercle. The mullerian tubercle must be canalized for a normal vagina to be formed. If this does not occur, this tissue may be left as a transverse vaginal septum that lies roughly at the junction between the lower two thirds and upper one third of the vagina. This occurs in approximately 1 in 75,000 females. Diagnosis is again made at the time of puberty with primary amenorrhea in the setting of menstrual symptoms. Surgical correction is the only form of treament.

Vaginal Agenesis

This may occur in Rokitansky-Kuster-Hauser (RKH) syndrome or testicular feminization. RKH syndrome is characterized by Müllerian agenesis or dysgenesis with aberrant development. Either complete agenesis of the Müllerian system occurs or only partial development of the corpus of the uterus. These patients may or may not have a rudimentary pouch of a vagina developed from the sinovaginal bulb. Testicular feminization syndrome occurs in 46,XY individuals who have an insensitivity to testosterone. Patients may have the beginning of a vagina as in RKH but will have undescended testes rather than the normal ovaries of the 46,XX RKH patient.

For both syndromes, the treatment involves surgical creation of a vagina or expansion of the short pouch with dilators. In addition, patients with testicular feminization should have surgical removal of the undescended testes, which are prone to development of seminomas.

Key Points

1. Labial fusion is often secondary to excess androgens, leading to ambiguous external genitalia.
2. Imperforate hymen and transvaginal septum both present with primary amenorrhea at puberty.
3. Vaginal agenesis can result in malformation in a genetic female or as a result of testosterone insensitivity in a genetic male.

► VULVAR DYSTROPHIES

These lesions range from hypertrophic to atrophic in etiology and must be differentiated from vulvar carcinoma. Hypertrophic lesions are often the result of chronic vulvar irritation. Initially, they are often an acute vulvitic lesion that is erythematous; however, over time and with chronic rubbing and itching, they may develop into raised white lesions.

Atrophic lesions are the result of decreased estrogenation to the local tissues. Thus, they are most common in postmenopausal women. The lesions can be erythematous in the setting of pure atrophy; however, these lesions too can become hyperkeratotic secondary to chronic scratching and rubbing, presenting as a mixed picture.

Diagnosis

Hypertrophic dystrophies often present with vulvar pruritus and either the acute erythematous moist lesion or a hyperkeratotic white lesion that develops as a result of chronic rubbing or itching of pruritic lesions. These lesions are called lichen simplex chronicus.

Atrophic lesions are seen in older patients, particularly those postmenopausal without estrogen supplementation. The decreased estrogenation of the tissues leads to atrophic changes such as the fusing of the labia minora and majora and thinning of the local tissues. Common presenting symptoms are dysuria, dyspareunia, vulvodynia, and pruritus. Lichen sclerosus and atrophicus is the most common cause of atrophic dystrophy (Fig. 11-1). It presents as above, and often the entire vulva and perineum is involved with atrophic changes that are often white secondary to the hyperkeratotic changes from chronic scratching of these lesions.

Neither change can be easily distinguished from vulvar cancers and occasionally from one another when a mixed picture of atrophic changes and hyperkeratotic lesions develop; therefore, all suspicious vulvar lesions need to be biopsied.

Treatment

The histologic diagnosis is the basis for treatment. Hypertrophic lesions are treated with hydrocortisone cream twice daily, which decreases the pruritus and local inflammation. Atrophic lesions are treated with hydrocortisone once a day to decrease inflammation and pruritus and once a day with 2% testosterone cream to build up the hypotrophic epithelium. Therapy usually takes 6 weeks to be effective, and patients may need oral antihistamines for their antipruritic effects to decrease irritation from scratching. Occasionally, patients may require steroid injections or stronger steroid creams, and they may be comanaged with dermatologists. Surgical therapy is rarely effective because local recurrence is common.

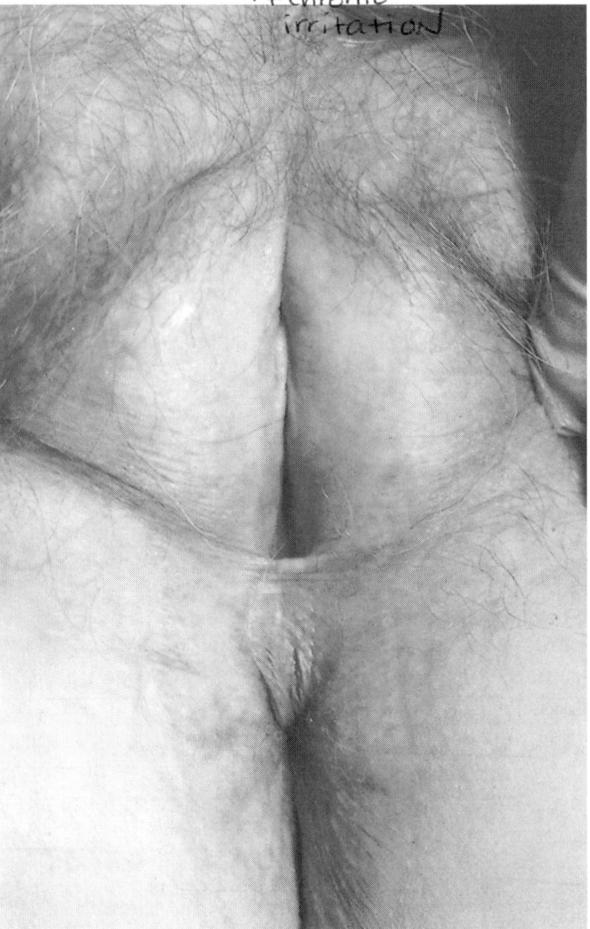

Figure 11-1 Lichen sclerosus and atrophicus. A late case, with loss of the labia.

Key Points

1. Hypertrophic lesions are secondary to chronic irritation and although initially erythematous, may evolve into white raised lesions.
2. Atrophic lesions are caused by decreased estrogen and are often erythematous because of the atrophic tissue; however, they can develop into white lesions with chronic scratching as well and may present as mixed lesions.
3. Diagnosis is made by biopsy.
4. Hypertrophic lesions are treated with hydrocortisone.

5. Atrophic lesions are treated with hydrocortisone and testosterone.

▶ BENIGN CYSTS

A variety of inclusion cysts can arise on the vulva. They can originate from occlusion of pilosebaceous ducts, sebaceous ducts, and apocrine sweat glands. They only need to be treated if they become symptomatic or infected.

Epidermal Cysts

These cysts usually result from occlusion of a pilosebaceous duct or a blocked hair follicle. They are lined with squamous epithelium and contain the tissue that would normally be exfoliated. These solitary lesions are normally small and asymptomatic; however, they can become superinfected and develop into abscesses. In this setting, incision (excision if possible) and drainage is the treatment.

Sebaceous Cysts

When the duct of a sebaceous gland becomes blocked, it results in a sebaceous cyst. The normally secreted sebum accumulates in this cyst. They are often multiple and asymptomatic. As with any cyst, they can become superinfected with local flora and need treatment with incision and drainage (I&D).

Apocrine Sweat Gland Cysts

These sweat glands are throughout the mons pubis and labia majora. They can become occluded and form occlusion cysts as well. **Fox-Fordyce** disease is a pruritic microcystic disease that results from occlusion of these sweat glands. As in the axillary region, if these cysts become infected and form multiple abscesses, hidradenitis suppurativa can result. Excision or incision and drainage is the treatment of choice. If the infection has an overlying cellulitis, often antibiotics are used as well.

Bartholin's Duct Cyst

An extensive discussion of Bartholin's duct cyst is in Chapter 14. These cysts arise when Bartholin's gland is obstructed. The location of this gland is at 4 and 8 o'clock on the labia majora. If asymptomatic, the cysts can be treated expectantly with sitz baths; however, in the case of infection, they are treated by I&D and insertion of a Word catheter. Recurrent Bartholin's abscesses are often treated with marsupialization.

Key Points

1. A variety of cysts from occlusion of ducts can be found on the vulva.
2. A solitary cyst is most likely epidermal in origin.
3. A collection of cysts that are asymptomatic are likely sebaceous cysts.
4. A collection of pruritic cysts is likely Fox-Fordyce disease, caused by occlusion of apocrine sweat glands.
5. Hidradenitis suppurativa is the result of abscess formation from superinfection of apocrine sweat glands and cysts.
6. Infection of any of these cysts is treated with I&D.

▶ BENIGN CERVICAL LESIONS

Congenital Anomalies

Isolated congenital anomalies of the cervix are rare. With uterine didelphys or double vagina, double cervix, or bicollis, may be found, but this does not arise on its own. However, women who were exposed in utero to diethylstilbestrol (last in the early 1970s) have some abnormality of the cervix approximately 25% of the time. These benign abnormalities include cervical collars, cervical hoods, cock's comb appearance, hypoplastic cervix, and pseudopolyps. Clear cell adenocarcinoma occurs in less than 0.1% of these patients but is a malignant process that can lead to untimely death.

Cervical Cysts

Most cysts of the cervix are dilated retention cysts called nabothian cysts. They are caused by blockage of an endocervical gland and expand to usually no more than 1 cm in diameter. They are more common in menstruating women. Nabothian cysts are usually asymptomatic, discovered on routine gynecologic examination, and require no treatment.

Cysts of the cervix can also be mesonephric cysts. These are remnants of the mesonephric (Wolffian) ducts that can become cystic. They differ from nabothian cysts in that they tend to lie deeper in the cervical stroma and on the external surface of the cervix. Finally, endometriosis can rarely implant on or near the cervix. These cysts tend to be red or purple in color and often the patient will have associated symptoms of endometriosis.

Cervical Polyps

True cervical polyps are benign growths that may be pedunculated or broad based; they can arise anywhere on the cervix and are often asymptomatic. Cervical polyps that do produce symptoms tend to be associated with intermenstrual or postcoital bleeding rather than pain of any kind, unless they are actually obstructing the cervical canal. Although cervical polyps are not usually considered a premalignant condition, they are generally removed, particularly those protruding from the cervical os. One reason for removal is that it can be difficult to determine whether a pedunculated polyp is actually uterine in origin that can be premalignant. Removal is often an office procedure with pedunculated polyps; however, dilatation and curettage may be required for broad-based polyps of the endocervix.

Cervical Fibroids

Leiomyomas (myomas or fibroids) are common benign tumors of the uterine corpus. They may also arise in the cervix. They can cause similar symptoms of intermenstrual bleeding that both uterine fibroids and cervical polyps can cause. However, depending on their location and size, they can also cause dyspareunia and bladder or rectal pressure. Once the possibility of cervical cancer is ruled out, an asymptomatic cervical fibroid can be followed with routine gynecologic care. Symptomatic fibroids can be surgically removed, but depending on their location, hysterectomy rather than myomectomy may be required.

Cervical Stenosis

Cervical stenosis can be congenital; a product of scarring after surgical manipulation or radiotherapy of the cervix; or secondary to obstruction with neoplasm, polyp, or fibroid. If cervical stenosis is asymptomatic and merely found on examination, it may be left alone. However, if egress from the uterus is blocked in a premenopausal woman, oligo/amenorrhea, dysmenorrhea, or an enlarged uterus may result. If there is an obstructive lesion, it should be removed. If the stenosis is secondary to scarring, the cervix should be gently dilated to allow the intrauterine contents to flow more easily.

Key Points

1. Cervical congenital anomalies are usually associated with abnormalities in the uterus.
2. Cervical polyps are rarely cancerous but should be removed if they are causing bleeding or obstruction of the cervical canal.
3. Fibroids of the cervix can be a problem in pregnancy and may lead to poor dilation of the cervix; nonpregnant patients may have problems with cervical stenosis due to external compression.

Uterine Fibroids — 20-30% of ♀; 3-9x ↑ in black ♀

- # cause of surgery in ♀ in U.S.
- proliferation of smooth muscle cells
- responsive to Estrogen ⇒ Grow a lot in pregnancy

50-60% are asymptomatic

- submucosal, intramural, & subserosal; intramural are most common.
- has a "pseudocapsule" of compressed smooth muscle cells w/ vessels & when they get large, they degenerate (hyaline Δ, cystic, hemorrhagic, calcific → any kind)
- hemorrhage + infarct in 20% of pregnancies

Sx = abnormal uterine bleeding

- cause 2-10% of infertility

Dx: u/s

Tx: Provera (progesterone) or Danazol, Lupron (GnRH agonist) } all shrink 'em, but they come back when meds stop

CHAPTER 12

Benign Disorders of the Upper Genital Tract

▶ ANATOMIC ANOMALIES OF THE UTERUS

Pathogenesis

The superior vagina, cervix, uterus, and fallopian tubes are formed by fusion of the paramesonephric (müllerian) ducts. Uterine anomalies arise during embryologic development, generally as a result of incomplete fusion of the ducts, incomplete development of one or both ducts, or degeneration of the ducts (müllerian agenesis). These anomalies can vary in scope and severity from the presence of simple septa or bicornuate uterus, to complete duplication of the entire female reproductive system (Fig. 12-1). The most common conditions result from malfusion of the paramesonephric ducts and result in varying degrees of septation. Many anatomical uterine abnormalities may also be associated with urinary tract anomalies.

Epidemiology

Anatomic anomalies of the uterus are extremely rare.

Clinical Manifestations

History

Some uterine anomalies are asymptomatic and may never be discovered, whereas others may not be recognized until the onset of menarche or attempts at childbearing. Some symptoms associated with anomalies of the uterus include dysmenorrhea, dyspareunia, cyclic pelvic pain, infertility, habitual abortion, spontaneous second trimester abortion, and premature labor.

Diagnostic Evaluation

The primary investigative tools for uterine abnormalities are pelvic ultrasound, hysterosalpingogram, and hysteroscopy.

Treatment

Many uterine anomalies require no treatment. However, when the defect causes significant symptoms or interferes with reproduction, treatment options should be explored. Uterine septa can be excised with operative hysteroscopy. Pregnancy has also been achieved with unification procedures.

Key Points

Anatomic anomalies of the uterus

1. Are extremely rare;
2. Result from problems in the fusion of the paramesonephric (müllerian) ducts;
3. May also be associated with urinary tract anomalies.

▶ UTERINE LEIOMYOMA

Uterine leiomyoma, also called fibroids or myomas, are local proliferations of smooth muscle cells of the uterus. Fibroids typically occur in women of childbearing age and then regress during menopause. These benign tumors constitute the most common cause for surgery for women in the United States. Most fibroids, however, cause no major symptoms and require no treatment. Generally, fibroids only become problematic when they become large enough to cause a mass effect on other pelvic structures, causing pelvic pain and pressure.

Pathogenesis

The cause of uterine leiomyomas is unclear. They are thought to develop from smooth muscle cells of the uterus or the uterine arteries, from metaplastic transformation of connective tissue cells, or from persistent embryonic nest cells.

These benign tumors are **hormonally responsive to estrogen**, especially during the late reproductive and perimenopausal years. Fibroids can grow quickly and to huge proportions during pregnancy or when exposed to exogenous estrogens. During menopause, the tumors usually stop growing and may atrophy in response to naturally lower endogenous estrogen levels.

Uterine leiomyomas are classified by their location on the uterus (Fig. 12-2). The typical classification of fibroids includes submucous, intramural, and subserosal. Intramural leiomyomas are the most common. A parasitic leiomyoma is a pedunculated fibroid that becomes attached to the pelvic viscera or omentum and develops its own blood supply.

Fibroids have a **"pseudocapsule"** of compressed smooth muscle cells that contain very few blood vessels and lymphatic vessels. Therefore, as leiomyomas enlarge, **degenerative changes** frequently occur, including hyaline, cystic, red (hemorrhagic), calcific, and sarcomatous degeneration. During pregnancy, the growth

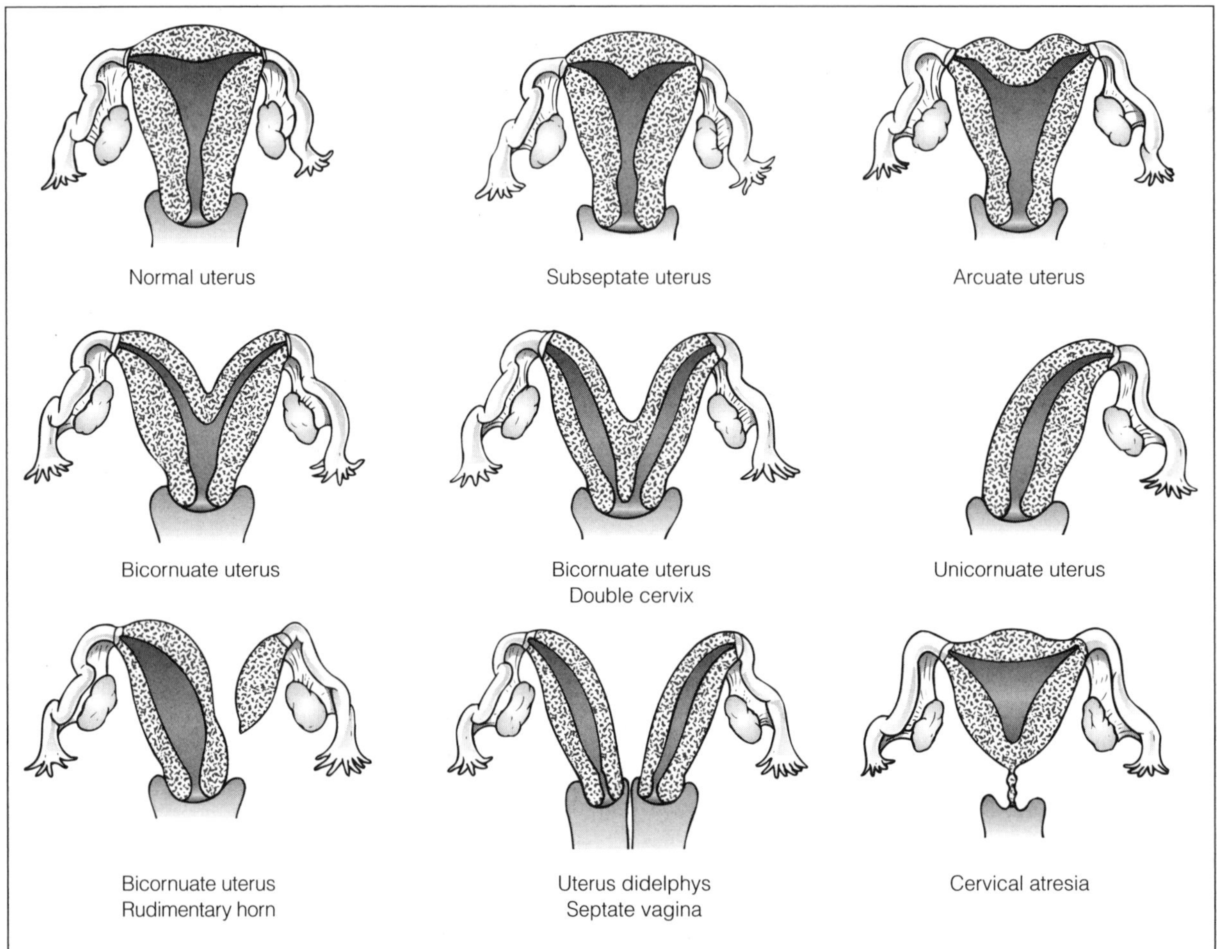

Figure 12-1 Anatomic anomalies of the uterus.

and degeneration of fibroids can lead to infarct and hemorrhaging (red degeneration) within the tumors in 50% of pregnancies.

It is unclear whether fibroids have any malignant potential. If they do, it is thought to be very minimal (perhaps 1 in 1,000 cases).

Epidemiology

It is estimated that 20 to 30% of American women develop leiomyoma by the age of 40.

Risk Factors

The incidence of leiomyomas is three to nine times higher in black women in the United States than in white women. The reason for this is not known.

Clinical Manifestations

History

Most women with fibroids (50 to 65%) have **no clinical symptoms**. Of those that do (Table 12-1), **abnormal uterine bleeding** is by far the most common presenting symptom. Bleeding typically presents as increasingly heavy periods of longer duration (menorrhagia). Blood loss from fibroids can lead to chronic iron deficiency anemia, weakness, and dizziness.

Pressure-related symptoms (pelvic pressure, fullness or heaviness) vary depending on the number and location of leiomyomas. If a fibroid impinges on nearby structures, patients may complain of constipation, urinary frequency, or even urinary retention as the space within the pelvis becomes more crowded. In general, pelvic pain is usually not part of the symptom complex unless vascular compromise is present.

Uterine myomas are also associated with an increased incidence of **infertility** but are solely responsible for infertility in only 2 to 10% of cases. Fibroids may distort the endocervical canal, fallopian tubes, or endometrial cavity, thus interfering with conception or implantation and sometimes causing spontaneous

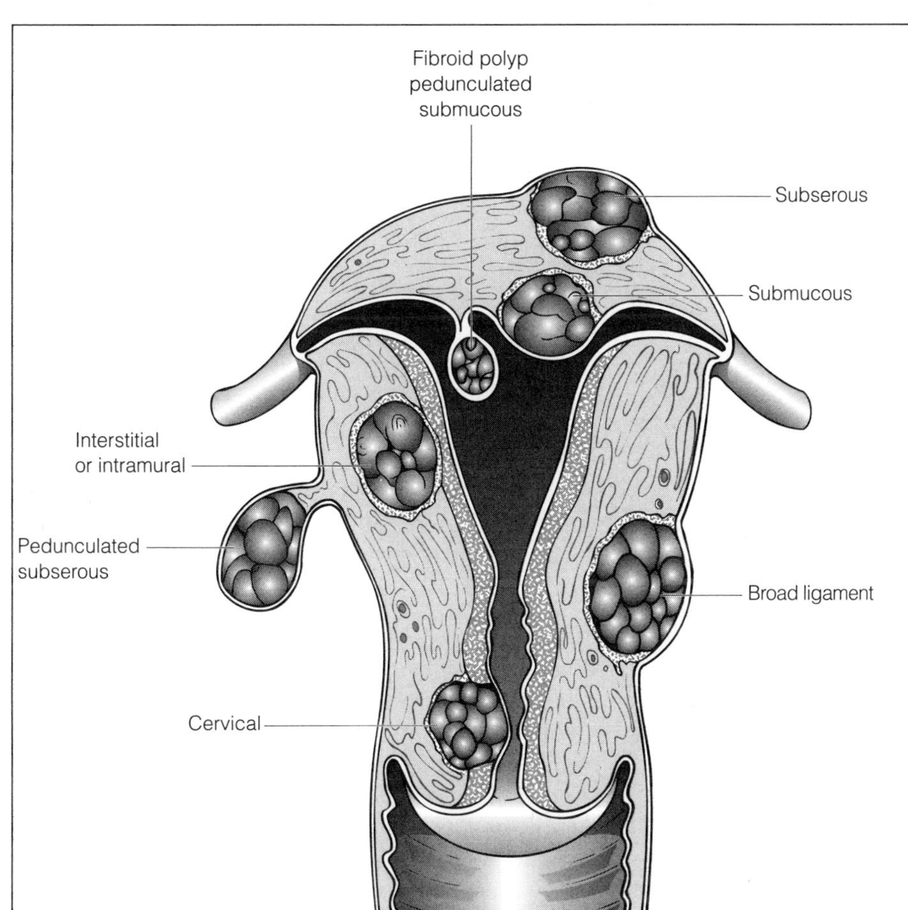

Figure 12-2 Common locations for uterine fibroids.

TABLE 12-1

Clinical Symptoms of Uterine Leiomyomas

Bleeding
Longer, heavier periods
Endometrial ulceration
Pressure
Pelvic pressure and bloating
Constipation and rectal pressure
Urinary frequency or retention
Pain
Secondary dysmenorrhea
Acute infarct (especially in pregnancy)
Dyspareunia
Reproductive difficulties
Infertility (failed implantation/spontaneous abortion)
Intrauterine growth restriction
Increased dystocia and cesarean sections

abortion. Most women with fibroids, however, are able to become pregnant. Because fibroids have the potential for excessive growth during pregnancy, they may contribute to intrauterine growth retardation, premature labor, or dystocia. They may also block the presenting part necessitating cesarean section.

Physical Examination

Depending on the location and size of uterine leiomyoma, they can sometimes be palpated on bimanual pelvic examination or on abdominal examination. Bimanual examination often reveals a nontender irregularly enlarged uterus with "lumpy-bumpy" or cobblestone protrusions that feel firm or solid on palpation.

Diagnostic Evaluation

The differential diagnosis for uterine leiomyoma depends on the patient's symptoms (Table 12-2). Malignancies of the ovaries and uterus represent potentially life-threatening differential diagnoses or coexistent diagnoses.

Because many women with leiomyomas are asymptomatic, the diagnosis is sometimes made only as an incidental finding on a pathology specimen. **Pelvic**

TABLE 12-2

Differential Diagnosis of Uterine Leiomyoma*

Abnormal bleeding
Endometrial hyperplasia
Endometrial carcinoma
Uterine sarcomas
Endometriosis
Adenomyosis
Exogenous estrogens
Uterine enlargement
Pregnancy
Adenomyosis
Endometrial carcinoma
Pelvic mass
Adenomyosis
Pregnancy
Ovarian cysts or neoplasm
Tubo-ovarian abscess

*Any of these conditions may **coexist** with leiomyomas.

ultrasound is the most common means of diagnosis. Myoma can be seen as areas of hypoechogenicity among normal myometrial material.

Treatment

Most cases of uterine fibroids do not necessitate therapy, and **expectant management** is appropriate. However, the diagnosis of leiomyoma must be unequivocal. Other pelvic masses should be ruled out, and the patient should be followed to monitor the size and growth of the leiomyomas.

When leiomyomas result in severe pain, infertility, urinary tract symptoms, or postmenopausal growth, treatment should be considered. The choice of treatment depends on the patient's age, pregnancy status, desire for future pregnancies, and on the size and location of the leiomyomas. Surgery is the most common treatment for leiomyomas.

Medical therapies for leiomyomas including medroxyprogesterone (Provera), danazol, and gonadotropin-releasing hormone agonists (naferelin acetate, Depot Lupron) have been found to shrink fibroids by decreasing circulating estrogen levels. Unfortunately, the tumors usually resume growth after discontinuation of these medications. For women nearing menopause, these treatments may be used as a temporizing measure until their own endogenous estrogens decrease naturally.

Hysterectomy is the definitive treatment for leiomyomas (vaginal hysterectomy for small myomas and total abdominal hysterectomy for large or multiple myomas). The indications for hysterectomy for fibroids are shown in Table 12-3. If the ovaries are diseased or if the blood supply has been damaged, then oophorectomy should be performed as well. Otherwise, the ovaries should be preserved in women under the age of 45. Surgical intervention should be avoided during pregnancy, although myomectomy or hysterectomy may be necessary after the pregnancy.

TABLE 12-3

Indications for Surgical Intervention for Uterine Leiomyomas

Abnormal uterine bleeding, causing anemia
Severe pelvic pain or secondary amenorrhea
Size > 12 weeks gestation obscuring evaluation of adnexae
Urinary frequency or retention
Growth after menopause
Infertility
Rapid increase in size

Adapted from Hacker N, Moore JG. Essentials of obstetrics and gynecology. Philadelphia: WB Saunders, 1992:351.

Follow-Up

When hysterectomy is not indicated for a patient with leiomyomas, careful follow-up should take place to monitor the size and location of the tumors. At no time should a myoma go untreated if it obscures the evaluation of the adnexae. Rapid growth of a tumor in postmenopausal women may be a sign of leiomyosarcoma and should be immediately investigated. Postmenopausal estrogens and premenopausal oral contraceptives at low current doses do not appear to pose a risk to the patient.

Key Points

Fibroids

1. Are benign, estrogen-sensitive, smooth muscle tumors of unclear etiology found in 20 to 30% of reproductive-aged women;
2. Have an incidence that is three to nine times higher in black women than in white women;
3. May be submucous, intramural, or subserosal and can grow to great size, especially during pregnancy;
4. Frequently show degeneration but malignancy is rare;
5. Are asymptomatic in 50 to 65% of patients; symptoms include bleeding (most common), pressure, pain, and infertility;
6. Are diagnosed with pelvic/abdominal examination and pelvic ultrasound;
7. Need no treatment in most cases;

8. Can be temporarily treated with Provera, danazol, gonadotropin-releasing hormone analogues to decrease estrogen and shrink the tumors;
9. Are treated surgically by hysterectomy for severe pain, size greater than 12 weeks gestation, urinary symptoms, and for postmenopausal or rapid growth.

▶ ENDOMETRIAL HYPERPLASIA

Pathogenesis

Endometrial proliferation is a normal part of the menstrual cycle that occurs during the follicular- or estrogen-dominant phase of the cycle. Simple proliferation is simply an overabundance of histologically normal endometrium. However, when the endometrium is exposed to continuous endogenous or exogenous sources of **estrogen in the absence of progesterone,** simple endometrial proliferation can advance to endometrial hyperplasia. **Endometrial hyperplasia** is the abnormal proliferation of glandular and stromal elements resulting in histologic alterations in the cellular architecture of the endometrium (Fig. 12-3).

The histologic variation of endometrial hyperplasia includes cystic hyperplasia, adenomatous hyperplasia, and atypical adenomatous hyperplasia. These changes do not necessarily involve the entire endometrium nor do they necessarily advance to carcinoma if left untreated. **Cystic hyperplasia** (also known as simple or mild hyperplasia) is the simplest form of hyperplasia. It represents a proliferation of both the stromal and glandular endometrial elements. These lesions rarely (<2%) progress to carcinoma. **Adenomatous hyperplasia** (also known as complex or moderate hyperplasia without atypia) represents abnormal proliferation of the glandular endometrial elements without proliferation of the stromal elements. In these lesions, the glands are crowded in a back-to-back fashion and are of varying shapes and sizes, but no cytologic atypia is present. Less than 5% of these lesions progress to carcinoma. **Atypical adenomatous hyperplasia** (also known as moderate hyperplasia with atypia) contains cellular atypia and mitotic figures in addition to glandular crowding and complexity. Atypical adenomatous hyperplasia has a 20 to 30% risk of malignant transformation. The more severe the atypia, the greater the risk.

Epidemiology

Endometrial hyperplasia typically occurs in the menopausal or perimenopausal woman but may also occur in the years immediately after menarche when ovulation may be infrequent.

Risk Factors

Patients at risk for endometrial hyperplasia, like those at risk for endometrial carcinoma, are also at risk for **unopposed estrogen exposure** (Table 12-4). This includes women with polycystic ovarian syndrome and estrogen-producing tumors, such as granulosa-theca cell tumors.

Clinical Manifestations

History

Endometrial hyperplasia typically presents with abnormal or excessive **uterine bleeding.** Uterine bleeding in a postmenopausal woman should raise high suspicion of endometrial hyperplasia or carcinoma.

Physical Examination

Occasionally, the uterus will be enlarged in endometrial hyperplasia. This is attributed both to the increase in the mass of the endometrium and to the growth of the myometrium in response to continuous estrogen stimulation.

Diagnostic Evaluation

Endometrial hyperplasia is diagnosed by **endometrial biopsy.** However, because the lesions may develop focally among normal endometrium, a dilation and curettage **(D&C)** procedure is required to rule out endometrial hyperplasia except in women under the age of 30.

Treatment

The treatment of endometrial hyperplasia depends on the histologic variant of the disease and on the age of the patient.

Simple, cystic, and adenomatous hyperplasia can be treated medically with the administration of **progesterone** (Provera) in doses that will inhibit and eventually reverse the endometrial hyperplasia. Atypical adenomatous hyperplasia is usually treated surgically by **hysterectomy** because most women with the disorder are either perimenopausal or postmenopausal. In younger patients with atypical adenomatous hyperplasia and chronic anovulation who wish to preserve fertility, endometrial curettage, longer-term progestin management, and ovulation induction may assist the patient in becoming pregnant.

Key Points

Endometrial hyperplasia

1. Represents a broad spectrum of abnormal proliferation of the endometrium accompanied by changes in the cellular architecture;

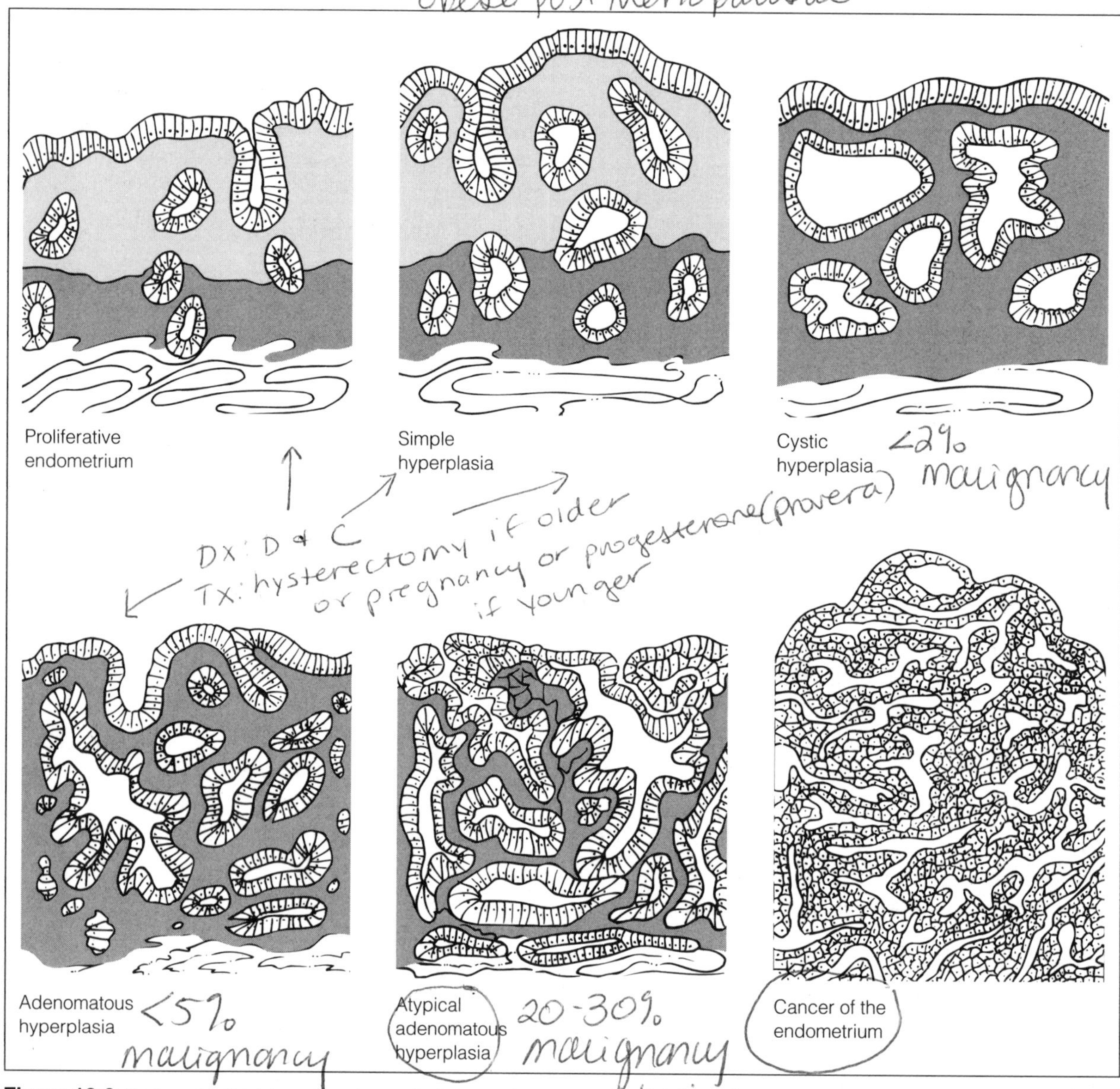

Figure 12-3 Endometrial histology from hyperplasia to carcinoma.

TABLE 12-4

Patients at Risk for Unopposed Estrogen Exposure

Patients using exogenous estrogen alone
Patients with a history of chronic anovulation
Obese postmenopausal patients
Patients with "late" menopause (>55 years old)

Reproduced with permission from Beckman CC, Ling F. Obstetrics and gynecology for medical students. Baltimore: Williams & Wilkins, 1992:407.

2. Has three types: cystic, adenomatous, and adenomatous with atypia;
3. Is caused by prolonged exposure to exogenous or endogenous estrogen in the absence of progesterone;
4. Has a <2% risk of malignant transformation in cystic hyperplasia and a <5% risk in adenomatous hyperplasia; atypical adenomatous hyperplasia has a 20 to 30% risk of malignant transformation;

5. Includes risk factors for unopposed estrogen exposure as seen in women using exogenous estrogen alone, women with chronic anovulation or late menopause, and obese postmenopausal women;
6. Is diagnosed by endometrial biopsy or D&C;
7. Is usually treated medically with progesterone if simple, cystic, or adenomatous in type and is managed with hysterectomy if it is of the atypical adenomatous type.

▶ OVARIAN CYSTS

Pathogenesis

In general, ovarian masses can be divided into functional cysts and neoplastic growths. Functional cysts of the ovaries result from normal physiologic functioning of the ovaries and are divided into follicular and corpus luteum cysts. Many cysts are small and clinically insignificant, but each could potentially represent an early form of a benign or malignant neoplasm.

Follicular cysts are those that arise after the failure of the follicle to rupture during follicular maturation. These may vary in size from 3 to 8 cm and are classically asymptomatic and usually unilateral. Large cysts can cause a tender palpable ovarian mass. Most will disappear spontaneously within 60 days.

Corpus lutein cysts are common functional cysts that occur during the luteal phase of the menstrual cycle. Most corpus lutein cysts are formed when the corpus luteum becomes cystic, or hemorrhagic (corpus hemorrhagicum), or fails to regress after 14 days. These cysts can cause a delay in menstruation and dull lower quadrant pain. Patients with corpus hemorrhagicum can present with acute pain and signs of hemoperitoneum late in luteal phase.

Theca lutein cysts are small bilateral cysts filled with clear straw-colored fluid. These ovarian cysts result from stimulation from abnormally high β-human chorionic gonadotropin (e.g., from a hydatidiform mole, choriocarcinoma, or clomiphene therapy).

Epidemiology

Seventy-five percent of ovarian masses in women of reproductive age are **functional cysts** and 25% are **nonfunctional neoplasms**. Although functional ovarian cysts can be found in females of any age, they most commonly occur between puberty and menopause.

Clinical Manifestations

History

Patients with functional cysts present with a variety of symptoms depending on the type of cyst. **Follicular cysts** tend to be asymptomatic and only occasionally cause menstrual disturbances such as prolonged intermenstrual intervals or short cycles. Larger follicular cysts can cause aching pelvic pain and dyspareunia. **Lutein cysts** may present with local pelvic pain and either amenorrhea or delayed menses. Bleeding from a hemorrhagic corpus luteum can result in acute abdominal pain as can a torsed or ruptured cyst.

Physical Examination

The findings on bimanual pelvic examination will vary with the type of cyst. Follicular cysts tend to be less than 8 cm and simple or unilocular in structure. Lutein cysts are generally larger than follicular cysts and often feel more firm or solid on palpation. A torsed or ruptured cyst will present with pain to palpation, acute abdominal pain, and rebound tenderness.

Diagnostic Evaluation

After a thorough history and physical, the primary diagnostic tool for the workup of ovarian cyst is the **pelvic ultrasound**. This study evaluates the structure of the growth as more cystic or solid in nature to guide further workup and treatment. A CA-125 level should be obtained from patients who are at high risk for ovarian cancer.

The differential for ovarian cysts include ectopic pregnancy, pelvic inflammatory disease, torsed adnexa, endometriosis, and ovarian neoplasm.

Treatment

Treatment of ovarian cysts depends on the age of the patient and the characteristics of the tumor. Table 12-5 shows the treatment options using these criteria. In general, a palpable ovary or adnexal mass in a **premenarchal or postmenopausal patient** is suggestive of an ovarian neoplasm rather than a functional cyst and

TABLE 12-5
Management of a Cystic Adnexal Mass

Age	Size of Cyst (cm)	Management
Premenarchal	>2	Exploratory laparotomy
Reproductive age	<6	Observe for 6 weeks
	6–8	Observe if unilocular; explore if multilocular or solid on ultrasound
	>8	Exploratory laparotomy
Postmenopausal	Palpable	Exploratory laparotomy

Reproduced with permission from Hacker N, Moore JG. Essentials of obstetrics and gynecology. Philadephia: WB Saunders, 1992:358.

exploratory laparotomy is in order. Likewise, reproductive age women with cysts **larger than 8 cm** that persist for longer than 60 days or are solid or complex on ultrasound probably do not have a functional cyst. These lesions should be closely investigated with **laparotomy**.

For patients of reproductive age with cysts less than 6 cm in size, **observation** with a follow-up ultrasound is the appropriate action. Most follicular cysts should spontaneously resolve within 60 days. As another alternative, patients are sometimes started on **oral contraceptives** during this observation period to suppress gonadotropin stimulation of the cyst. Cysts that do not resolve within 60 days despite observation and gonadotropin suppression require evaluation with a pelvic ultrasound.

Key Points

1. Functional cysts result from normal physiologic functioning of the ovaries.
2. Follicular cysts result from unruptured follicles. They are usually asymptomatic unless torsion occurs. Management includes observation for 6 to 8 weeks with or without oral contraceptives followed by pelvic ultrasound.
3. Lutein cysts result from an enlarged and/or hemorrhagic corpus luteum. They may cause a missed period or dull lower quadrant pain. They should resolve spontaneously or may be suppressed with oral contraceptives if recurrent.
4. Any palpable ovary or adnexal mass in a premenarchal or postmenopausal patient is suggestive of ovarian neoplasm and should be investigated with exploratory laparotomy.

Cysts: before menarche → laparoscopy/laparotom. to explore

Reproductive age

<6 cm - reeval. in 6wks

6-8cm observe if unilocular
explore multilocular or cystic

Postmenopausal : >8 cm → laparotomy

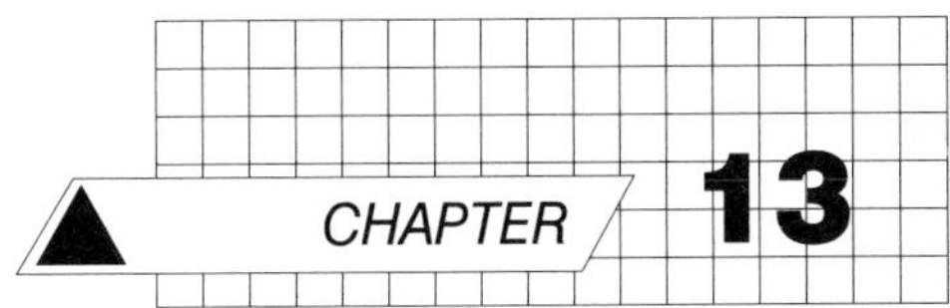

Endometriosis and Adenomyosis

▶ ENDOMETRIOSIS

Pathogenesis

Endometriosis is the presence of endometrial glands and stroma outside the endometrial cavity. An endometrioma is a cystic collection of endometriosis in the ovary. Although endometrial tissue can be found anywhere in the body, the most common sites are the ovary and the pelvic peritoneum. Other common sites include the pouch of Douglas, the round ligament, the fallopian tubes, and the sigmoid colon (Fig. 13-1).

There are three main theories about the etiology of endometriosis. The Halban theory proposes that endometrial tissue is transported via the **lymphatic system** to ectopic sites in the pelvis where it grows ectopically. Meyer proposes that multipotential cells in peritoneal tissue undergo **metaplastic transformation** into functional endometrial tissue. Finally, Sampson suggests that endometrial tissue is transported through the fallopian tubes during **retrograde menstruation**, resulting in intra-abdominal pelvic implants.

Epidemiology

The incidence of endometriosis is estimated to be between 10 and 15%. It is found almost exclusively in women of reproductive age, and it is the single most common reason for hospitalization of women in this age group.

Risk Factors

Women with first-degree relatives with endometriosis have a **genetic predisposition** (7 to 9%) to develop the disorder. Endometriosis is identified less often in black women.

Clinical Manifestations

History

The symptoms associated with endometriosis are dysmenorrhea, dyspareunia, infertility, abnormal bleeding, and pelvic pain. Interestingly, the severity of symptoms does not necessarily correlate with the amount of endometriosis. Women with widely disseminated endometriosis or a large endometrioma may have little pain, whereas women with minimal disease in the cul de sac may suffer with severe pain.

The symptoms of endometriosis vary depending on the area involved. Dysmenorrhea usually begins in the third decade and worsens with age. Dyspareunia is usually associated with deep penetration, which aggravates endometriosis lesions in the cul de sac or on the uterosacral ligament. Patients with endometriosis may also experience premenstrual and postmenstrual spotting, menorrhagia, ovulatory pain, midcycle bleeding, or dyschezia (rare).

Endometriosis is also believed to contribute to **infertility**. Many theories have been postulated for this association, including distortion of the pelvic architecture, interference with tubal mobility, and tubal obstruction from dense adhesions.

Physical Examination

The physical findings associated with early endometriosis may be subtle or nonexistent. When more disseminated disease is present, the physician may find **uterosacral nodularity** on rectovaginal examination or a **fixed or retroverted uterus**. When the ovary is involved, a tender, fixed, adnexal mass may be palpable on bimanual examination.

Diagnostic Evaluation

Direct visualization with diagnostic laparoscopy or laparotomy is required for a definitive diagnosis of endometriosis. Endometriosis may appear as rust-colored to dark brown "powder burns" or raised blue-colored "mulberry" or "raspberry" lesions. The areas may be surrounded by reactive fibrosis that can lead to dense adhesions in extensive disease. The ovary itself can develop large cystic collections of endometriosis filled with thick, dark, old blood. These are known as "chocolate cysts."

Once the diagnosis of endometriosis is made, the anatomic location and extent of the disease can be used to properly classify the operative findings. The American Fertility Society's revised classification schema is shown in Table 13-1.

Differential Diagnosis

The most common disorders confused with endometriosis are chronic pelvic inflammatory disease, recurrent acute salpingitis, a hemorrhagic corpus luteum,

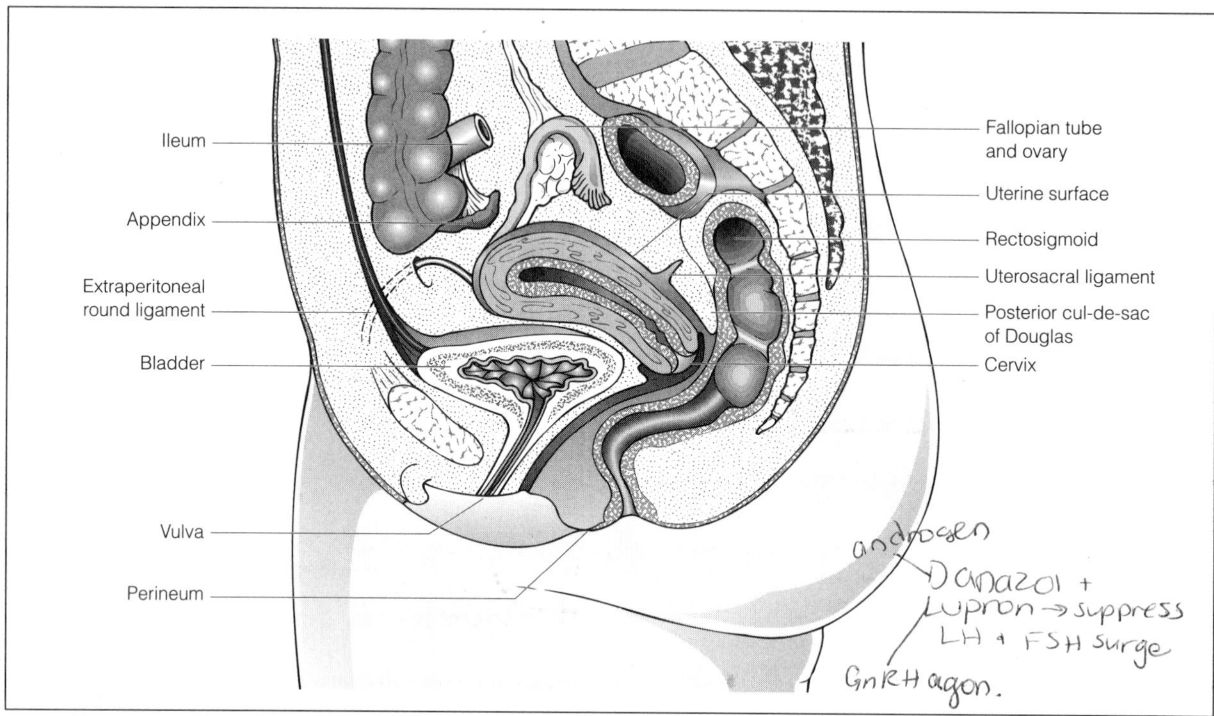

Figure 13-1 Potential sites for endometriosis.

an ectopic pregnancy, or benign or malignant ovarian neoplasms.

Treatment

The treatment choice for patients with endometriosis depends on the extent and location of disease, the severity of symptoms, and the desire for future fertility. Although both surgical and medical options are available for the treatment of endometriosis, all medical options are **temporizing measures** rather than permanent treatments. Expectant management may be used in patients with minimal or nonexistent symptoms and in patients attempting to conceive.

Medical treatment for endometriosis is aimed at suppression and atrophy of the endometrial tissue. Current regimens include either continuous administration of oral contraceptives or Provera (medroxyprogesterone). These treatments induce a state of **"pseudopregnancy"** by suppressing both ovulation and menstruation, thereby avoiding dysmenorrhea. This therapy is best for patients with milder endometriosis who are not currently seeking to conceive.

Patients can also be placed in a reversible state of **"pseudomenopause"** with the use of danazol, an androgen derivative, or gonadotropin-releasing hormone (GnRH) agonists such as Lupron. Both methods suppress follicle-stimulating hormone and luteinizing hormone midcycle surges. As a result, the ovaries do not produce estrogen, which stimulates endometriosis. Existing endometrial implants atrophy, and new implants are prevented. However, these effects are temporary, and the endometriosis usually eventually recurs after cessation of therapy. The drawback to danazol is that the patients may experience some androgen-related, anabolic side effects including acne, oily skin, weight gain, edema, hirsutism, and deepening of the voice. The side effects of GnRH agonists include hot flashes and bone loss.

Surgical treatment for endometriosis can be classified as either conservative or definitive. **Conservative therapy** typically involves ablation, electrocauterization, or excision of visible endometriosis during laparoscopy while preserving the reproductive organs to allow for future fertility. The success rate of conservative therapy depends on the extent of the disease (Table 13-2).

Definitive therapy includes total abdominal hysterectomy and bilateral salpingo-oophorectomy (TAHBSO), lysis of adhesions, and removal of endometriosis lesions. This therapy is reserved for cases in which fertility is

TABLE 13-1

Revised American Fertility Society Classification of Endometriosis

Endometriosis	Less Than 1 cm	1–3 cm	More Than 3 cm
Peritoneum			
Superficial	1	2	4
Deep	2	4	6
Ovary*			
Superficial	1	2	4
Deep	4	16	20
		Partial	Complete
Posterior cul-de-sac obliteration		4	40
Adhesions	Less Than ⅓ Enclosure	⅓–⅔ Enclosure	More Than ⅔ Enclosure
Ovary*			
Filmy	1	2	4
Dense	4	8	16
Uterine tube*			
Filmy	1	2	4
Dense	4†	8†	16

Scoring: Stage 1 disease (minimal) = 1–5, stage 2 (mild) = 6–15, stage 3 (moderate) = 16–40, stage 4 (severe) = more than 40.

*Each ovary and uterine tube is scored separately.

†If the fimbriated end of the tube is completely enclosed, the score is 16.

Reproduced with permission from DeCherney A, Pernoll M. Current obstetric and gynecologic diagnosis and treatment. Norwalk, CT: Appleton and Lange, 1994:806.

TABLE 13-2

Conception Rates After Conservative Treatment of Endometriosis

Extent of Disease	Conception Rates (%)
Mild	75
Moderate	50–60
Severe	30–40

not an issue and for women with severe disease or symptoms that are refractory to conservative medical or surgical treatment.

Key Points

Endometriosis

1. Is the presence of endometrial glands and stroma outside the endometrial cavity, most often in the ovary or pelvic peritoneum;
2. Is estimated to occur in between 10 and 15% of women of reproductive age;
3. Has symptoms (dysmenorrhea, dyspareunia, abnormal bleeding, infertility, and pelvic pain) that do not correlate with extent of disease;
4. Requires direct visualization with diagnostic laparoscopy or laparotomy for a definitive diagnosis;
5. Can be treated medically (OCPs, danazol, GnRH agonists) to reduce pain, but these methods have lower pregnancy rates (20 to 40%), and are used mainly as temporizing agents;
6. Can be treated surgically with conservative therapy to ablate implants and adhesions and to preserve reproductive organs with 50 to 60% post-therapy pregnancy rates;
7. Can be treated with definite surgery including TAHBSO, lysis of adhesions, and removal of endometriosis lesions.

▶ ADENOMYOSIS

Pathogenesis

Adenomyosis is the extension of endometrial glands and stroma into the uterine musculature. The cause of adenomyosis is not known.

The development of adenomyosis causes the uterus to become diffusely enlarged and globular due to the **hypertrophy and hyperplasia** of the myometrium adjacent to the ectopic endometrial tissue. Rarely, adenomyosis may also present as a well-circumscribed, isolated region known as an **adenomyoma**. Unlike endometriosis, the endometrial tissue in adenomyosis does not undergo the proliferative and secretory cycles induced by the ovary. Unlike uterine myoma, adenomyoma does not have a distinct capsular margin.

Epidemiology

The incidence of adenomyosis in women is 15%. The disease generally develops in parous women in their late 30s or early 40s. The disease occurs very infrequently in nulliparous women.

Risk Factors

About 15% of patients with adenomyosis also have associated **endometriosis** and 50 to 60% will have submucous leiomyoma as well as adenomyosis.

Clinical Manifestations

History

The most common symptoms of adenomyosis are secondary dysmenorrhea (30%), menorrhagia (50%), or both (20%). The typical presentation is increasingly severe secondary dysmenorrhea before and during menstruation and menorrhagia (heavy or prolonged menstrual flow). Others may only experience pressure on the bladder or rectum due to an enlarged uterus. As many as 30% of patients are **asymptomatic**, and the disease is only discovered incidentally.

Physical Examination

The pelvic examination of a patient with adenomyosis may reveal a symmetrically enlarged uterus with a consistency softer than uterine myoma that are typically more nodular and irregular.

Diagnostic Evaluation

Hysterectomy is the only definitive means of diagnosing adenomyosis. MRI can sometimes identify adenomyosis, but the cost can be prohibitive.

Treatment

The treatment for adenomyosis depends on the severity of the dysmenorrhea and menorrhagia. Women with minimal symptoms or those near menopause may be managed with analgesics alone. **Hysterectomy** is the only definitive treatment for adenomyosis.

Key Points

Adenomyosis

1. Is the presence of endometrial glands and stroma in the myometrium, making the uterus symmetrically enlarged and globular;
2. Occurs in 15% of women, most of whom are parous and in their late 30s or early 40s;
3. Occurs in 15% of women who also have endometriosis;
4. Is typically presented as increasing secondary dysmenorrhea (30%), menorrhagia (50%), or both (20%); 30% of patients are asymptomatic;
5. May be treated for minimal symptoms with analgesia;
6. Is treated definitively by hysterectomy.

CHAPTER 14

Infections of the Lower Female Reproductive Tract

THE EXTERNAL ANOGENITAL REGION

There are a variety of infectious diseases that affect the external genitalia. In the female patient, the entire perianal and pubic regions should be considered in addition to the vulva. The skin overlying these areas is subject to the same infections that can occur anywhere on the epidermis, but the exposure and environment differ and must be considered when discussing these infections. There are also a variety of focal and systemic processes that can present with lesions or symptoms in this region. Anogenital lesions are usually categorized as ulcerating or nonulcerative, and common symptoms include pain and itching.

ULCERATED LESIONS

Many primary vulvar ulcers are caused by sexually transmitted diseases (Table 14-1) such as **herpes, syphilis, chancroid,** and **lymphogranuloma venereum.** However, even with a diagnosis of an infectious process, these lesions can be associated with malignant processes as well.

There are other conditions that can lead to vulvar ulcerations. Crohn's disease can have linear "knife cut" vulvar ulcers as its first manifestation and can precede gastrointestinal or other systemic manifestations by months to years. Behçet's disease has vulvar lesions that are tender and highly destructive often causing fenestrations in the labia and extensive scarring.

Vulvitis

The most common cause of vulvitis and usually vulvar pruritus is candidiasis. There is usually noticeable erythema on the vulva, pruritus, and small satellite lesions. If the vulvitis does not respond to the usual treatment of candidiasis with antifungals, one must consider other sources of the symptoms such as allergic reaction, chemical or fabric irritants, and the vulvar dystrophies. Malignancy should always be ruled out in the case of chronic vulvar irritation.

Syphilis

The spirochete *Treponema pallidum* causes the chronic systemic infection of **syphilis.** It is primarily transmitted through sexual contact. In 1988, the incidence of primary and secondary syphilis in the United States was 16.7 cases per 100,000 persons with a total of 40,000 cases reported. Currently, the incidence is rising in heterosexual men and women with a decline among the gay population, likely secondary to safe sexual practices in this population.

T. pallidum likely enters the body through minute abrasions in the skin or mucosal surface and replicates locally. Thus, initial lesions commonly occur on the vulva, vagina, cervix, anus, nipples, or lips. The initial lesion that characterizes the primary stage is a painless, red, round, firm ulcer approximately 1 cm in size with raised edges known as **chancre** (Fig. 14-1). It develops approximately 3 weeks after inoculation and is usually associated with concomitant regional adenopathy. Material from the chancre will usually reveal motile spirochetes under dark-field microscopy.

The secondary stage of syphilis occurs as *T. pallidum* disseminates. Between 1 and 3 months after the primary stage resolves, the secondary stage presents with a maculopapular rash and/or moist papules on the skin or mucous membranes. Classically, the rash appears on the palms of the hands or soles of the feet. The dermatologic manifestations of secondary syphilis are manifest and have led syphilis to be known as the "great imitator." There may be other organ involvement with meningitis, nephritis, or hepatitis. All lesions resolve spontaneously, and this stage can be entirely asymptomatic. After resolution of this stage, the infection can enter a latent phase that can last for years.

Tertiary syphilis is quite uncommon today but is characterized by granulomas (gummas) of the skin and bones; cardiovascular syphilis with aortitis; and neurosyphilis with meningovascular disease, paresis, and tabes dorsalis.

Diagnosis

T. pallidum is commonly screened via a nonspecific antibody test. Either the rapid plasmin reagin (RPR) or the Venereal Disease Research Laboratory (VDRL) test can be used to screen and then follow treatment course. The diagnosis is confirmed with more specific testing: either the microhemagglutination assay for antibodies to *T. pallidum* (MHA-TP) or the fluorescent

TABLE 14-1

Infectious Causes of Ulcerated Lesions

Characteristic	Syphilis	Herpes	Chancroid	LGV
Incubation period	7 to 14 days	2 to 10 days	4 to 7 days	3 to 12 days
Primary lesion	Papule	Vesicle	Papule/pustule	Papule/vesicle
Number of lesions	Single	Multiple	1 to 3, occasionally more	Single
Size	5 to 15 mm	1 to 3 mm	2 to 20 mm	2 to 10 mm
Painful	No	Yes	Yes	No
Diagnostic test	Dark field Mic. RPR/MHATP/ FTA-ABS	Viral culture	Gram stain with "school of fish" appearance	Complement fixation
Treatment	Penicillin	Acyclovir	Ceftriaxone or azithromycin	Doxycycline

Figure 14-1 (A) Slightly indurated primary of 2 days' duration. It was neither painful nor tender. It points to the need for a high index of suspicion concerning all genital lesions. Dark field microscopy prevents diagnostic error and embarrassment. (B) Papulosquamous secondary syphilis involving the palm.

A

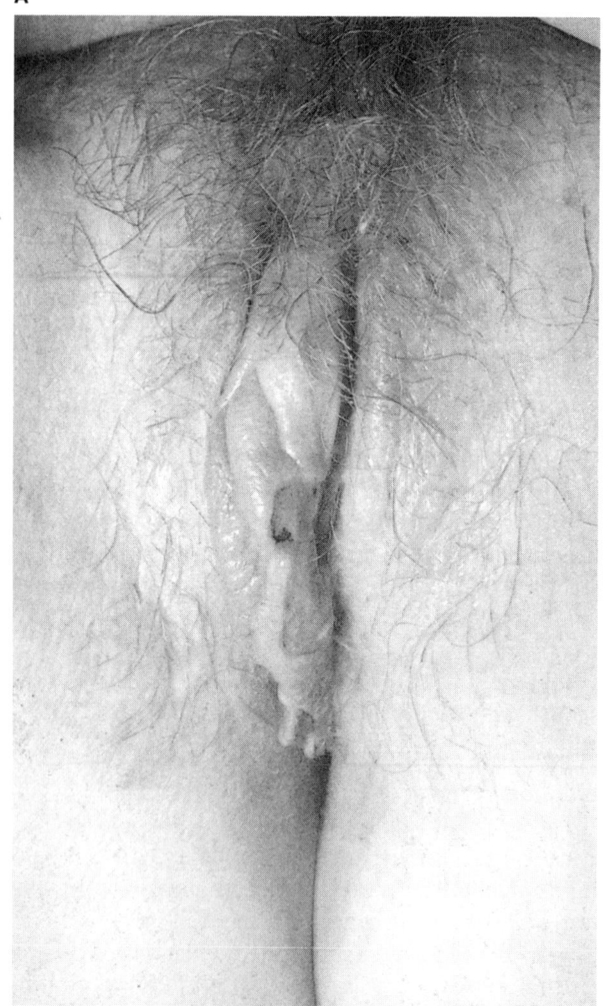

B

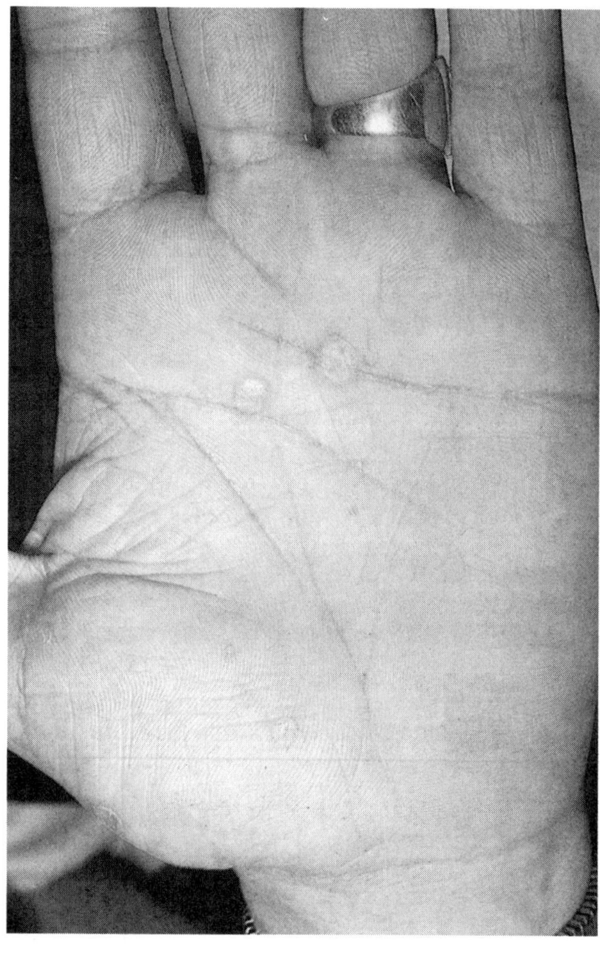

treponemal antibody-absorption (FTA-ABS) technique. False-positive rates in these latter two tests occur less than 1% of the time.

Treatment

Penicillin is still the drug of choice when treating syphilis. Early syphilis can be treated with benzathine penicillin G, 2.4 million units intramuscularly one time. For syphilis of more than a year's duration, the same dose can be given once a week for 3 weeks. Neurosyphilis is a more serious infection and requires aqueous crystalline penicillin G, 2 to 4 million units intravenously every 4 hours for 10 to 14 days, followed by three weekly doses of benzathine penicillin. Alternative regimens to penicillin include tetracycline 500 mg orally QID or doxycycline 100 mg orally BID. Early syphilis should be treated for 2 weeks and syphilis of more than a year's duration for 4 weeks. There is no recommended treatment alternative for neurosyphilis. Treatment can be verified by following RPR or VDRL titers, which should decline fourfold in 3 to 6 months.

Key Points

1. The painless chancre is the initial lesion of syphilis.
2. Syphilis is screened for with the RPR and VDRL tests and confirmed with either the MHA-TP or FTA-ABS.

Figure 14-1 (*continued*) (C) Typical coppery-red papules in secondary syphilis. (D) Healing gumma. Delay in diagnosis is suggested by widespread pigmentation and scarring. Response to treatment was slow and the final scarring led to permanent edema of the foot, sometimes called "paradoxical healing."

C

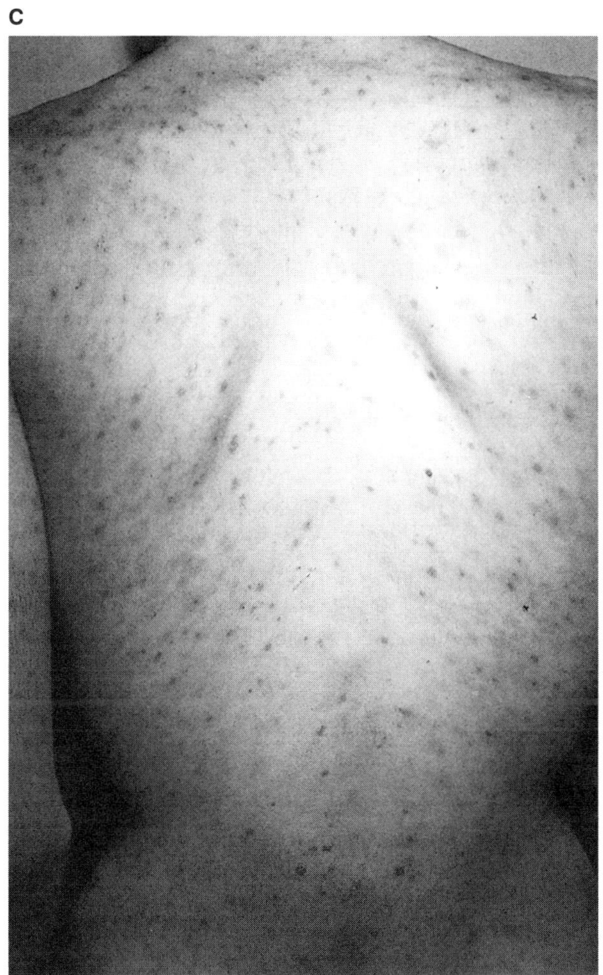

D

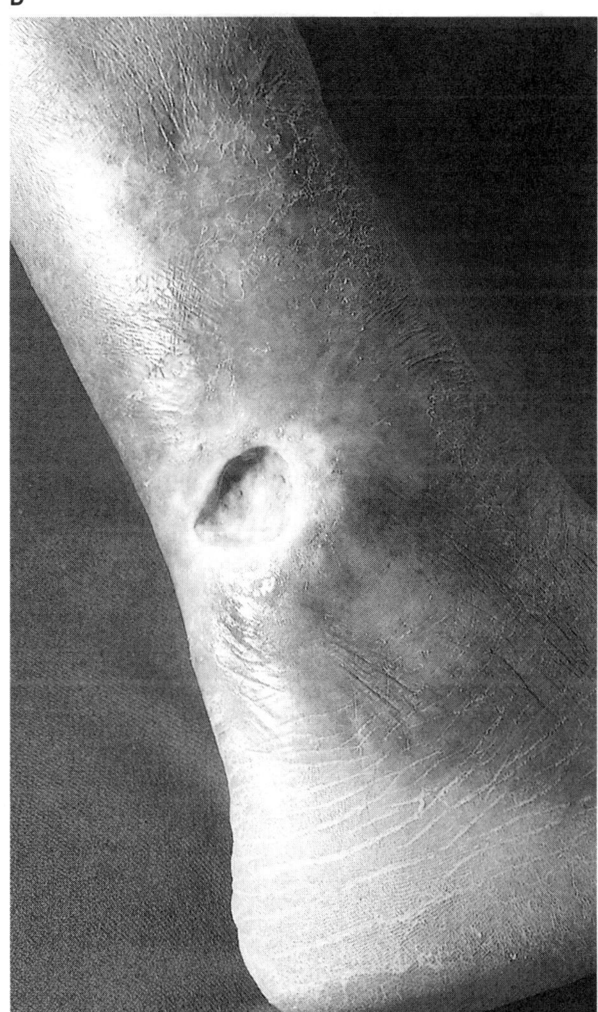

3. Benzathine penicillin is the first drug of choice for syphilis. Neurosyphilis requires intravenous penicillin.

Herpes

Genital herpes simplex virus (HSV) infections are quite common. Although only about 5% of women report a history of genital herpes infection, as many as 25 to 30% test antibody positive. In those individuals with a history of genital herpes, approximately 63% of the causative organism is shown to be HSV-2 and the remaining 37% is HSV-1.

Thus, although some women have the classic "severe" presentation of genital herpes with painful genital ulcers, many women have a mild initial presentation or are entirely asymptomatic. Initial infections usually present with flu-like symptoms including malaise, myalgias, nausea, diarrhea, and fever. Vulvar burning and pruritus precede the multiple vesicles that appear next and usually remain intact for 24 to 36 hours before evolving into painful genital ulcers (Fig. 14-2). These ulcers can require a mean of 10 to 22 days' healing time. After this initial herpes outbreak, recurrent episodes can occur, often one to six times per year. Because of the possibility of frequent recurrence and the devastation of neonatal herpes, pregnant women should have careful vaginal examinations around the time of delivery. Those with lesions should be delivered via cesarean section.

Diagnosis

Diagnosis is made clinically with an examination of the vesicles and ulcers and with a good sexual history. A Tzanck smear can be made from one of the lesions and examined for multinucleated giant cells with a characteristic appearance. Viral cultures may also be used to garner the specific diagnosis, and specific antibody titers may be used to determine whether one is having a primary infection and by what serotype.

Figure 14-2 Herpes labialis. Typical recurrent lesion on upper lip.

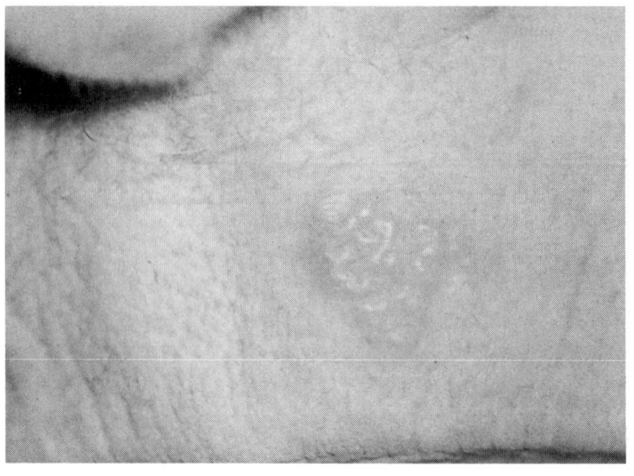

Treatment

Although many palliative treatments have evolved over the years such as sitz baths for comfort and analgesics to reduce the pain, the only antiviral agent available is acyclovir. For a **primary infection**, acyclovir 200 mg every 4 hours or 400 mg TID can reduce the length of infection and the length of time a patient is shedding the virus. With severe HSV infections, such as those that occur in immunocompromised patients, intravenous acyclovir should be used at a dose of 5 mg/kg every 8 hours. For individuals with frequent recurrences, prophylactic or suppression therapy of 400 mg orally QD can be used.

Key Points

1. Genital herpes infections are caused by HSV-2 63% of the time and the remaining 37% are caused by HSV-1.
2. Presentation of herpes is often multiple vesicles that develop into painful ulcers.
3. Treatment is usually palliative, although acyclovir can reduce the length of primary infection and suppressive therapy may decrease the number of recurrences.

Chancroid

Chancroid is caused by *Haemophilus ducreyi*. It is a common sexually transmitted disease around the world, although the incidence in North America has just started rising over the past decade. The male to female incidence around the world ranges from 3:1 to 25:1.

Chancroid presents with a painful, demarcated, nonindurated ulcer located anywhere in the anogenital region. There is often concomitant painful inguinal lymphadenopathy. Usually, just a single ulcer is present, but multiple ulcers and occasionally extragenital infections have been known to occur.

Diagnosis

Diagnosis is difficult because *H. ducreyi* is difficult to culture. Often, transporting the culture swab in Amies or Stuart transport media or chocolate agar can aid in the culture. Direct Gram stains have not been a consistent method of diagnosis; thus, the diagnosis is often made clinically and by ruling out other sources of infection.

Treatment

Treatment regimens include ceftriaxone 250 mg intramuscularly once, azithromycin 1 g orally once, and erythromycin 500 mg QID for 7 days. Alternative regimens include ciprofloxacin 500 mg orally BID for 3 days and Bactrim DS 1 orally BID for 7 days. As with most other sexually transmitted diseases, sexual partners should be treated as well.

Key Points

1. Chancroid presents with a painful genital ulcer and usually concomitant lymphadenopathy.
2. The diagnosis of chancroid is difficult to make and neither cultures or Gram stains have been particularly consistent.
3. Treatment regimens have included many antibiotics, the easiest are single doses of PO azithromycin or IM ceftriaxone.

Lymphogranuloma Venereum

The L-serotypes of *Chlamydia trachomatis* can cause the systemic disease lymphogranuloma venereum (LGV). The primary stage of this illness is often a local lesion that may be a papule or a shallow ulcer, which is often painless, transient, and can go unnoticed. The secondary stage (inguinal syndrome) is characterized by painful inflammation and enlargement of the inguinal nodes. Systemic manifestations include fever, headaches, malaise, and anorexia. The tertiary stage (anogenital syndrome) of this disease is characterized by proctocolitis, rectal stricture, rectovaginal fistula, and elephantiasis. Initially, an anal pruritus will develop with a concomitant mucous rectal discharge.

Treatment

Treatment of LGV is with doxycycline, 100 mg orally BID for 21 days. With persistent illness, the antibiotic regimen can be repeated. If the external genitalia and rectum are disfigured and scarred, surgical measures may be required.

▶ NONULCERATIVE LESIONS

One of the most common nonulcerative lesions is the condyloma (Fig. 14-3). Condyloma acuminata are "warty" lesions that occur anywhere in the anogenital region and are considered a sexually transmitted disease. Other nonulcerative lesions include those caused by **molluscum contagiosum;** ***Phthirus pubis***, the crab louse, and ***Sarcoptes scabiei***, the itch mite.

Finally, when considering nonulcerative lesions, folliculitis should always be included in the differential. The skin in the pubic region has hair follicles and there is always a risk of folliculitis. In rare cases, this can lead to larger lesions such as boils, carbuncles, and abscesses. The usual source of these infections are skin flora, primarily *Staphylococcus aureus*.

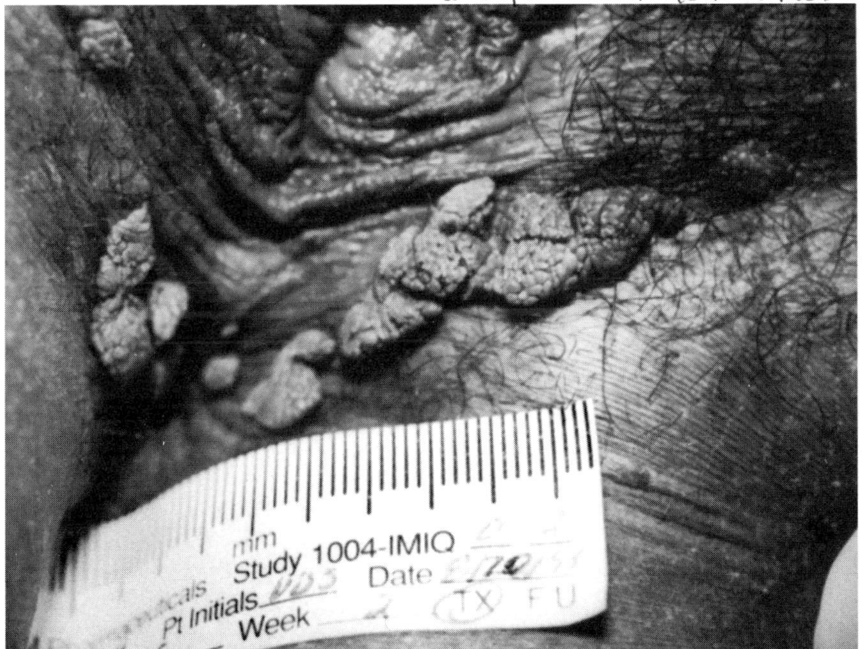

Figure 14-3 Extensive external condylomata acuminata. These fleshy, exophytic growths are covered with small, papillary surface projections. Some of the lesions are pedunculated; others are sessile.

Factors contributing to these lesions in the anogenital region include tight undergarments, sanitary pads, lack of cleanliness, diabetes, and immunosuppression.

Human Papilloma Virus

The most obvious gross results of human papilloma virus (HPV) infection are **condyloma acuminata** or genital warts. However, of more significance in terms of morbidity and mortality, HPV has been correlated with cervical cancer and more recently with other squamous cell malignancies of the female and male reproductive tracts. There has been an increasing incidence of HPV infections in the United States to over 3 million reported cases per year. It is clearly a sexually transmitted disease with 60 to 80% of partners being affected.

Although genital warts are often throughout the lower reproductive tract, patients usually present with anogenital lesions that they have identified or have become pruritic or caused bleeding. The condyloma acuminata are most commonly caused by serotypes 6 and 11, whereas cervical cancer is more often associated with serotypes 16, 18, and 31.

Diagnosis

Diagnosis of condyloma acuminata is usually made via clinical examination. The wart has a raised papillomatous or spiked surface. Initially, the lesions are small, 1 to 5 mm diameter lesions, but they can evolve into larger pedunculated lesions and eventually into cauliflower-like growths. In addition to the vulva, perineal body, and anogenital region, they can also arise in the anal canal, on the walls of the vagina, and on the cervix. When uncertain of diagnosis or for lesions that are unresponsive to therapy, a biopsy of the lesion can be made for definitive diagnosis.

Treatment

Treatment of the lesions includes cryotherapy, topical trichloroacetic acid, topical 25% podophyllin, and 5-fluorouracil cream (Efudex 5%). These treatments are usually repeated until all lesions are gone. For larger condylomas or those unresponsive to medical treatment, the CO_2 laser may be used to vaporize the lesion. Regardless of treatment modality, a recurrence rate of approximately 20% is seen in all patients.

Key Points

1. HPV causes condylomata, but more seriously some serotypes are the likely etiology of cervical cancer.
2. Genital warts are usually diagnosed by appearance but can be confirmed with biopsy.
3. Treatment is usually with cryotherapy or topical medications; larger lesions are usually excised or vaporized with the CO_2 laser.

Molluscum Contagiosum

Molluscum contagiosum is caused by a pox virus that is spread via close contact with an infected person or autoinoculation. The lesion is a small, 1 to 5 mm, domed papule with an umbilicated center (Fig. 14-4). Also known as "water warts," these lesions contain a waxy material that reveals intracytoplasmic molluscum bodies under microscopic examination when stained with Wright's stain or Giemsa stain. Molluscum lesions can occur anywhere on the skin except on the palms and soles of the feet. These lesions are often asymptomatic and generally resolve on their own. They can be removed via local excision and/or treatment of the nodule base with trichloroacetic acid or cryotherapy.

Phthirus pubis and *Sarcoptes scabiei*

The nonulcerative lesions caused by *Phthirus pubis*, the crab louse, and *Sarcoptes scabiei*, the itch mite are similar. Signs and symptoms for these two infections include pruritus, irritated skin, vesicles, and burrows. The primary difference is that lesions from *P. pubis*, or **pediculosis**, are usually confined to the pubic hair, whereas **scabies** may infect throughout the entire

Figure 14-4 Two typical molluscum lesions, one of which shows a mosaic appearance.

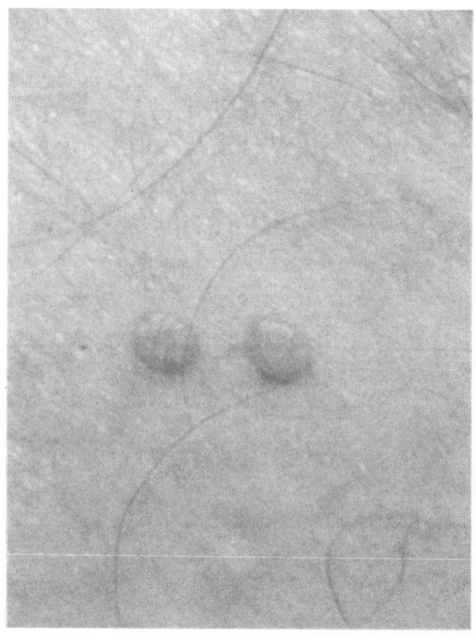

body. Thus, when treating with lindane (Kwell) shampoo, pediculosis can be cured by applying to the specific areas, whereas it is more effective to treat scabies by using lindane lotion over the entire body.

Bartholin's Abscess

The Bartholin's gland is located bilaterally at approximately 4 and 8 o'clock on the labial majora (Fig. 14-5). It is a mucus-secreting gland that has a duct that opens just external to the hymenal ring. This duct can become obstructed and lead to an enlarged Bartholin's cyst. If the cyst remains small (1 to 2 cm) and is not causing any symptoms, it can be left alone and will often resolve on its own. However, some of the cysts can become quite large and cause pressure symptoms such as local pain, dyspareunia, and even difficulty walking.

Figure 14-5 Gross clinical appearance of a Bartholin cyst of the vulva.

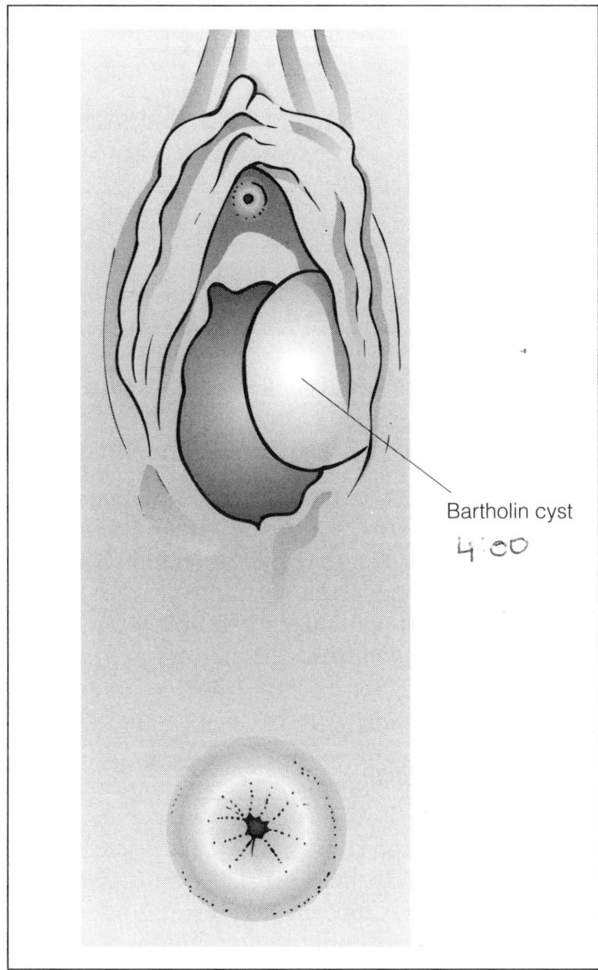

When the cysts do not resolve, they can become infected and lead to Bartholin's gland abscesses. These abscesses can range in size and can be quite large, causing exquisite pain and tenderness and associated cellulitis. Bartholin's abscesses or symptomatic cysts should be treated similarly to any abscess by drainage. However, simple incision and drainage can often lead to recurrence, so one of two methods is often used:

1. A small incision (5 mm) is made to drain and irrigate the abscess. A Word catheter, which has a balloon tip, is placed inside the remaining cyst and inflated to fill the space. It is left in place for 4 to 6 weeks while epithelialization of the cyst and tract occurs.
2. Marsupialization of the abscess where the entire abscess is incised and sewn open (Fig. 14-6). Epithelialization can then occur and there is no closed space for recurrence to ensue.
3. With either treatment, warm sitz baths several times per day is recommended for both pain relief and to decrease healing time. Adjunct antibiotic therapy is only recommended when the drainage is cultured for *Neisseria gonorrhoeae*, which is approximately 10% of the time. Concomitant cellulitis or an abscess that seems refractory to simple surgical treatment should also be treated with antibiotics that cover skin flora, primarily *Staphylococcus aureus*.

Key Points

1. Bartholin's cysts and abscesses are located at 4 and 8 o'clock on the labia majora.
2. When uninfected, Bartholin's cysts often resolve on their own.
3. Bartholin's abscesses can be treated similarly to other abscesses with I&D.
4. Antibiotic therapy is only recommended for abscesses with cultures positive for *N. gonorrhoeae* or concomitant cellulitis.

▶ VAGINAL INFECTIONS

Symptoms related to vaginal infections are the number one cause of visits to a gynecologist. The vagina provides a warm, moist environment that can be colonized by a variety of organisms. When anything upsets the balance of microflora in the vagina such as

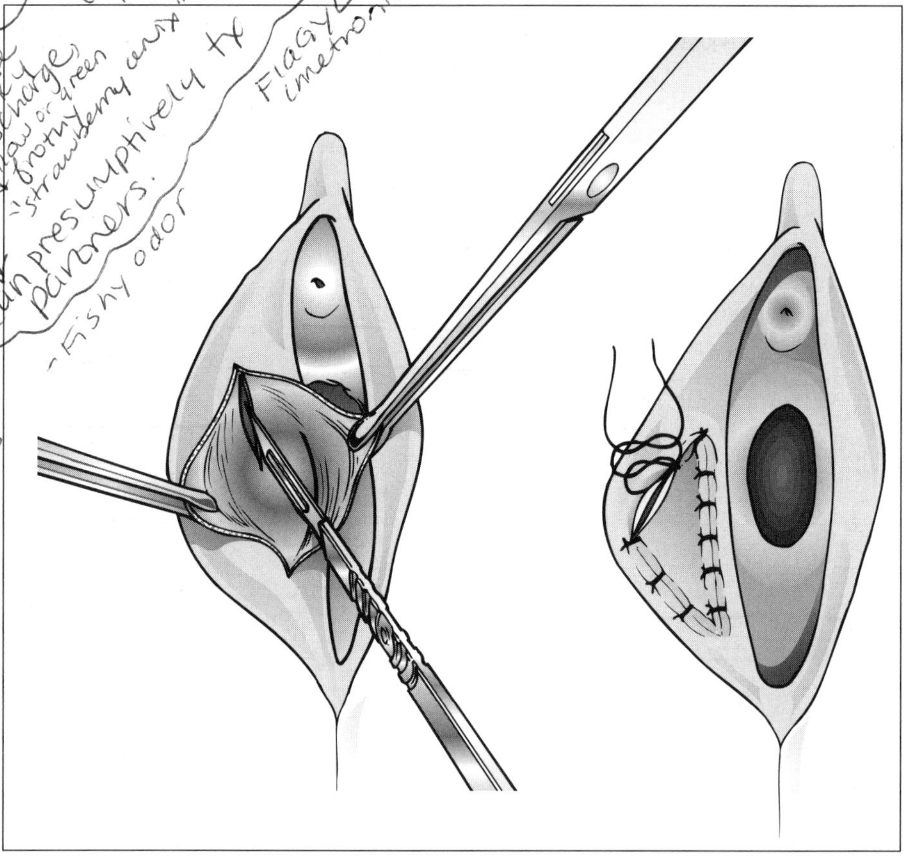

Figure 14-6 Incision, drainage, and marsupialization of a Bartholin abscess.

antibiotics, diet, systemic illness, or the introduction of a pathogen, overgrowth of one variety of organism can lead to symptoms including itching, pain, discharge, burning, and odor. Common organisms that cause symptoms with overgrowth include *Candida, Trichomonas*, and *Gardnerella* (Fig. 14-7). These can each be easily diagnosed and treated quite effectively with antimicrobials. However, any chronic vaginitis with pruritus, pain, bleeding, and/or ulcerated lesions that does not respond to drug therapy should be investigated to rule out malignancy.

Yeast Infections

Candidiasis probably causes 30% of the vaginitis that leads women to be seen by a gynecologist. Many more of these infections are treated by women using over-the-counter (OTC) preparations. It is caused by *Candida albicans* in 80 to 90% of all cases, with the remaining cases caused by other candidal species. Predisposing factors for candidal overgrowth include the use of broad-spectrum antibiotics, diabetes mellitus, and decreased cellular immunity as in AIDS patients or those on immunosuppressive therapies. Yeast infections are also associated with intercourse and increase during the late luteal phase of the menstrual cycle.

Diagnosis

Typical symptoms of genital candidiasis include vulvar and vaginal pruritus, burning, dysuria, dyspareunia, and vaginal discharge. On physical examination there is vulvar edema and erythema with a scant vaginal discharge. Only approximately 20% of patients display the characteristic white plaques adherent to the vaginal mucosa or the cottage cheese-like discharge. Diagnosis is usually made by microscopic examination of a KOH prep of the vaginal discharge that reveals characteristic branching hyphae and spores. Although the KOH preparation is estimated to have a sensitivity of 25 to 80%, the Gram stain is almost 100% sensitive for yeast infections. The most sensitive test is culture on Sabouraud's agar. Clinically, treatment is often instituted on the basis of clinical signs and symptoms.

Treatment

Treatment includes any of the azole agents via topical applications, typically Monistat-7 as an OTC preparation or terazole cream by prescription. Nystatin

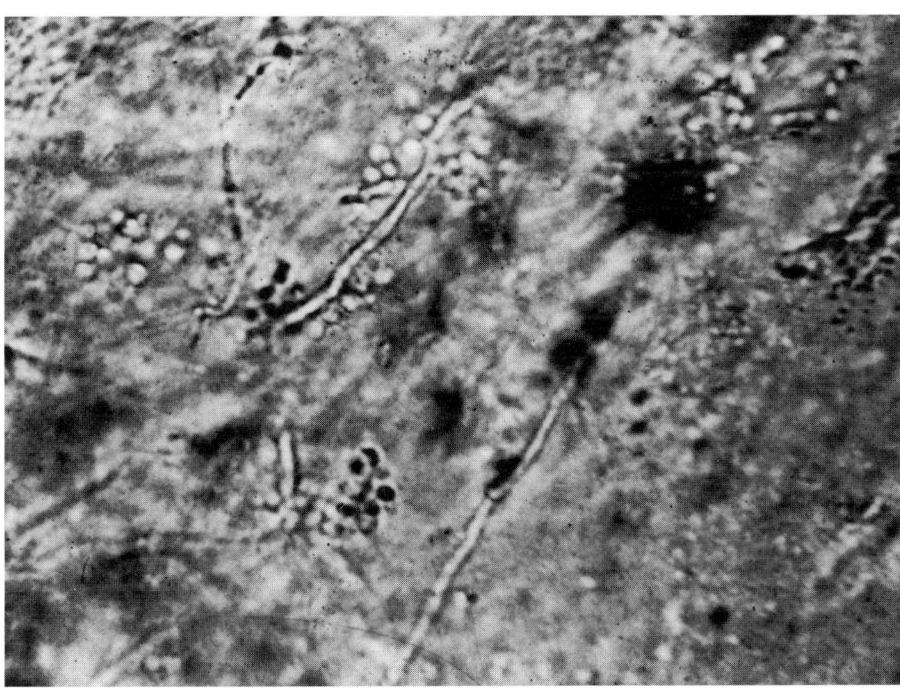

Figure 14-7 *Candida albicans*, KOH mount of skin scraping.

suppositories or powder may prove to be effective as well. Other local therapies include boric acid capsules 600 mg every day for 2 weeks or the application of 1% aqueous solution of gentian violet. More recently, fluconazole (Diflucan) 150 mg orally once has been shown to be as effective as any of the local treatments. For chronic recurrent candidal infections, ketoconazole 400 mg orally every day for 1 to 2 weeks has been shown to be effective.

Key Points

1. As with vulvitis, the number one cause of vaginitis is candida.
2. Diagnosis is often made with a wet prep (trich and BV) or KOH prep (yeast).
3. In the absence of microscopic evidence, symptoms and type of discharge should dictate the treatment.

Trichomonas vaginalis

Trichomonas vaginalis is a unicellular anaerobic flagellated protozoan that can cause vaginitis. It inhabits the lower genitourinary tracts of women and men, and there are approximately 3 million cases diagnosed annually in the United States. The disease is sexually transmitted with 75% of sexual partners of those colonized also culture positive.

The signs and symptoms of *T. vaginitis* include a profuse discharge with an unpleasant odor. The discharge may be yellow, gray, or green in coloration and may be frothy in appearance. Vulvar erythema, edema, and pruritus can also be noted. The characteristic erythematous, punctate epithelial papillae, or "strawberry" appearance of the cervix is apparent in only 10% of cases. Symptoms are usually worse immediately after menses because of the transient increase in vaginal pH at that time.

Diagnosis

Diagnosis of *Trichomonas* is made via microscopic examination of wet preps of vaginal swabs. The protozoan is slightly larger than a white blood cell count; three to five flagella, often active movement of the flagella, and propulsion of the organism can be seen (Fig. 14-8). The diagnosis can be confirmed when necessary with culture, but this not commonly used.

Treatment

The mainstay of treatment for *T. vaginalis* infections is metronidazole (Flagyl) 2 g orally once. The single-dose regimen has been found to be as effective as the more traditional 250 mg orally TID for 7 days. When giving Flagyl, patients need to be reminded of its Antabuse effect when taken with alcohol. Alternative treatment to metronidazole is clotrimazole cream topically for 7

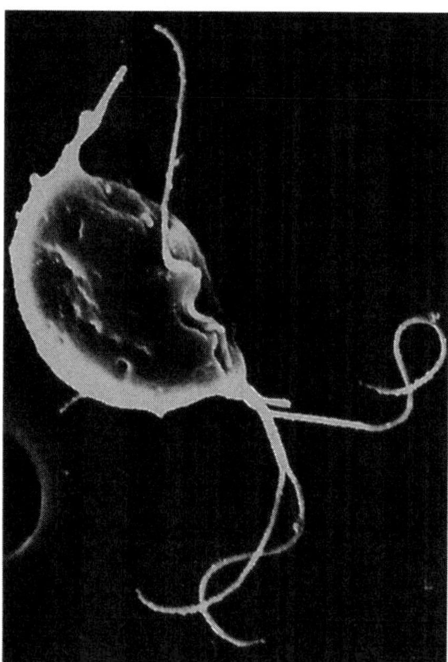

Figure 14-8 Scanning electronmicrograph of *Trichomonas vaginalis*. The undulating membrane and flagellae of *Trichomonas* are its characteristic features.

days; however, it is unclear whether this regimen is particularly effective. Because of the high rate of concomitant infections in sexual partners, both should be treated to prevent reinfection.

Key Points

1. Seventy-five percent of sexual partners of those with *Trichomonas* will also be colonized and should be presumptively treated.
2. Diagnosis is made via wet prep but is usually presumed with a profuse, malodorous, gray-green frothy discharge.
3. Treatment is metronidazole 2 g orally one time.

Gardnerella vaginalis

Although bacterial vaginosis is likely to be polymicrobial, one of the most common organisms present in culture is *G. vaginalis.* Bacterial vaginosis is quite common, with prevalence rates of 5% of college populations and as high as 60% in sexually transmitted disease clinics. Risk factors include lower socioeconomic status, IUD usage, multiple sexual partners, and smoking.

Diagnosis

Many patients with bacterial vaginosis may be asymptomatic or have just an increase in discharge. However, symptomatic patients will complain of a profuse nonirritating discharge often with a malodorous "fishy" amine odor. Diagnosis is made most commonly with microscopic examination of a wet prep of a vaginal swab that reveals clue cells. These are vaginal epithelial cells that are diffusely covered with bacteria. The amine odor of bacterial vaginosis can be enhanced by adding KOH to a vaginal prep (**the whiff test**), and this is considered pathognomonic for the syndrome. Vaginal cultures can be done as well and may often reveal *G. vaginalis*, but the simple clinical diagnosis made from vaginal swabs are more often used in the clinical setting.

Treatment

Treatment of bacterial vaginosis is usually with either Flagyl 500 mg orally BID for 7 days or clindamycin 300 mg TID for 7 days. Both antibiotics are also available in gel or cream and can be used topically. Similarly to *Trichomonas* infections, because it is likely that untreated sexual partners may cause reinfection, they should be treated presumptively.

Key Points

1. Bacterial vaginosis is polymicrobial but usually attributed to *Gardnerella*.
2. The discharge is usually less than with *Trichomonas* but has a characteristic "fishy" amine odor; the whiff test exaggerates this odor with KOH.
3. Diagnosis is made formally with clue cells on wet prep.
4. First-line treatment is metronidazole (Flagyl) for a 7-day course.

▶ INFECTIONS OF THE CERVIX

The organisms that most commonly cause cervicitis and infections of the upper reproductive tract are different from those most commonly causing infections of the lower reproductive tract. ***Neisseria gonorrhoeae*** and ***Chlamydia trachomatis*** are the two most common organisms causing cervicitis and the only organisms shown to cause mucopurulent cervicitis. Clinically, cervicitis is diagnosed as cervical motion tenderness in the absence of other signs of pelvic inflammatory disease (PID).

Other organisms can cause infections of the cervix including HSV, HPV, mycoplasma hominis, and ureaplasma ureolyticum. HSV causes either herpes lesions or a white plaque that resembles cervical cancer. Infection with HPV leads to condyloma and is also thought to be the etiology of cervical cancer. Neither mycoplasma or ureoplasma have been shown to be correlated with active disease but may be a cause of nonmucopurulent cervicitis and bacterial vaginosis.

Neisseria gonorrhoeae

Gonococcal infections remain today one of the most commonly reported sexually transmitted infections, with approximately 2 million cases reported annually in the United States. Most cases occur in the 15- to 29-year-old age group. Among sexually active women, 15 to 19 year olds have two times the incidence of the 20 to 24 year olds. However, the highest overall prevalence is in the 20- to 24-year-old age group because they have the highest percentage of sexually active individuals.

Multiple risk factors have been associated with gonococcal infections, including low socioeconomic status, urban residence, nonwhite and non-Asian ethnicity, early onset of sexual activity, early age of first sexual activity, illicit drug use, prostitution, unmarried marital status, and previous gonococcal infections. Condoms, diaphragms, and spermicides decrease risk of transmission. There are also seasonal variations in the incidence of gonorrhea in the United States with a peak seen in late summer.

Transmission between the sexes is unequal with male to female transmission estimated at 80 to 90% compared with an estimated 20 to 25% female to male transmission rate after a single sexual encounter. This difference in transmission is likely related to the type of epithelium exposed in the different sexes. In males, this is primarily keratinized epithelium on the external surface of the penis, whereas females receive primary contact with mucosa of the vagina and the nonkeratinized epithelium of the cervix. Furthermore, male ejaculation increases the amount of exposure time in women, which supports the use of condoms as an exceptional prophylactic measure against gonococcal transmission.

Gonococcus can infect the anal canal, the urethra, the oropharynx, and Bartholin's glands, in addition to the more commonly reported cervicitis and PID. In neonates, gonococcal conjunctivitis is an issue. As much as 1% of recognized gonococcal infections may proceed to a disseminated infection. This infection begins with fevers and erythematous macular skin lesions and proceeds to a tenosynovitis and septic arthritis.

Diagnosis

Identification of the causative organism, *N. gonorrhoeae*, a Gram-negative diplococcus resembling paired kidney beans is necessary for the definitive diagnosis. Isolation using the modified Thayer-Martin chocolate agar has a sensitivity of 96% in endocervical cultures. Recently, many hospitals and health care facilities have begun using a gonococcal DNA probe similar to that used to diagnose chlamydia.

Treatment

The recommended treatment is ceftriaxone 250 mg intramuscularly once. Therapy should be followed by a week-long course of doxycycline 100 mg orally BID or a 1-g dose of azithromycin to treat likely concomitant chlamydial infections. Ofloxacin may be used as a single agent to treat both organisms.

Key Points

1. *N. gonorrhoeae* causes a reported 2 million infections per year.
2. Common diseases caused include cervicitis, PID, tubo-ovarian abscess (TOA), and Bartholin's abscess.
3. Diagnosis can be made with culture, Gram stain, or DNA probe.
4. Treatment for uncomplicated infections is ceftriaxone 250 mg intramusculary once.
5. Treatment for *N. gonorrhoeae* should always include doxycycline 100 mg orally BID for a week to treat likely concomitant chlamydial infections.

Chlamydia trachomatis

Chlamydia trachomatis is a pathogen that causes ocular, respiratory, and reproductive tract infections. In the United States, its transmission is primarily via sexual contact, although vertical transmission from a mother to a newborn is also seen. Epidemiologically, *C. trachomatis* infections are parallel to those of *N. gonorrhoeae,* although they have been more difficult to diagnose because they are obligate intracellular bacteria and difficult to culture. With the advent of a genetic probe, more isolated chlamydial infections are being diagnosed. Prevalence is estimated at 3 to 5% in asymptomatic women, and 5 to 7% of pregnant women have had positive chlamydiazyme tests.

Women with chlamydial infections may be entirely asymptomatic. Common sites of infection include the endocervix, urethra, and rectum. Clinical manifestations of symptomatic chlamydial infections are often quite similar to those of *N. gonorrhoeae* and include symptoms of cervicitis, urethritis, and PID. The L-serotypes of *C. trachomatis* can cause the systemic disease LGV.

Treatment

Treatment of choice of chlamydial infections is doxycycline 100 mg orally BID for 1 week or a one time 1-g dose of azithromycin. Alternative regimens include tetracycline 500 mg orally QID and for the pregnant patient, erythromycin 500 mg orally QID. For LGV, the treatment regimen should be extended to 3 weeks. When treating chlamydial infections, most physicians also treat for *N. gonorrhoeae* with a single intramuscular shot of 250 mg ceftriaxone.

Key Points

1. Chlamydial infections tend to coincide with gonorrhea infections.
2. Many chlamydial infections are entirely asymptomatic.
3. Treatment is with doxycycline 100 mg BID; alternatively, azithromycin, a one time 1-g dose, is used.
4. LGV is caused by the L-serotypes of chlamydia.

Gonorrhea

- 15-29 y/o (15-19 > 20-24 ♀)
- condoms, spermicides, diaphragms ↓ risk
- incidence peaks in summer

♂ → ♀ 90% transmission

- Gram ⊖ diplococci in pairs; Thayer-Martin chocolate Agar

Tx: ceftriaxone 250 mg IM x 1

cervicitis, urethritis, PID

Chlamydia

CHAPTER 15

Upper Female Reproductive Tract and Systemic Infections

▶ ENDOMETRITIS

An infection of the uterine endometrium is **endometritis**; if the infection invades into the myometrium, it is known as **endomyometritis**. Endometritis and endomyometritis are most common after instrumentation or disruption of the intrauterine cavity. It is seen most commonly after cesarean section but also after vaginal deliveries, dilatation and evacuation or curettage, and intrauterine device (IUD) placement. Nonpuerperal endometritis is not commonly recognized but is probably coexistent with 70 to 80% of pelvic inflammatory disease (PID). Its etiology is related to ascent of infection from the cervix that then proceeds to the fallopian tubes to cause acute salpingitis and eventually widespread PID.

Chronic endometritis is often asymptomatic but is clinically significant as it leads to other pelvic infections and uncommonly endomyometritis. The diagnosis can be made in a nonpuerperal patient with endometrial biopsy and endocervical cultures. It is often a polymicrobial infection with a variety of pathogens, including skin and gastrointestinal flora in addition to the usual flora colonizing the lower reproductive tract. A clinical diagnosis is made in anyone with uterine tenderness, fever, and elevated white blood cell (WBC) count.

Treatment of severe endomyometritis is usually clindamycin 900 mg intravenously (IV) every 8 hours and gentamycin loaded with 2 mg/kg IV and then maintained with 1.5 mg/kg IV every 8 hours. Less severe endometritis is often treated with a cephalosporin such as cefoxitin 2 g IV every 6 hours or cefotetan 2 g IV every 12 hours. Treatment course is given until asymptomatic and/or afebrile for 48 hours.

Key Points

1. Endomyometritis is most common after a delivery or instrumentation of the endometrial cavity.
2. Diagnosis is made with uterine tenderness, fever, and elevated WBC count.
3. In a nonpuerperal patient, the diagnosis can be made with endometrial biopsy.
4. Treatment is broad spectrum with intravenous clinda and gent, with less severe infections treated with intravenous cephalosporins.

▶ ACUTE SALPINGITIS AND PID

Acute salpingitis, or more generally PID, is the most common serious complication of sexually transmitted diseases. Approximately 1 million cases occur annually in the United States. The economic costs for initial treatment are estimated at greater than $3.5 billion, which is in addition to the treatment for the principal sequelae, including infertility and increased ectopic pregnancies. Infertility is estimated to occur in 20% of all PID patients, and the risk of ectopic pregnancy is increased as much as 10-fold. Other sequelae, including chronic pelvic pain, dyspareunia, and pelvic adhesions, may also require surgical therapy, lending greater weight to the economic costs and patient morbidity of this disease.

Among sexually active women, the incidence of this disease is higher in the 15- to 19-year-old age group (three times greater than the 25- to 29-year-old age group). This may be attributed to higher risk behavior in this age group. It may also be related to decreased immunity to sexually transmitted disease agents in younger women, although the pathophysiologic mechanisms are unclear. Finally, the younger age group is less likely to have a regular gynecologist or seek medical attention until bacterial vaginosis or cervicitis has progressed to the more symptomatic PID.

Other risk factors for PID include nonwhite and non-Asian ethnicity, unmarried marital status, recent history of douching, and cigarette smoking. Barrier contraceptives have been shown to decrease the incidence of PID, whereas IUDs are considered a risk factor for PID.

The principal symptom of acute salpingitis is abdominal or pelvic/adnexal pain. The character of the pain can range (burning, cramping, stabbing) and can be unilateral or bilateral. It may also be pain free in what has been deemed "silent" PID. Other associated symptoms include increased vaginal discharge, abnormal odor, abnormal bleeding, gastrointestinal disturbances, and urinary tract symptoms. Fever is a less common symptom seen in only 20% of women with PID.

Clinical Manifestations

Diagnosis is made clinically with an elevated WBC count, fever, pelvic pain, cervical motion tenderness, and adnexal tenderness (Fig. 15-1). Cervical cultures are done to find a causative organism but, due to its polymicrobial nature, should not dictate the treatment regimen. The definitive diagnosis is made via laparoscopy. In practice, this is only used when appendicitis cannot be ruled out by clinical examination. Ultrasonography is not useful in the diagnosis of PID but is helpful after the treatment of tubo-ovarian abscesses.

The principal organisms suspected to cause PID are *Neisseria gonorrhoeae* and *C. trachomatis*. However, cultures from the upper reproductive tract have shown that most PID is likely to be polymicrobial, including anaerobic organisms such as *Bacteroides* spp. and facultative bacteria such as *Gardnerella, Escherichia coli, H. influenzae,* and streptococci.

Treatment

Because of the high rate of ambulatory treatment failures and the seriousness of sequelae, patients are now usually hospitalized for treatment of PID. Because of its polymicrobial nature, PID is usually treated with a broad-spectrum cephalosporin plus doxycycline. A typical regimen is cefoxitin 2 g IV every 6 hours or cefotetan 2 g IV every 12 hours given until the patient is asymptomatic for 48 hours with a concomitant 10- to 14-day course of doxycycline 100 mg orally BID. As an outpatient, ceftriaxone 500 mg IM every day or cefoxitin 2 g intramuscularly (IM) plus 1 g of probenecid orally is used with close follow-up for resolution of symptoms.

Figure 15-1 Intra-abdominal spread of gonorrhea and other pathogenic bacteria.

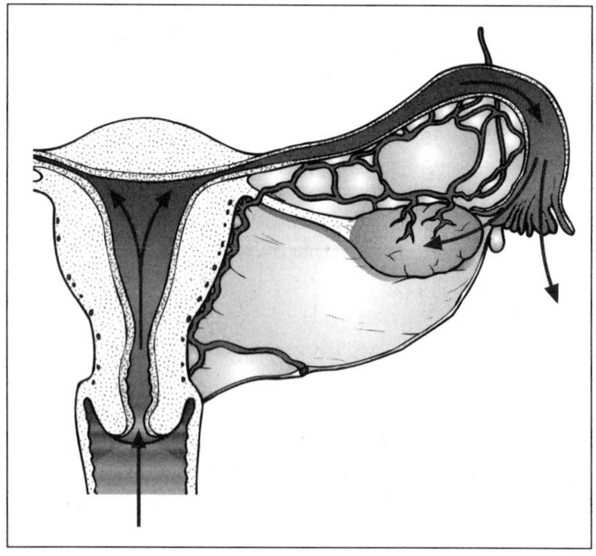

Key Points

1. There are approximately 1 million cases of PID annually.
2. Twenty percent of patients with PID will go on to have infertility.
3. PID can be diagnosed with uterine and adnexal tenderness, fever, elevated WBC count, and cultures or tests for gonorrhea and chlamydia.
4. Because of the seriousness of this disease and its sequelae, patients should be hospitalized and treated with IV antibiotics.

▶ TUBO-OVARIAN ABSCESS

Persistent PID can lead to the development of a **tubo-ovarian abscess** (TOA) (Fig. 15-2). Most so-called TOAs are actually tubo-ovarian complexes, the difference being that complexes are not walled off like the true abscess and thus more responsive to antimicrobial therapy. Estimates of the progression from PID to TOA range from 3 to 16%; thus, any PID not responsive to therapy should be investigated further to rule out TOA.

Diagnosis

The diagnosis of TOA can be made clinically in the setting of PID and the appreciation of an adnexal or posterior cul-de-sac mass or fullness. WBC count is usually elevated with a left shift and the erythrocyte sedimentation (ESR) is often elevated as well. Cultures should include endocervical swabs and blood

Figure 15-2 Findings associated with chronic pelvic inflammatory disease, including tubo-ovarian abscess, adhesions, pyosalpinx, and an abscess located in the posterior cul-de-sac.

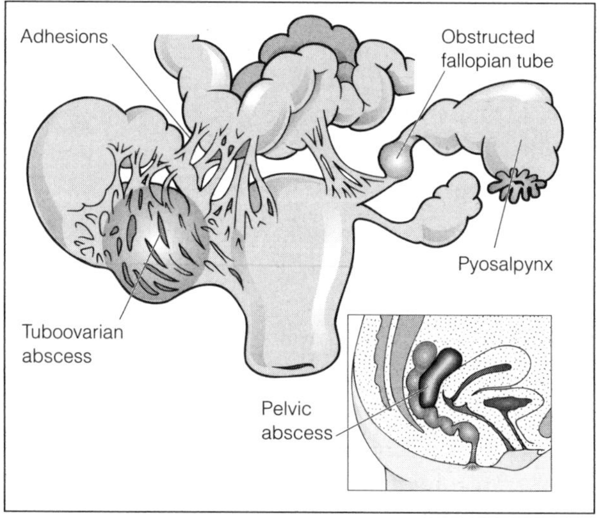

cultures to rule out sepsis. Culdocentesis that reveals gross pus is diagnostic but has been used less as imaging studies have been used more. Ultrasound diagnosis of pelvic abscess has increased as this modality has been refined. Pelvic computed tomography may be required, particularly in obese patients where ultrasound use is limited. Finally, laparoscopy can lead to a definitive diagnosis but is usually only used when the clinical picture is unclear.

Treatment

Unless the abscess is ruptured, causing peritoneal signs, surgical treatment can be avoided and patients can be treated with antibiotics. The standard of care is to hospitalize any patient with a TOA/TOC and treat with broad-spectrum antibiotics. The first-line choice is often cefoxitin 2 g IV every 6 hours with doxycycline 100 mg orally BID. If there is no response to this therapy, coverage can be expanded to triple antibiotic therapy such as ampicillin, gentamycin, and clindamycin or metronidazole. The course of the disease can be followed by symptoms, clinical examination, temperature, WBC count, and, if these are equivocal, imaging studies.

For more serious TOAs, those unresponsive to antibiotic therapy, or with gross rupture, surgical intervention is necessary. Usually unilateral adnexectomy is curative for the unilateral TOA. For bilateral TOAs, often a bilateral salpingo-oophorectomy (BSO) or a total abdominal hysterectomy (TAH) is performed.

Key Points

1. Chronic or acute PID can lead to TOAs or TOCs.
2. Diagnosis is made in the setting of PID with an adnexal mass, confirmation is usually with an imaging study, and CT is the "gold standard."
3. Treatment includes hospitalization and IV antibiotics. For TOAs not responsive to antibiotics, adnexal surgery is the definitive cure.

▶ TOXIC SHOCK SYNDROME

Toxic shock syndrome (TSS) reached its peak in the United States in 1980 when the case rate was 3 in every 100,000 menstruating women. Since 1984, there have been fewer than 300 cases per year. Initially, TSS was correlated with high absorbency tampons and menstruation. Nonmenstrually related TSS has been associated with vaginal infections, vaginal delivery, cesarean section, postpartum endometritis, miscarriage, and laser treatment of condylomata.

Diagnosis

TSS is caused by colonization or infection with specific strains of *Staphylococcus aureus* that produce an epidermal toxin–toxic shock syndrome toxin-1 (TSST-1). This toxin and other staphylococcal toxins are likely to cause most of the symptoms of TSS. Symptoms include high fever (>102°F), erythematous rash, desquamation of the palms and soles 1 to 2 weeks after the acute illness, and hypotension. Gastrointestinal disturbances, myalgias, mucous membrane hyperemia, increased blood urea nitrogen (BUN), and creatinine (Cr) platelet count less than 100,000, and alteration in consciousness can also be seen. Often blood cultures are negative because it is thought that the exotoxin is absorbed through the vaginal mucosa.

Treatment

Because of the seriousness of the disease (2 to 8% mortality rate), hospitalization is always indicated. For more severe patients who are hemodynamically unstable, admission to an intensive care unit may be necessary. Of highest priority is treatment of hypotension with IV fluids and pressors if needed. Because the disease is caused by the exotoxin, treatment with IV antibiotics often does not shorten the length of the acute illness. However, it does decrease the risk of recurrence, which has been as high as 30% in women who continued to use high absorbent tampons.

Key Points

1. TSS peaked in 1984; now there are less than 300 cases per year in the United States.
2. Symptoms including fever, rash, desquamation of palms and soles are likely caused by an *S. aureus* toxin TSST-1.
3. Because of the seriousness of this illness, patients are hospitalized, treated with IV antibiotics, and, if necessary, hemodynamic support.

▶ HUMAN IMMUNODEFICIENCY VIRUS

The human immunodeficiency virus (HIV) is the causative agent of acquired immunodeficiency syndrome (AIDS). HIV is transmitted via sexual contact, via parenteral inoculation, and vertically from mothers to infants via a transplacental route, during birth, and via breast milk. Currently, there are an estimated 1 to 2 million HIV carriers in the United States. Although women account for only 7% of AIDS cases in the United States, they are one segment of the population that are currently rising quite quickly. Worldwide, women represent a much more substantial segment of those affected with HIV.

Infection with HIV, a retrovirus, leads to decreased cellular immunity because of infection of a variety of cells carrying the CD4 antigen, including helper T cells, B cells, monocytes, and macrophages. Initially, the infection is entirely asymptomatic, although the individual is a carrier of the disease; this stage can last for 5 to 7 years on the average. The disease can present initially with the AIDS-related complex, lymphadenopathy, night sweats, malaise, diarrhea, weight loss, and unusual recurrent infections such as oral candidiasis, varicella-zoster, or herpes simplex. As the infection further decreases cellular immunity, full-blown AIDS develops with opportunistic infections such as *Pneumocystis carinii* pneumonia, toxoplasmosis, mycobacterium avium intracellulare, cytomegalovirus, and various malignancies such as Kaposi's sarcoma and non-Hodgkin's lymphoma.

Diagnosis

The diagnosis of HIV infection is made initially via a screening test. The test is an enzyme-linked immunosorbent assay (ELISA) using HIV antigens to which patient serum is added. A positive test results when antigen-antibody complexes form. The test does have false-positive results, which in low-risk populations may occur more often than true positive results. Thus, positive tests are always confirmed by a Western blot.

Treatment

There is no effective treatment nor cure for HIV or AIDS. Thus, great efforts are being directed toward prevention of HIV transmission by encouraging the change of risky behavior. Condoms are recommended for sexually active patients. IV drug users can avoid sharing needles and use clean needles. For those requiring a blood transfusion, the risk of HIV infection is currently estimated at less than 1 in 200,000.

Therapy for HIV and AIDS centers around prophylaxis and treatment for the opportunistic infections that occur and a variety of antiretroviral nucleoside analogues [AZT, deoxyadenosine (DDI), dideoxycytidine (DDC)] that theoretically may delay the progression of the disease. Recently protease inhibitors have been added to the medical armamentarium and have been effective in increasing CD4 counts and decreasing viral load. Although specific treatments are not discussed, there are two key points in the management of HIV infection in women that deserve special emphasis. The first concerns obstetric care of the HIV patient and the second relates to the high incidence of invasive cervical cancer in this population.

Approximately 25% of infants born to HIV-infected mothers become infected with HIV. Current evidence suggests that zidovudine (AZT) administration during the antepartum (after the first trimester), intrapartum, and neonatal period can reduce the risk of maternal-fetal HIV transmission by two thirds in women with mildly symptomatic HIV disease.

The high incidence of invasive cervical cancer in HIV-infected women is also an important issue in gynecologic outpatient management. Studies have confirmed the synergistic association of HIV and human papilloma virus (HPV), the causative agent in squamous cell carcinoma of the cervix, and the Centers for Disease Control and Prevention currently recommends routine pap smears at initial evaluation and 6 months later. Thereafter, yearly evaluations are sufficient if results are negative unless there is documentation of previous HPV infection, squamous intraepithelial lesion, or symptomatic HIV disease, in which case the pap smear should be repeated at 6-month intervals.

Key Points

1. HIV is transmitted via sexual contact, sharing IV needles, and any activity where infected blood is introduced to a noninfected host.
2. HIV infection is screened for with the ELISA test and confirmed with a Western blot.
3. There is currently no cure for HIV infection so treatment centers around AZT once the CD4 count has dropped and treatment of the multiple opportunistic infections.
4. Prenatal and peripartum treatment with AZT has been shown to decrease vertical transmission during pregnancy.

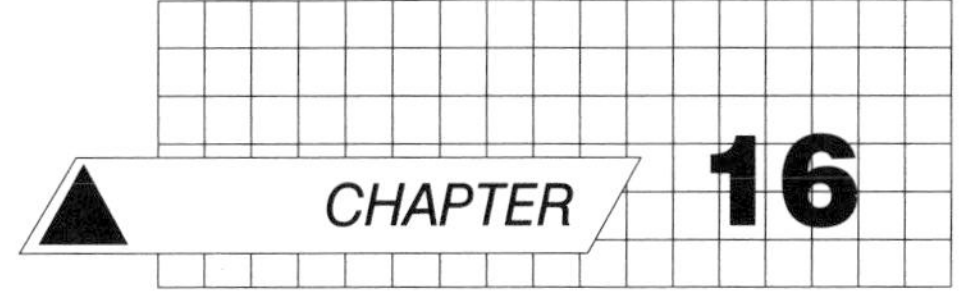

Pelvic Relaxation

▶ PATHOGENESIS

As shown in Figure 16-1, normal support of the pelvic organs is provided by a complex network of muscles (e.g., levator muscles), fascia (e.g., urogenital diaphragm, endopelvic fascia), and ligaments (e.g., uterosacral and cardinal ligaments). Damage to any one of these structures can potentially result in a weakening or loss of support to the pelvis and pelvic organs (Fig. 16-2). Damage to the anterior vaginal wall can result in herniation of the bladder (**cystocele**) or urethra (**urethrocele**) into the vaginal vault. Injuries to the endopelvic fascia of the rectovaginal septum can result in herniation of the rectum (**rectocele**) or small bowel (**enterocele**) into the vaginal vault. And injury or stretching of the cardinal ligaments can result in descensus, or prolapse, of the uterus (**uterine prolapse**).

Pelvic relaxation can cause pelvic pressure and pain, dyspareunia, bowel and bladder dysfunction, and urinary incontinence. The causes for loss of support include birth trauma; chronic increases in intraabdominal pressure from obesity, chronic cough, or heavy lifting; intrinsic weakness; and atrophic changes due to aging or estrogen deficiency.

▶ EPIDEMIOLOGY

The problem of pelvic relaxation is increased in postmenopausal women as tissues become less resilient and the accumulative stresses on the pelvis take effect. Black women and Chinese women have a much lower rate of uterine prolapse than do white women.

▶ RISK FACTORS

The incidence of pelvic relaxation is increased for patients with **chronically increased abdominal pressure** due to chronic cough, straining, ascites, and large pelvic tumors. Obstructed labor and traumatic delivery are also risk factors for pelvic relaxation as are **aging and menopause**.

▶ CLINICAL MANIFESTATIONS

History

The symptoms reported with pelvic relaxation vary depending on the structures involved and the degree of prolapse. With small degrees of pelvic relaxation, patients are often asymptomatic. With more extensive relaxation, patients often complain of **pelvic pressure** or heaviness in the lower abdomen that may be worse at night or aggravated by prolonged standing, vigorous activity, or lifting heavy objects. Urinary incontinence and other urinary symptoms, including frequency, urgency, and retention, may also be reported by patients with pelvic relaxation. Other symptoms are listed in Table 16-1.

Physical Examination

Pelvic relaxation is best observed by separating the labia and viewing the vagina while the patient strains or coughs. A **urethrocele or cystocele** may cause a downward movement of the anterior vaginal wall when the patient strains (Fig. 16-3). **Rectoceles and enteroceles** are best visualized by using a Sims speculum or the lower half of a Grave's speculum to provide better visualization of the anterior and posterior vaginal walls individually (Fig. 16-4). A **prolapsed uterus** can also be viewed using either or these methods or by palpation.

The degree of pelvic relaxation is determined by the amount of descent of the structure. In first-degree pelvic relaxation, the structure is in the upper two thirds of the vagina. In second-degree pelvic relaxation, the structure has descended to the level of the introitus, and in third-degree, the structure protrudes outside of the vagina.

▶ DIAGNOSTIC EVALUATION

The diagnosis of pelvic relaxation depends primarily on the history and physical examination. Other tools that may be useful in the diagnosis of cystocele and urethrocele include urine cultures, cystoscopy, urethroscopy, and urinary dynamic studies if indicated. When rectocele is suspected from a history of chronic constipation and difficulty passing stool, obstructive lesions should be ruled out using anoscopy or sigmoidoscopy. A barium enema study may also help to show a rectocele or enterocele but is not always essential to diagnosis.

▶ DIFFERENTIAL DIAGNOSIS

Although rare, the differential diagnosis for cystocele and urethrocele includes urethral diverticula and

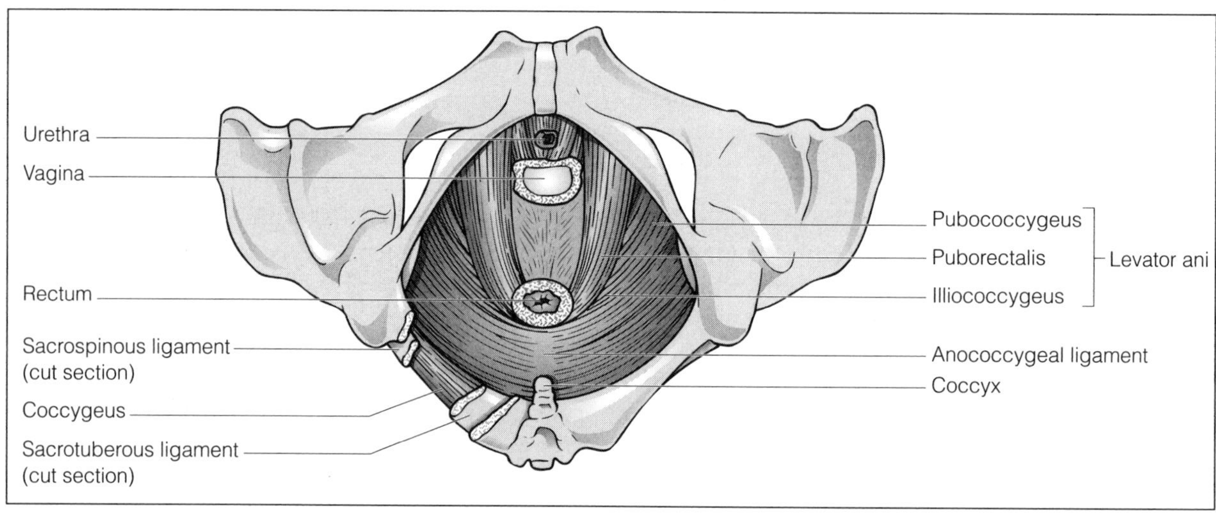

Figure 16-1 Normal structural support of the pelvis.

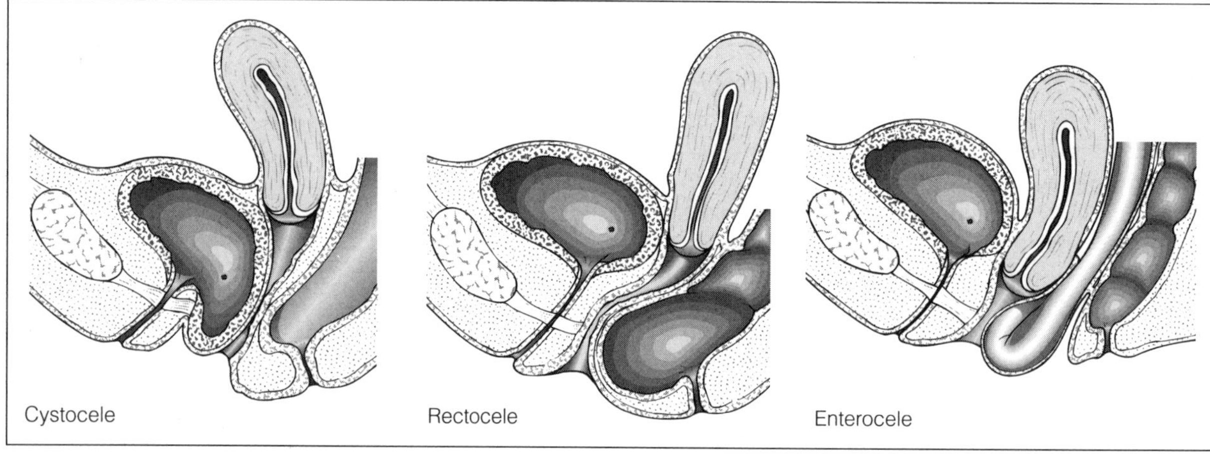

Figure 16-2 Anatomic defects in pelvic relaxation.

TABLE 16-1

Symptoms of Pelvic Relaxation

Pelvic pressure or heaviness
Backache
Dysparunia
Urinary incontinence
Other urinary symptoms
- Frequency
- Hesitancy
- Incomplete voiding
- Recurrent infection

Rectal symptoms
- Constipation
- Painful defecation
- Incomplete defecation

Skene's glands abscess. When a rectocele is suspected, obstructive lesions of the colon and rectum (lipomas, fibromas, sarcomas) should be investigated. Cervical elongation, prolapsed cervical polyp, and prolapsed cervical and endometrial tumors may be mistaken for uterine prolapse.

▶ TREATMENT

Pelvic relaxation is essentially a structural problem and therefore requires therapies that reinforce the lost support to the pelvis. These include exercises to strengthen the pelvic musculature, mechanical support devices, and surgical repair of the defect.

In postmenopausal women, **estrogen replacement** (systemic or vaginal) can be an important supplemental

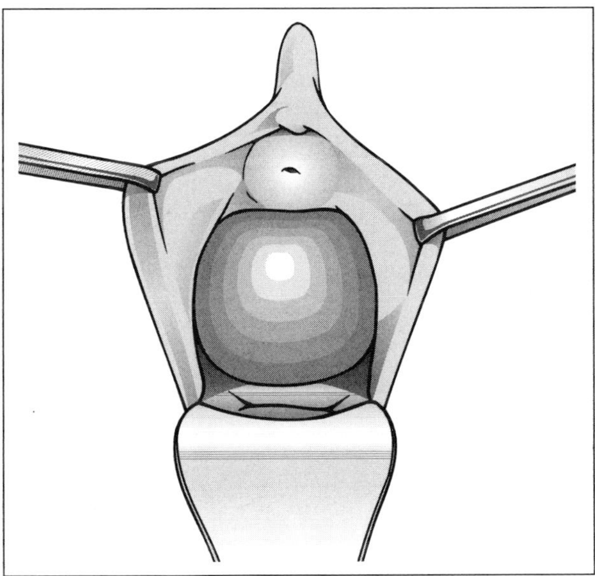

Figure 16-3 Cystocele.

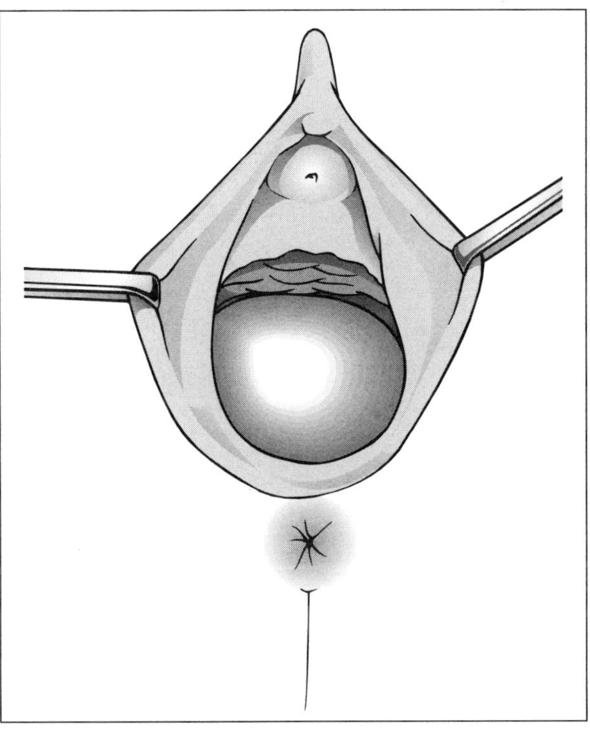

Figure 16-4 Rectocele.

treatment by improving tissue tone and facilitating reversal of atrophic changes in the vaginal mucosa.

In motivated patients with less severe symptoms, a first attempt at treatment may involve the use of Kegel peritoneal exercises to strengthen the pelvic musculature. These exercises involve the tightening and releasing of the pelvic muscles repeatedly throughout the day.

Mechanical support devices for pelvic relaxation involve the use of **vaginal pessaries** to replace the lost structural integrity of the pelvis or to diffuse the forces of descent over a wider area. Pessaries are indicated for patients in whom surgery is contraindicated but whose symptoms are severe enough to require treatment and in pregnant and postpartum women. These devices are placed in the vagina similar to the positioning of a diaphragm and serve to hold the pelvic organs in their normal position (Fig. 16-5). The use of vaginal pessaries requires a highly motivated patient and close initial follow-up to avoid vaginal trauma and necrosis and to ensure appropriate placement and proper hygiene to avoid infections and leukorrhea.

Patients who are not helped by nonoperative approaches may require **surgical correction**. In general, surgical repair for pelvic relaxation produces very good results. The type of repair varies with the type of defect and can range from hysterectomy to a variety of supportive sling procedures. The degree of success depends on the skill of the surgeon; the degree of pelvic relaxation; and the age, weight, and lifestyle of the patient.

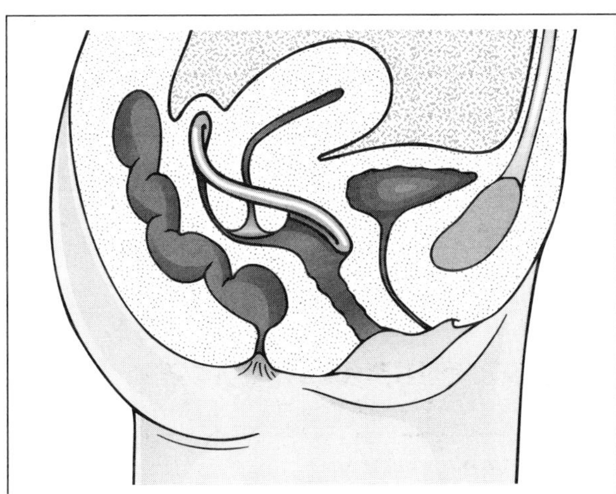

Figure 16-5 Placement of a vaginal pessary to treat pelvic relaxation.

▶ KEY POINTS

Pelvic relaxation

1. Can result in descent or prolapse of the bladder (cystocele), urethra (urethrocele), rectum (rectocele), small bowel (enterocele), or uterus (uterine prolapse) into the vaginal vault;

2. Is caused by birth trauma, chronic increases in intra-abdominal pressure, intrinsic weakness, and change due to aging;
3. Can result in pelvic pressure and pain, dyspareunia, bowel and bladder dysfunction, and urinary incontinence;
4. Is diagnosed primarily by history and physical examination but may also include urine cultures, cystoscopy, urethroscopy, urinary dynamic studies, anoscopy, sigmoidoscopy, and barium enema as indicated;
5. Is treated by Kegel exercises, vaginal pessaries, a variety of surgical sling procedures, or hysterectomy.

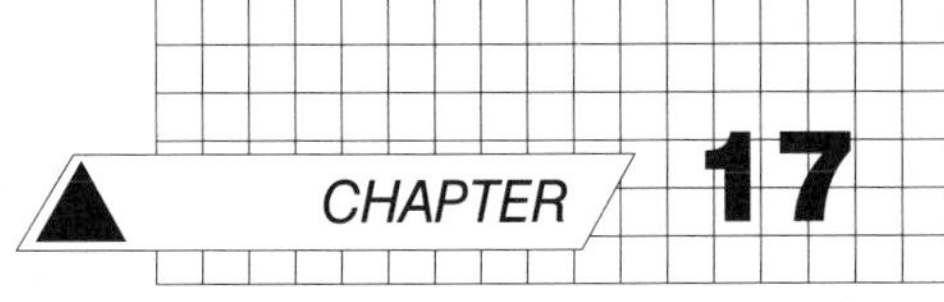

CHAPTER 17 Urinary Incontinence

▶ EPIDEMIOLOGY

The involuntary loss of urine is common, affecting an estimated 25 million Americans of all ages. Nearly 50% of all women experience occasional urinary incontinence and 20% of women over the age of 75 are affected daily. Thirty percent of nursing home residents suffer from urinary incontinence, and it is often a major reason for placing individuals in nursing homes. The incidence of urinary incontinence increases with age and with increasing degrees of **pelvic relaxation**.

The four most common types of urinary incontinence are described in Table 17-1. **Stress incontinence** is characterized by urine loss with exertion or straining (coughing, laughing, exercising) and is typically associated with pelvic relaxation and displacement of the urethrovesical junction. This differs from **urge incontinence,** also known as detrusor instability, where urine leakage is due to involuntary and uninhibited bladder contractions. **Total incontinence** results from urinary fistula and presents with continuous urine leakage. In the United States, almost all cases of total incontinence result from pelvic surgery or pelvic radiation. Finally, **overflow incontinence** is urine loss due to poor or absent bladder contractions. This can lead to urinary retention with overdistention of the bladder.

TABLE 17-1
Common Types of Urinary Incontinence

Type	Description
Stress incontinence	Urine loss with exertion or straining (coughing, laughing, exercising) typically associated with pelvic relaxation and displacement of the urethrovesical junction.
Urge incontinence	Urine leakage due to involuntary and uninhibited bladder contractions known as detrusor instability.
Total incontinence	Continuous urine leakage due to urinary fistula resulting from pelvic surgery or pelvic radiation.
Overflow incontinence	Incontinence due to poor or absent bladder contractions that lead to urinary retention with overdistention of the bladder and overflow incontinence.

▶ ANATOMY

Understanding the anatomy and physiology of the lower urinary tract and pelvic floor is crucial to understanding the mechanism behind each type of urinary incontinence (Fig. 17-1). The detrusor muscle is a meshwork of smooth muscle layers ending in the trigone area at the base of the bladder. The internal sphincter is at the urethrovesical junction. The urethra is made of smooth muscle. It is suspended by the pubourethral ligaments that originate at the lower pubic bone and extend to the middle third of the urethra to form the external sphincter.

Urinary continence at rest is possible because the **intraurethral pressure** exceeds the **intravesical pressure**. Continuous contraction of the internal sphincter is one of the primary mechanisms for maintaining continence at rest. The external sphincter provides about 50% of urethral resistance and is the second line of defense against incontinence. This multifaceted system allows a sudden increase in intra-abdominal pressure to be transmitted equally to the bladder and proximal third of the urethra, thus preserving continence.

In addition to the internal and external sphincters, continence is also maintained through the action of the submucosal vasculature of the urethra. When this vasculature complex fills with blood, the intraurethral pressure is increased, thus preventing involuntary loss of urine (Fig. 17-2). The filling mechanism of this system, known as **mucosal coaptation,** is estrogen sensitive, which explains why the estrogen-deficient postmenopausal state can lead to incontinence.

Neurologic control of the bladder and urethra is provided by both the **autonomic and somatic nervous systems** (Fig. 17-3). The parasympathetic nervous system allows micturition to occur. Parasympathetic control of the bladder is supplied by the pelvic nerve derived from S2, S3, and S4 of the spinal cord.

The sympathetic nervous system prevents micturition by contracting the bladder neck and internal sphincter. Sympathetic control of the bladder is achieved via the hypogastric nerve originating from T10 to L2 of the spinal cord.

Internal sphincter
Trigonal ring
Loop of Heiss
Posterior loop
External sphincter
Sphincter urethrae muscle
Compressor urethrae muscle
Urethrovaginal muscle
Urethra
Vagina
Perineal body
Ureter

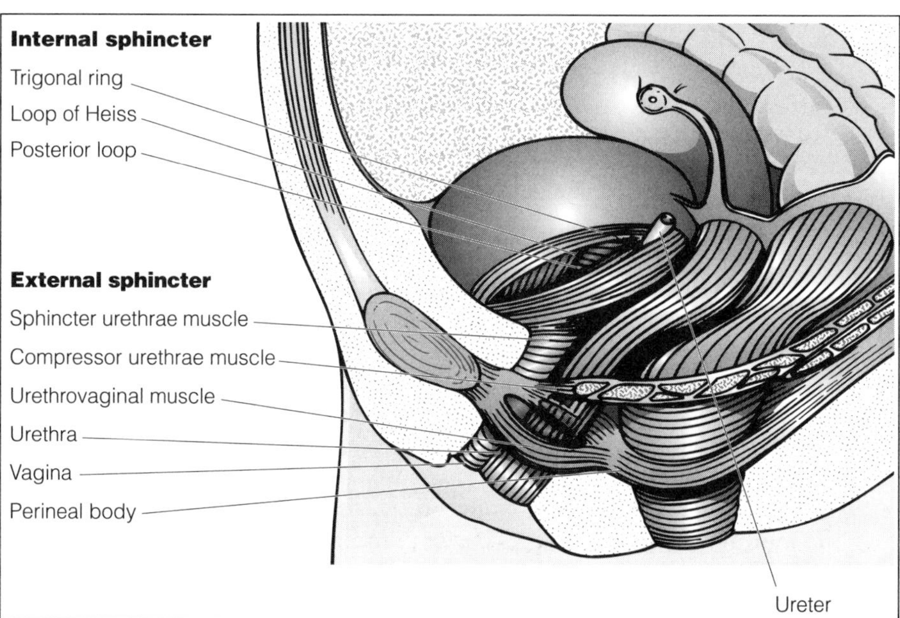

Figure 17-1 Anatomy of the lower urinary tract.

Figure 17-2 Urethral mucosal coaptation.

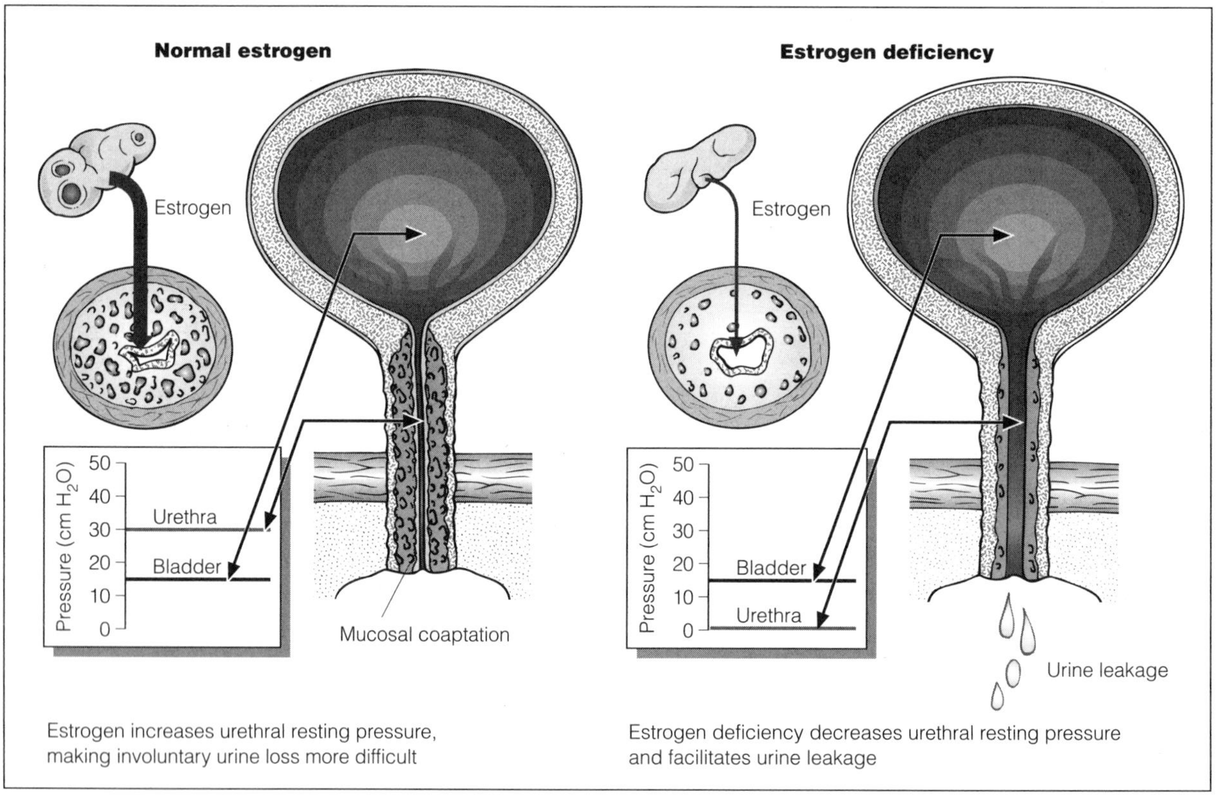

Normal estrogen
Estrogen
Pressure (cm H_2O)
50
40
30
20
10
0
Urethra
Bladder
Mucosal coaptation
Estrogen increases urethral resting pressure, making involuntary urine loss more difficult
Estrogen deficiency
Estrogen
Pressure (cm H_2O)
50
40
30
20
10
0
Bladder
Urethra
Urine leakage
Estrogen deficiency decreases urethral resting pressure and facilitates urine leakage

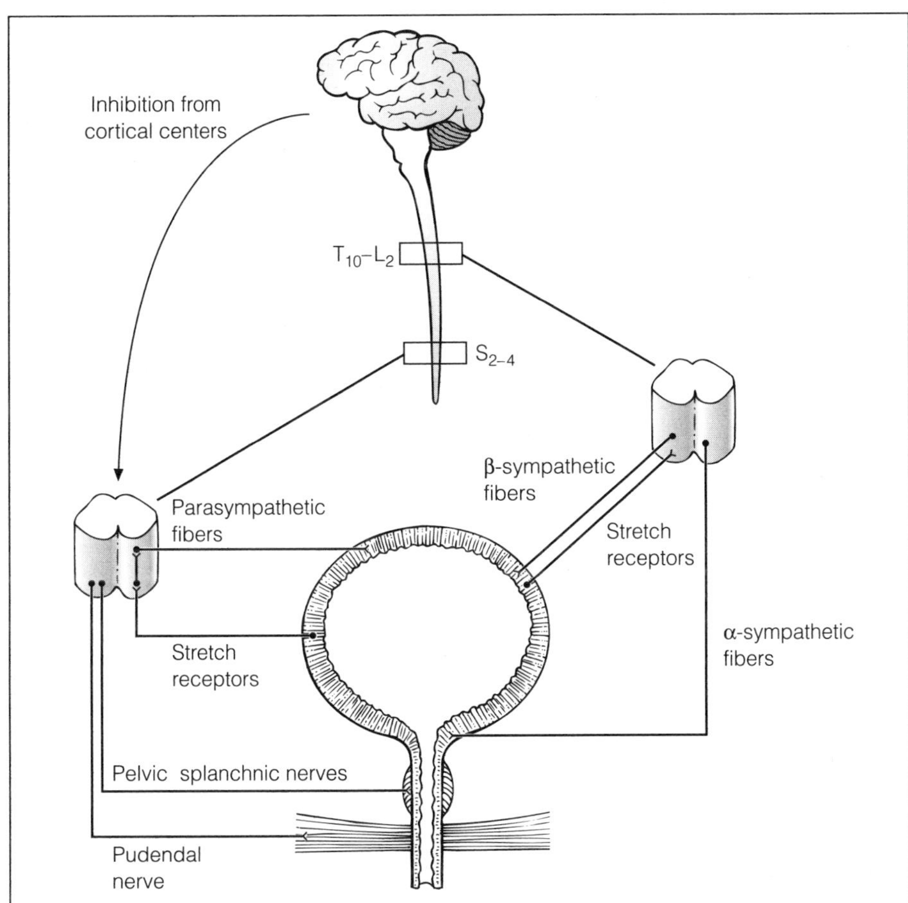

Figure 17-3 Innervation of the lower urinary tract.

Finally, the somatic nervous system aids in voluntary prevention of micturition by innervating the striated muscle of the external sphincter and pelvic floor through the pudendal nerve.

During micturition, the bladder releases its contents under voluntary control through a series of coordinated activities by the urethra and detrusor muscle. Stretch receptors in the bladder wall send a signal to central nervous system to begin voluntary voiding. This triggers inhibition of the sympathetic sacral and pudendal nerves, thus causing relaxation of the urethra, external sphincter, and levator ani muscles. This is closely followed by activation of the parasympathetic pelvic nerve resulting in contraction of the detrusor muscle and micturition begins.

▶ PHYSICAL EXAMINATION

All patients presenting with urinary incontinence should receive thorough medical and surgical history. The physical examination should include both internal and external **pelvic examinations**. Because the innervation of the lower urinary tract is closely associated with the innervation of the lower extremities and rectum, patients should receive a thorough **neurologic examination**. In particular, deep tendon reflexes, anal reflex, pelvic floor contractions, and the bulbocavernosus reflex (contraction after gentle tapping or squeezing the clitoris) should be elicited.

▶ DIAGNOSTIC EVALUATION

Fortunately, a variety of diagnostic tests are available for the evaluation of urinary incontinence. A **urinalysis and urine culture** should be obtained to rule out infection as a cause of incontinence. The scope of this text precludes an exhaustive compilation of every diagnostic modality, the most common are the standing stress test, the cotton-swab test, cystometrogram, and uroflowmetry.

A **standing stress test** is performed by having the patient with a full bladder stand over a towel or sheet with feet shoulder-distance apart. The patient is asked to cough, and the physician observes to verify a loss of urine. As an alternative, the physician can ask the patient to cough while in the lithotomy position. Either method may be used to document stress incontinence. The stress test has low specificity and sensitivity.

The purpose of the **cotton-swab test** is to diagnose a hypermobile bladder neck associated with genuine stress incontinence. The physician inserts a lubricated cotton swab into the urethra to the angle of the urethrovesical junction. When the patient strains as if urinating, the urethrovesical junction descends and the cotton swab moves. The change in cotton-swab angle is normally less than 30 degrees but will range from 30 to 60 degrees with a hypermobile bladder neck (Fig. 17-4).

The purpose of the **cystometrogram** is to distinguish between genuine stress incontinence and detruser instability. Pressure sensors are used to determine bladder and sphincter tone as the bladder is filled with fluid. Observations can be made about the bladder filling capacity, the presence or absence of a detrusor reflex, and the patient's ability to control or inhibit the strong desire to void.

Uroflowmetry measures the rate of urine flow through the urethra when a patient is asked to spontaneously void while sitting on a uroflow chair. This is particularly useful in patients complaining of hesitancy, incomplete bladder emptying, poor stream, and urinary retention.

Key Points

Urinary incontinence

1. Has an incidence that increases with age and with increasing degrees of pelvic relaxation;
2. Can be classified into four primary types: stress incontinence, urge incontinence, total incontinence, and overflow incontinence;
3. May have a variety of causes including pelvic relaxation, detrusor instability or insufficiency, and urinary fistulas;
4. Is avoided under normal circumstances due to the complex system of muscles, ligaments, sphincters, and nerves that keeps the intraurethral pressure greater than the intravesical pressure;

Figure 17-4 Cotton-swab test.

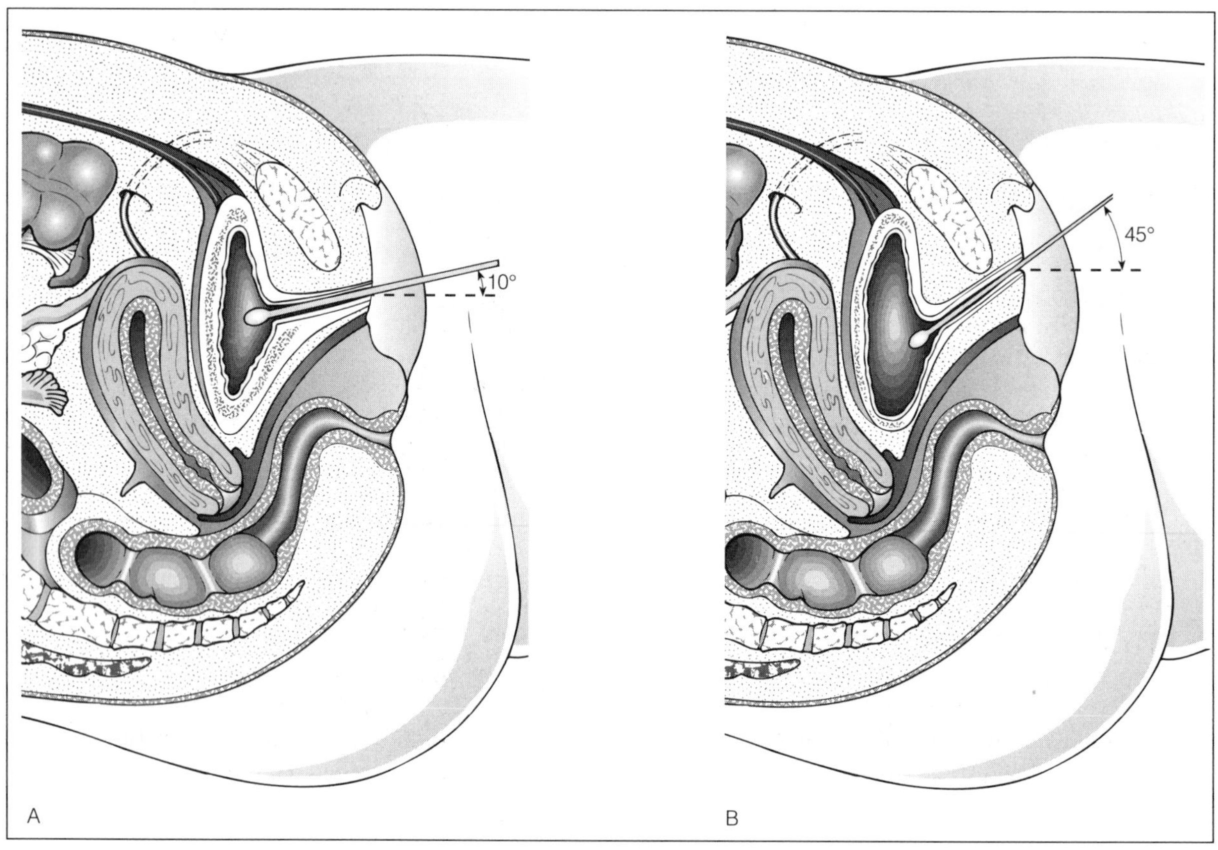

5. Can be diagnosed using the history and physical examination, urinalysis, urine culture, standing stress test, cotton-swab test, cystometrography, and uroflowmetry as needed.

▶ STRESS INCONTINENCE

Pathogenesis

Stress incontinence, also known as genuine stress incontinence and true stress incontinence, is the involuntary release of urine through the intact urethra in response to a sudden increase in **intra-abdominal pressure** such as coughing or exercise. In most cases, pelvic relaxation causes the bladder neck to become hypermobile so increases in intra-abdominal pressure are no longer transmitted equally to the bladder and urethra. Instead, increases in intra-abdominal pressure are transmitted primarily to the bladder. Therefore, as intravesical pressures exceed intraurethral pressure, stress urinary incontinence occurs (Fig. 17-5).

Risk Factors

The risk factors for stress urinary incontinence include factors that affect the normal transmission of intra-abdominal pressure and those that result in an increase in intravesical pressure or a decrease in intraurethral

Figure 17-5 Patient with stress urinary incontinence.

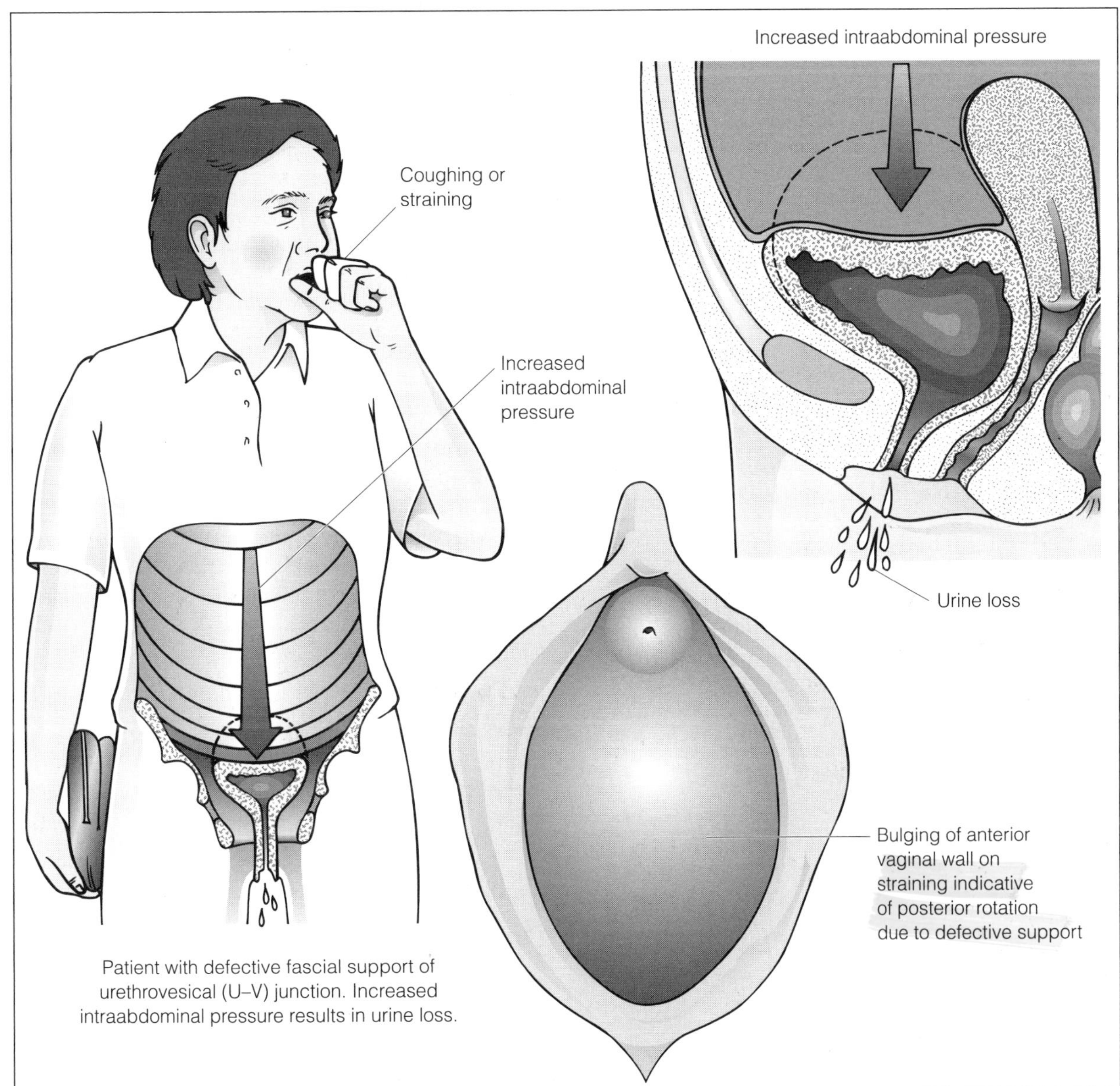

TABLE 17-2

Risk Factors for Stress Urinary Incontinence

Conditions causing pelvic relaxation
- Vaginal childbirth
- Aging
- Genetic factors

Conditions causing chronic increases in intra-abdominal pressure
- Constipation
- Chronic coughing from lung disease, smoking
- Chronic heavy lifting
- Obesity (doesn't cause incontinence but worsens it)

Conditions that weaken the urethral closing mechanism
- Estrogen deficiency
- Scarring
- Denervation
- Medications

TABLE 17-3

Gradations of Urinary Stress Incontinence

Grade I	Incontinence only with severe stress such as coughing, sneezing, or jogging.
Grade II	Incontinence with moderate stress such as rapid moving or walking up and down stairs.
Grade III	Incontinence with mild stress such as standing. The patient is continent in the supine position.

Adapted from Hacker N, Moore JG. Essentials of obstetrics and gynecology. Philadelphia: WB Saunders, 1992:400.

TABLE 17-4

Criteria and Tools for Diagnosing of Stress Incontinence

Normal urinalysis

Negative urine culture

Normal neurologic examination

Poor anatomic support (suggesting pelvic relaxation)
- Cotton swab test
- X-ray
- Urethroscopy

Demonstrable leakage with stress
- Stress test
- Pad test

Normal cystometrogram or urethrocystometry
- Normal residual urine volume
- Normal bladder capacity and sensation
- No involuntary detrusor contractions

Adapted from De Cherney A, Pernoll M. Current obstetric and gynecologic diagnosis and treatment. Norwalk, CT: Appleton and Lange, 1994:837.

pressure. The three major risk factors for stress urinary incontinence include **pelvic relaxation** (affects transmission), chronically **increased intra-abdominal pressure** (increases intravesical pressure), and **menopause** (decreases intraurethral pressure). Other risk factors are shown in Table 17-2.

History

Stress urinary incontinence may present with a sole complaint of involuntary loss of urine with coughing, laughing, sneezing, and straining. With more severe stress incontinence, urine leakage may be experienced with activities that cause even small increases in intra-abdominal pressure, such as walking or changing positions. Table 17-3 shows the grading system for stress incontinence.

Diagnostic Evaluation

Table 17-4 contains the criteria for diagnosing stress urinary incontinence.

Treatment

Pelvic diaphragm exercises (Kegel exercises) result in an increase in resting and active muscle tone and thereby increase urethral closing pressure in cases of mild incontinence.

Medical therapies including estrogen replacement therapy and alpha-adrenergic agonists (Propadrine and pseudoephedrine) work to increase urethral sphincter tone and enhance urethral closure.

Pessaries and other intravaginal devices are used to physically elevate and support the bladder neck, which restores normal anatomic relationships. As a result, increases in intra-abdominal pressures are transmitted equally to the bladder and urethra. Although pessaries are noninvasive, they preclude sexual intercourse and require close medical supervision.

Surgery aims to restore normal anatomy by returning the hypermobile bladder neck to its original position. Disadvantages of surgery include the risks of an invasive procedure and the risk of failure with resumption of symptoms over time.

Key Points

Stress incontinence

1. Is the involuntary loss of urine with exertion or straining (e.g., laughing, coughing, exercising);
2. Is usually due to pelvic relaxation (e.g., with aging or after childbirth) that results in a hypermobile bladder neck;
3. Can be treated with pelvic exercises, medication to enhance urethral sphincter closure (estrogen, Propadrine), or surgery to restore the intra-abdominal position of the proximal urethra.

▶ DETRUSOR INSTABILITY

Pathogenesis

Detrusor instability, also known as **urge incontinence**, is usually caused by involuntary and uninhibited detrusor contractions during the filling phase of bladder function. Under normal circumstances, these contractions should not occur.

Most detrusor instability is **idiopathic**. Some known causes are conditions that stimulate receptors in the bladder wall causing involuntary detrusor contraction, including urinary tract infections, bladder stones, bladder cancer, suburethral diverticula, and foreign bodies (Fig. 17-6). Detrusor overactivity, or detrusor hyperreflexia, may also be due to neurologic disease such as stroke, Alzheimer disease, Parkinson disease, multiple sclerosis, and diabetes mellitus (Table 17-5).

Epidemiology

The incidence of detrusor instability is 10 to 15% in the general population.

Clinical Manifestations

History

Patients with urge incontinence will usually present with a history of involuntary urine loss whether the bladder is full or not. Many women will complain of not being able to reach the bathroom in time or dribbling or leakage from just seeing a bathroom.

Physical Examination

Detrusor instability presents with symptoms that suggest bladder overactivity, including urinary urgency, frequency (more than seven times a day), stress incontinence, and nocturia (more than one time per night). Given the wide differential for detrusor instability, patients should also be asked about neurologic symptoms, history of previous anti-incontinence surgery, and hematuria (suggestive of cancer, stones, or infection).

Figure 17-6 Causes of detrusor instability.

Secondary detrusor instability
Bladder stones
Infection
Bladder tumors
Foreign bodies
Suburethral diverticulum with stone
Many conditions stimulate receptors in bladder wall. Reflex causes involuntary detrusor contraction and urine loss.
Urethal compression
Bladder neck suspension procedures compress urethra, causing detrusor instability if done too tightly.
Vagina

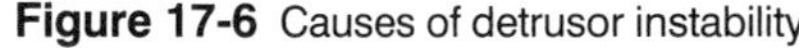

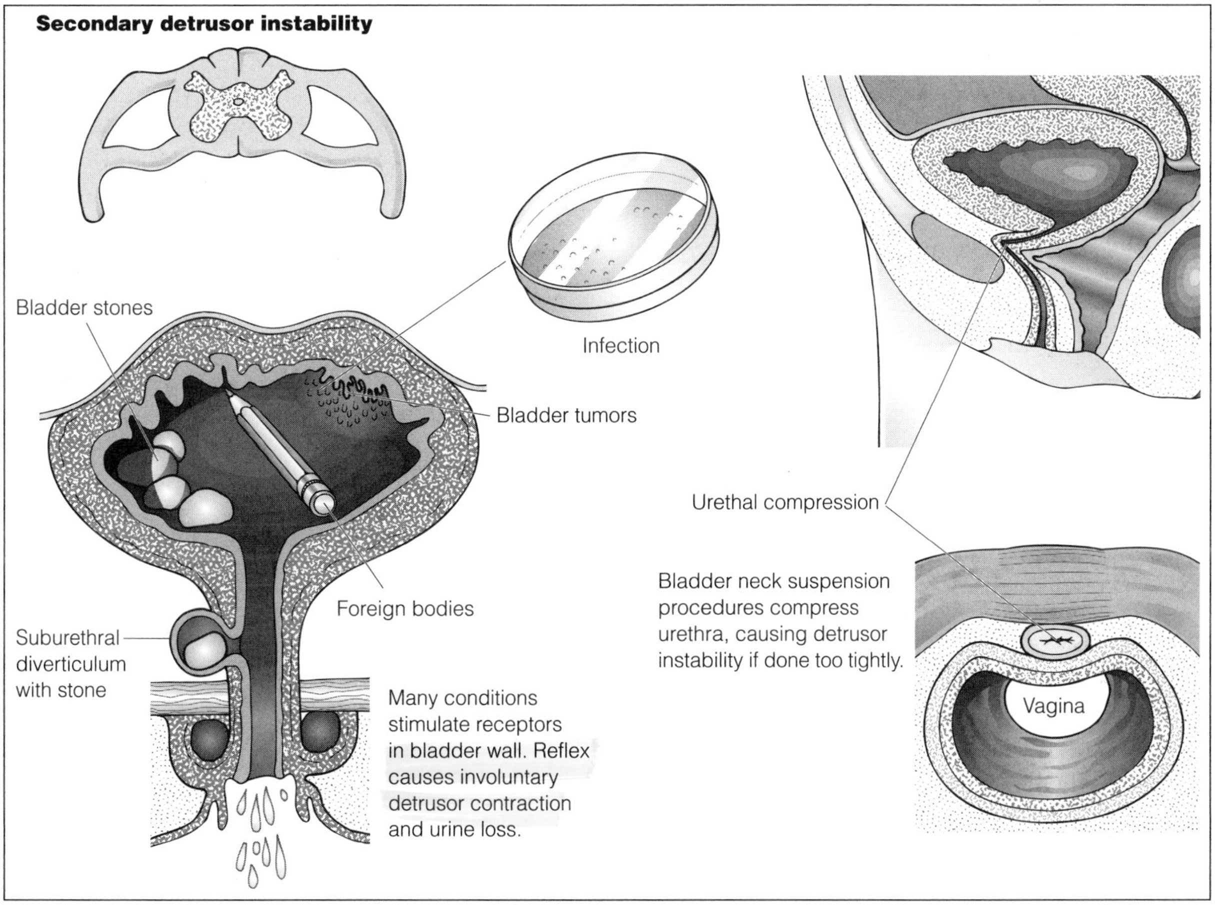

TABLE 17-5
Common Causes of Urge Incontinence

Detrusor instability
Urinary tract infections
Urethral obstruction
Urethral compression (previous surgery)
Bladder stones
Bladder cancer
Suburethral diverticula
Foreign bodies
Detrusor hyperreflexia
Cerebrovascular accident
Alzheimer's disease
Parkinsonism
Multiple sclerosis
Diabetes
Peripheral neuropathies
Autonomic neuropathies
Cauda equina lesions

Treatment

The treatment of urge incontinence will depend on the etiology of disease. The most frequently used and most effective medications for urge incontinence are anticholinergics (e.g., Pro-Banthine, Ditropan) that inhibit the cholinergically innervated detrusor muscle. Beta-adrenergic agonists (e.g., Alupent) work on beta-adrenergic receptors on the detrusor to relax it. Smooth muscle relaxants (e.g., Urispas) and tricyclic antidepressants (e.g., Tofranil) also relax the detrusor muscle. Fifty to 80% of patients will respond to these medications used alone or in combination.

Bladder training, Kegel exercises, biofeedback, hypnosis, and psychotherapy are methods of behavior modification that have met with moderate success in controlling urge incontinence. Bladder training begins by establishing a regular voiding schedule that is modified to gradually lengthen the intervals between voiding until the patient reestablished cortical control over the voiding reflex.

There are no effective surgical procedures to treat detrusor instability.

Key Points

Detrusor instability

1. Results from involuntary and uninhibited detrusor contractions caused by urinary tract infection, bladder stones, cancer, diverticula, and neurologic disorders (stroke, multiple sclerosis, Alzheimer's), although most cases are idiopathic;
2. Symptoms include urinary urge, frequency, and nocturia;
3. Can be treated with medication (especially anticholinergics), bladder training, or a variety of behavior modification strategies.

► TOTAL INCONTINENCE

Pathogenesis

Total urinary incontinence (bypass incontinence) is typically the result of a **urinary fistula** formed between the bladder and the vagina (vesicovaginal fistula), as shown in Figure 17-7, or between the ureter and the vagina (ureterovaginal fistula) or the urethra and the vagina (urethrovaginal fistula).

In developing countries, the most common cause of urinary fistulas is **obstetric trauma** from a prolonged second stage or operative procedures (e.g., forceps). However, in the United States, genitourinary fistulas are most often caused by **pelvic radiation** or **pelvic surgery**. Ectopic ureters and urethral diverticula may also produce total incontinence.

Epidemiology

Pelvic radiation and pelvic surgery account for over 95% of total urinary incontinence cases in the United States. In particular, simple abdominal hysterectomy and vaginal hysterectomy alone account for over 50% of vesicovaginal fistulas. Urethrovaginal fistulas may

Figure 17-7 Vesicovaginal fistula.

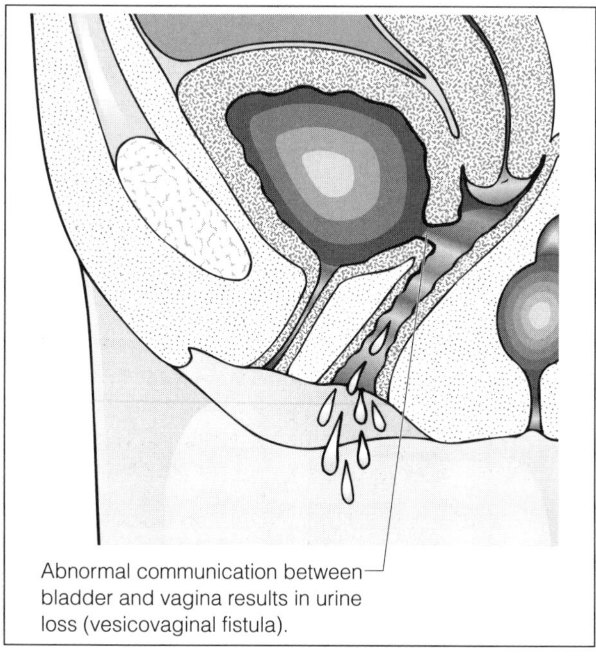

also occur as complications of surgery for urethral diverticula, anterior vaginal wall prolapse, or stress urinary incontinence. Ureterovaginal fistula, as seen after 1 to 2% of radical hysterectomies, are usually due to devascularization rather than direct injury. **Obstetric injuries** associated with operative deliveries were once the leading cause of urinary fistulas but are now rare causes of total urinary incontinence in the United States, Canada, and Western Europe.

Risk Factors

The incidence of fistula formation after surgery is higher if the patient has a history of preoperative radiation, endometriosis, pelvic inflammatory disease, or previous pelvic surgery.

History

Urinary fistula usually presents with a history of **painless and continuous loss of urine** from the vagina, usually after pelvic surgery or radiation. Fistulas after surgery become clinically apparent in 5 to 14 days.

Diagnostic Evaluation

Methylene blue dye instilled into the bladder will leak onto a vaginal pad if a vesicovaginal fistula is present. To diagnose a ureterovaginal fistula, **indigo carmine** is given intravenously. As the compound is filtered through the kidney and passes through the ureters, it will stain the vaginal pad. If a ureterovaginal fistula is present, the methylene blue test will be negative and the indigo carmine test will be positive. **Cystourethroscopy** can then be used to identify the number and location of fistula. Intravenous pyelogram and retrograde pyelogram may also be used to localize ureterovaginal fistulae.

Treatment

Surgery is the main mode of treatment of urinary fistula. Most obstetric fistulas can be repaired immediately; however, it is typical to wait 3 to 6 months before attempting to repair postsurgical fistulas. This waiting period allows inflammation to decrease and vascularity and pliability of the area to increase. **Antibiotics** for urinary infection and **estrogen** for postmenopausal women are also used during this period. Steroids have been used to decrease inflammation, although their use is still controversial.

Key Points

Total incontinence

1. Is usually due to vesicovaginal or ureterovaginal fistulas;
2. Symptoms include painless continuous urine leakage from the vagina;
3. Is caused by pelvic radiation and pelvic surgery in over 95% of cases in the United States;
4. In developing countries is attributable to obstetric trauma, often leading to urinary fistula;
5. Is treated surgically.

▶ OVERFLOW INCONTINENCE

Pathogenesis

Overflow incontinence in women is usually due to **detrusor insufficiency** (bladder hypotonia) or **detrusor areflexia** (bladder acontractility). As a result, bladder contractions are weak or nonexistent, causing incomplete voiding, urinary retention, and overdistention of the bladder (Fig. 17-8). The causes of overflow incontinence due to detrusor insufficiency vary widely from

Figure 17-8 Overdistended bladder inducing overflow incontinence.

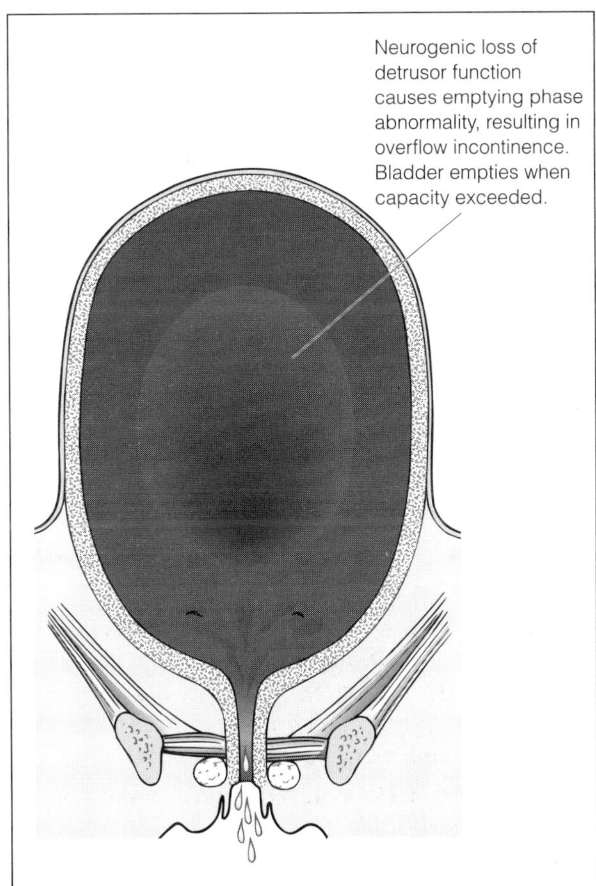

fecal compaction, to use of certain medications, to neurological diseases including lower motor neuron disease, autonomic neuropathy (diabetes), spinal cord injuries, and multiple sclerosis (Table 17-6).

Outflow obstruction, typically due to surgical procedures that result in urethral kinking, stenosis, or obstruction, can also cause bladder overdistention and overflow incontinence but is rarely seen in women. **Postoperative overdistention** of the bladder due to unrecognized urinary retention and the use of epidural anesthesia are common causes of overflow incontinence.

Clinical Manifestations

Overflow incontinence may present with a wide variety of symptoms including frequent or constant urinary dribbling along with the symptoms of stress incontinence and urge incontinence. Outflow obstruction (rare) presents with a history of straining to void, poor stream, urinary retention, and incomplete emptying.

TABLE 17-6

Causes of Overflow Incontinence

Causes
Neurogenic causes
Lower motor neuron disease
Autonomic neuropathy (diabetes mellitus)
Spinal cord injuries
Multiple sclerosis
Obstructive causes
Postsurgical urethral obstruction
Postoperative overdistention (rare)
Pelvic masses
Pharmacologic causes
Anticholinergic drugs
Alpha-adrenergic agonists
Epidural and spinal anesthesia
Other causes
Psychogenic (psychosis or severe depression)
Idiopathic
Fecal impaction

Treatment

Treatment strategy in overflow incontinence is geared toward relieving urinary retention, increasing bladder contractility, and decreasing urethral closing pressure.

Medical management for overflow incontinence includes the use of **alpha-adrenergic** agents (prazosin, terazin, phenoxybenzamine) to reduce urethral closing pressure and the use of **striated muscle relaxants** (diazepam, dantrolene) to reduce bladder outlet resistance. **Cholinergic** agents (bethanechol) are used to increase bladder contractility. Intermittent **self-catheterization** may also be used in overflow incontinence to avoid chronic urinary retention and infection.

Patients with overflow incontinence due to **urinary obstruction** may benefit from surgical correction of the obstruction. Postoperative overdistention of the bladder is typically temporary and may be managed by continuous bladder drainage for 24 to 48 hours.

Key Points

Overflow incontinence

1. Is most commonly due to detrusor insufficiency caused by medications or neurologic disease; obstruction and postoperative overdistention occur less frequently;
2. Is usually treated with self-catheterization and/or medications to increase bladder contractility (cholinergic agents) and lower urethral resistance (alpha-adrenergic agents).

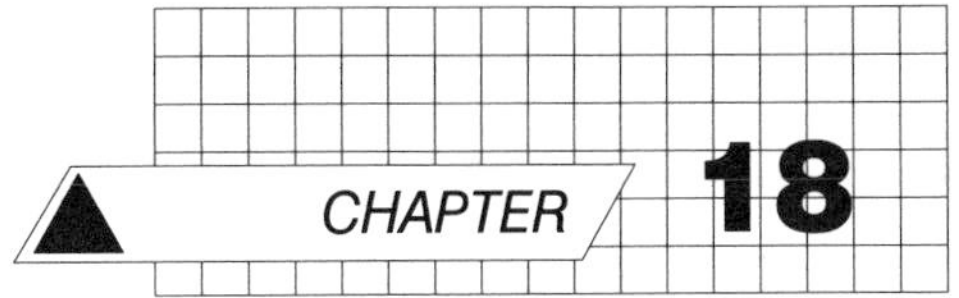

CHAPTER 18

Puberty, the Menstrual Cycle, and Menopause

▶ PUBERTY

Puberty describes the series of events in which a child matures into a young adult. These changes include the development of secondary sex characteristics, the growth spurt, and achievement of fertility. Before any perceived phenotypic change, adrenarche occurs with regeneration of the zona reticularis in the adrenal cortex. Gonadarche follows with pulsatile gonadotropin-releasing hormone (GnRH) secretion stimulating the anterior pituitary to produce luteinizing hormone (LH) and follicle-stimulating hormone (FSH). Subsequently, breast development (thelarche), development of pubic and axillary hair (pubarche), the growth spurt (peak height velocity), and onset of menstruation (menarche) all occur, usually in this order (Fig. 18-1).

Adrenarche and Gonadarche

Adrenarche occurs between the ages of 6 and 8. The adrenal gland begins regeneration of the zona reticularis of the adrenal gland, which had regressed shortly after birth, with concomitant enhancement of the P450 microsomal enzymes. This inner layer of the adrenal cortex is responsible for the secretion of sex steroid hormones. As a result, the adrenal androgenic steroid hormones, dehydroepiandrosterone sulfate (DHEAS), DHEA, and androstenedione, are increasingly produced from ages 6 to 8 up until ages 13 to 15.

Gonadarche begins around the age of 8, when pulsatile GnRH secretion from the hypothalamus is increased. This leads to stimulation of the gonadotrophs in the anterior pituitary with subsequent secretion of LH and FSH. Initially, these increases occur mostly during sleep and fail to lead to any phenotypic changes. As the girl enters early puberty, the LH and FSH elevations eventually lead to stimulation of the ovary and subsequent estrogen release.

Thelarche

The first stage of thelarche, the development of breast buds, usually occurs around age 11. Thelarche is usually the first phenotypic sign of puberty and occurs in response to the increase in levels of circulating estrogen. Concomitantly, there is estrogenation of the vaginal mucosa and growth of the vagina and uterus. Further development of the breast will continue

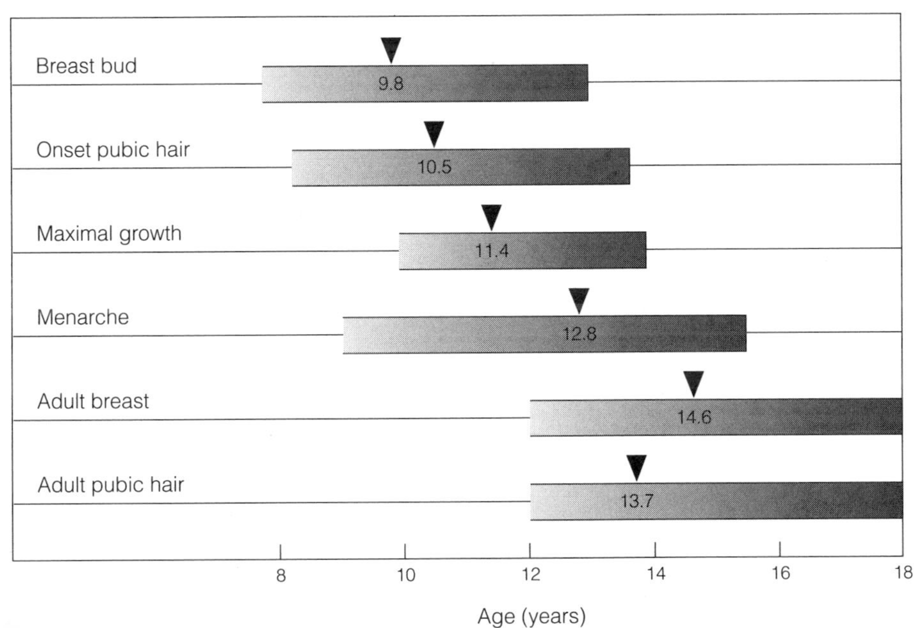

Figure 18-1 Average age of onset and range given for the events of puberty.

throughout puberty and adolescence as described by Marshall and Tanner (Table 18-1 and Fig. 18-2).

Pubarche

The onset of growth of pubic hair (Fig. 18-3) usually occurs around age 12 and is often accompanied by growth of axillary hair. Pubarche usually follows thelarche, but a normal variant in order is seen with pubarche preceding thelarche, particularly in African-American girls. The growth of pubic and axillary hair is likely secondary to the increase in circulating androgens.

Peak Height Velocity

The growth spurt is characterized by an acceleration in growth rate around age 9 to 10, leading to a peak height velocity around age 12 to 13. The increased rate of growth is likely secondary to the increased level of growth hormone (GH) and somatomedin-C (S-C), which increases in response to increasing levels of estrogen. However, this relationship is dose related and excess levels of estrogen will lead to decreased GH and S-C. Furthermore, because estrogen causes fusion of the epiphyseal plate in long bones, a rapid growth spurt may be followed by growth cessation.

Menarche

The average age of onset of menstruation is between 12 and 13. The menstrual cycle is usually irregular, reflecting anovulatory cycles, for the first 6 months to a year after menarche. It will take an average of 2 years after menarche before regular ovulatory cycles are achieved. Menarche is often delayed in gymnasts, distance runners, and ballet dancers. Some theories propose that this is due to an insufficient amount of percent body fat that may be required to have menstrual cycles. However, it is unclear whether it is the percent body fat or the exercise and stress on the body that interferes with menarche.

TABLE 18-1

The Tanner Stages of Breast Development

Stage 1: Preadolescent: elevation of papilla only
Stage 2: Breast bud stage: elevation of breast and papilla, areolar enlargement
Stage 3: Further enlargement of breast and areola without separation of contours
Stage 4: Projection of areola and papilla to form a secondary mound
Stage 5: Mature stage: projection of papilla only as areola recesses to breast contour

Adapted from Speroff L, Glass RH, Kase NG. Clinical gynecologic endocrinology and infertility. 5th ed. Baltimore: Williams and Wilkins, 1994:377.

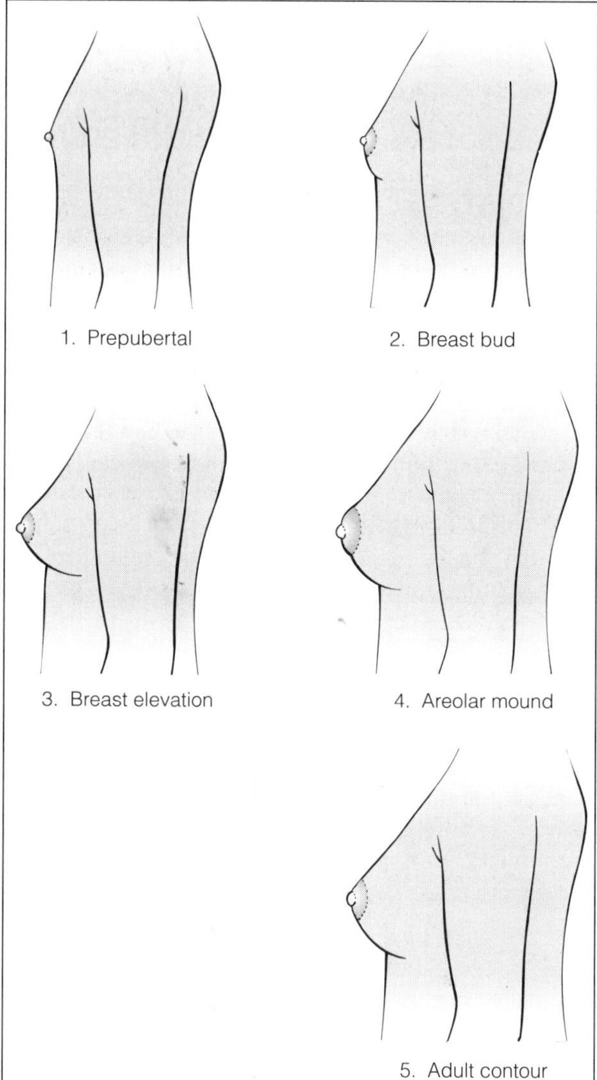

Figure 18-2 Tanner stages of thelarche.

► THE MENSTRUAL CYCLE

The hypothalamus, pituitary, ovaries, and uterus are all involved in maintaining the menstrual cycle (Fig. 18-4). During the **follicular phase**, release of FSH from the pituitary results in development of a primary ovarian follicle. The ovarian follicle produces estrogen, which causes the uterine lining to proliferate. At midcycle, approximately day 14, there is a surge in LH, which stimulates ovulation, the release of the ovum from the follicle. After ovulation the **luteal phase** begins. The remnants of the follicle left behind in the ovary develop into the corpus luteum. It is responsible for the secretion of progesterone, which maintains the endometrial lining in preparation to receive a fertilized ovum. If fertilization does not occur, the corpus luteum degenerates and progesterone levels fall. Without progesterone, the endometrial lining is sloughed off, which is known as menstruation.

Follicular Phase

The withdrawal of estrogen and progesterone during the luteal phase of the prior cycle causes a gradual increase in FSH. In turn, FSH stimulates growth of approximately 5 to 15 primordial ovarian follicles, initiating the follicular phase. Of these primordial follicles, one becomes the dominant follicle and develops and matures until ovulation. The developing follicle destined to ovulate produces estrogens, which enhances its own maturation and increases the production of FSH and LH receptors in an autocrine fashion.

Figure 18-3 Tanner stages of pubarche.

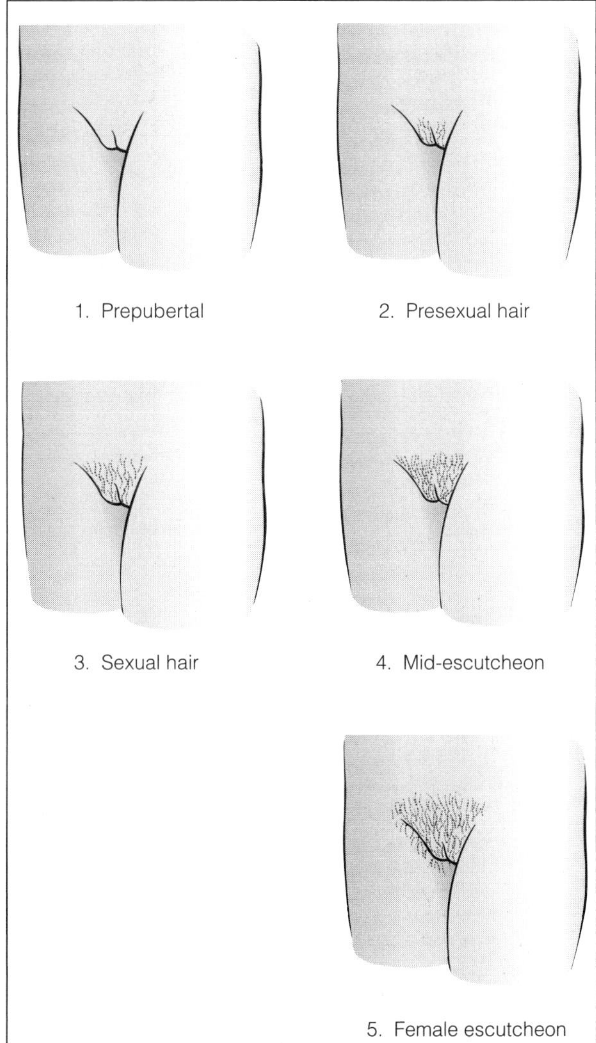

The estrogen is produced in a two-cell process with the theca interna cells producing androstenedione in response to LH stimulation and the granulosa cells converting this androstenedione to estradiol when stimulated by FSH. LH also rises and stimulates the synthesis of androgens, which are converted to estrogen. As rising estrogen levels negatively feed back on pituitary FSH secretion, the dominant follicle is protected from the decrease in FSH by its increased number of FSH receptors (Fig. 18-5).

Ovulation

Toward the end of the follicular phase, estrogen levels eventually reach a critical level that triggers the anterior pituitary to release an LH surge. Ovulation occurs as the LH surge causes the follicle to rupture and release the mature ovum (Fig. 18-6). The ovum usually passes into the adjoining fallopian tube and is swept down to the uterus by the cilia lining the tube. This process takes 3 to 4 days. Fertilization of the ovum must occur within 24 hours or it degenerates.

Luteal Phase

After ovulation, the luteal phase ensues. The **granulosa** and **theca interna cells** lining the wall of the follicle form the corpus luteum under stimulation by LH. The corpus luteum synthesizes estrogen and significant quantities of progesterone, which causes the endometrium to become more glandular and secretory in preparation for implantation of a fertilized ovum. If fertilization occurs, the developing trophoblast synthesizes **human chorionic gonadotropin** (hCG), a glycoprotein very similar to LH, which maintains the corpus luteum so that it can continue production of estrogen and progesterone to support the endometrium until the placenta develops its synthetic function. If fertilization, with its concomitant rise in hCG, does not occur, the corpus luteum degenerates, progesterone levels fall, the endometrium is not maintained, and menstruation occurs.

Menstruation

The endometrium of the uterus undergoes cyclical changes during the menstrual cycle. During the follicular phase, the endometrium is in the **proliferative phase**, growing in response to estrogen. During the luteal phase, the endometrium enters the **secretory phase** as it matures and is enabled to support implantation. If the ovum is not fertilized, the corpus luteum degenerates after approximately 14 days, leading to a fall in estrogen and progesterone levels. The withdrawal of progesterone causes the endometrium to slough, initiating the

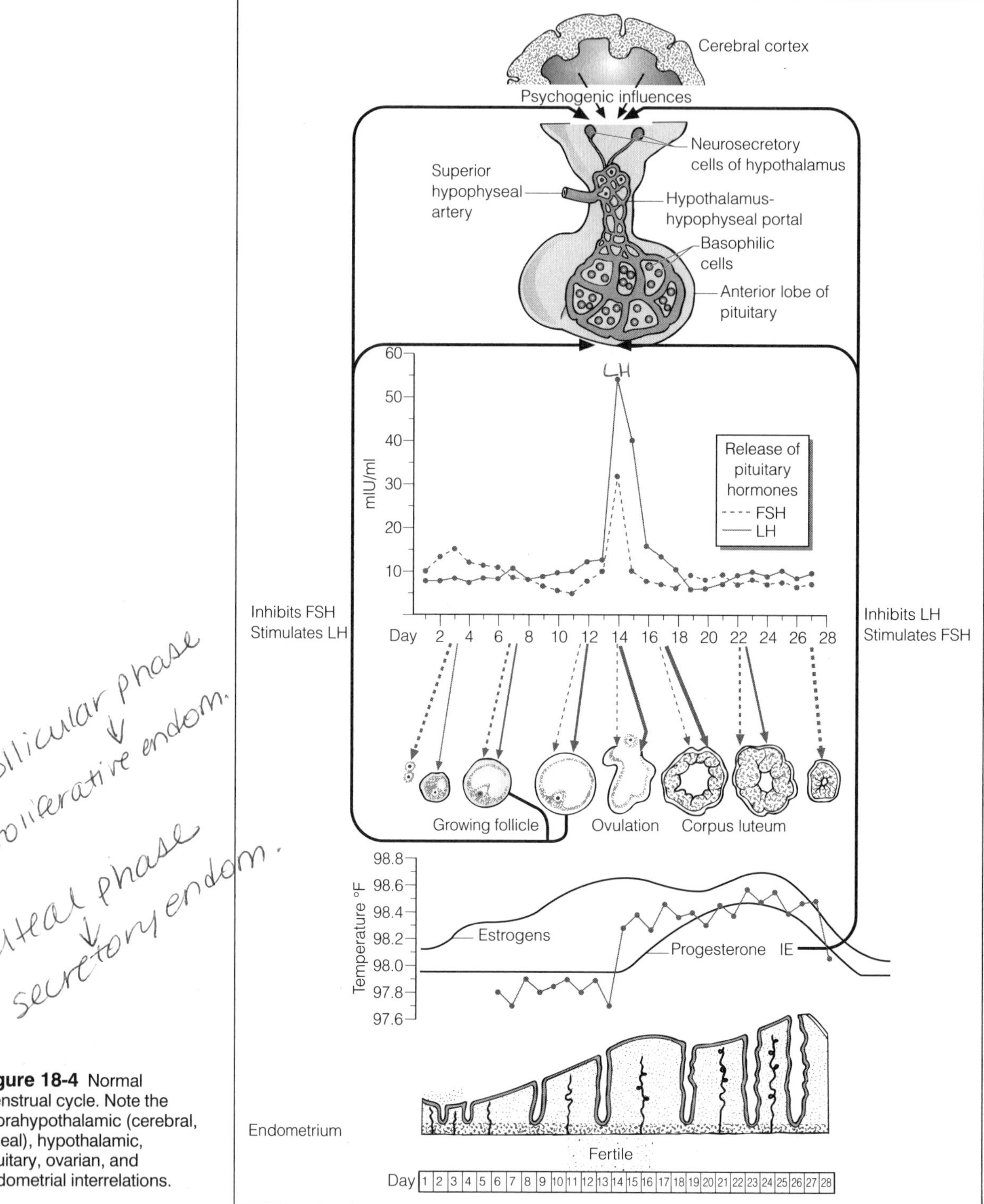

Figure 18-4 Normal menstrual cycle. Note the suprahypothalamic (cerebral, pineal), hypothalamic, pituitary, ovarian, and endometrial interrelations.

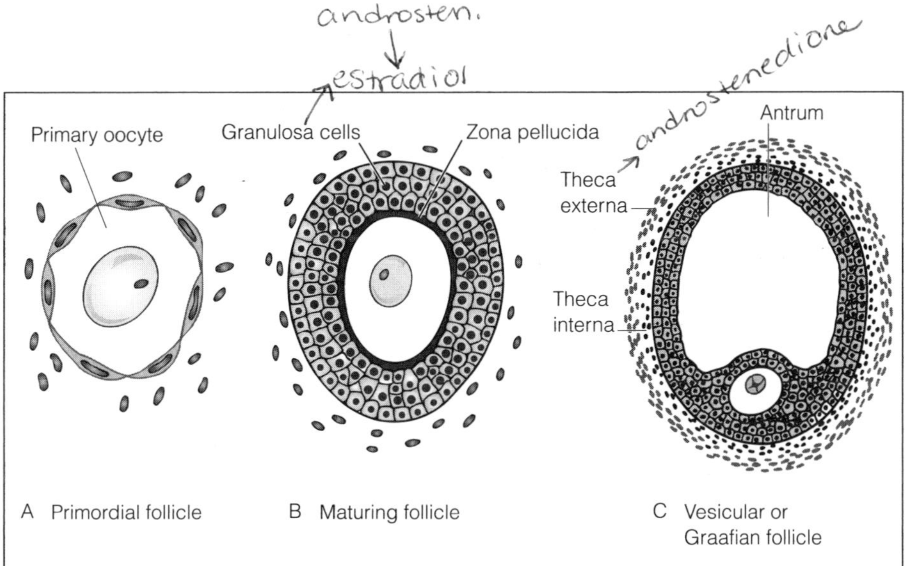

Figure 18-5 Drawing of the changes occurring in the primordial follicle during the first half of the ovarian cycle. Under influence of FSH the primordial follicle (A) matures into the graafian follicle (C). The oocyte remains a primary oocyte in the diplotene stage until shortly before ovulation. During the last few days of the growing period the estrogens produced by the follicular and theca cells stimulate the formation of LH in the pituitary.

menstrual phase. At the same time, FSH levels begin to slowly rise in the absence of negative feedback and the follicular phase starts again.

▶ MENOPAUSE AND POSTMENOPAUSE

The "climacteric" marks the termination of the reproductive phase in a woman's life. At this point, nearly all the oocytes have undergone atresia, although a few remain and can be found on histologic examination. The term "menopause" denotes the final menstruation and marks the cornerstone event during the climacteric. The average age of menopause in the United States is 50 to 51 years. Various physiologic and hormonal changes occur during this period, including a decrease in estrogen, increase in FSH, and classic symptoms such as "hot flashes." If menopause occurs before the age of 40, it is considered premature.

Etiology

Menopause is generally heralded by menstrual irregularity as the number of oocytes capable of responding to FSH and LH decrease and anovulation becomes more frequent. During this period, LH and FSH levels gradually rise because of decreased negative feedback from diminished estrogen production. The fall in estradiol levels leads to the symptoms of vasomotor flushing, sweats, mood changes, and depression. Early menopause is associated with cigarette smoking. Premature menopause is often a result of premature ovarian failure that is usually idiopathic. If it occurs before age 35, chromosomal studies are sent to rule out a genetic basis (e.g., mosaicism).

Diagnosis

The diagnosis of menopause can usually be made by history and physical and confirmed, if necessary, by

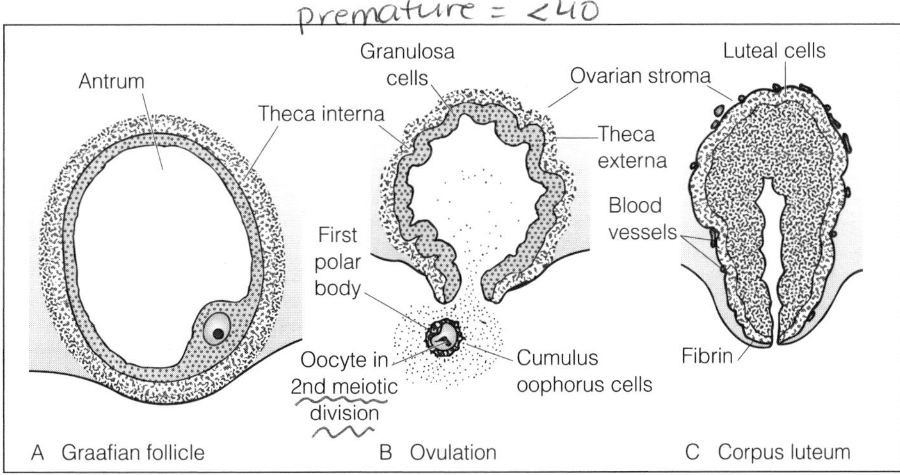

Figure 18-6 (A) The graafian follicle just before rupture. (B) Ovulation. The oocyte, beginning its second meiotic division, is discharged from the ovary, together with a large number of cumulus oophorus cells. The follicular cells remaining inside the collapsed follicle differentiate into luteal cells. (C) Corpus luteum. Note the large size of the corpus luteum caused by hypertrophy and accumulation of lipid in the granulosa and theca interna cells. The remaining cavity of the follicle is filled with fibrin.

hormonal tests. Patients will classically present between the ages of 48 and 52 with complaints of oligomenorrhea and vasomotor instability, sweats, mood changes, depression, dyspareunia, and dysuria. These symptoms generally disappear within 12 months, although a substantial proportion of women can remain symptomatic for years.

On physical examination there may be decrease in breast size and change in texture. Vaginal, urethral, and cervical atrophy may all be seen, which are consistent with decreased estrogenation. An elevated FSH is diagnostic of menopause.

Pathogenesis

Although menopause is a naturally occurring event, there are two important pathophysiologic consequences of the estrogen decrease. From a cardiovascular standpoint, the protective benefit of estrogen on lipids [increased high density lipoprotein (HDL), decreased low density lipoprotein (LDL)] and the vascular endothelium (prevents atherogenesis, increases vasodilatation, inhibits platelet adherence) is lost and women are at increased risk for coronary artery disease. With menopause, there is an acceleration in bone resorption because estrogen plays an important role in regulating osteoclast activity. The increased bone resorption leads to osteopenia and finally osteoporosis.

Hormone Replacement Therapy

The benefits of postmenopausal **hormone replacement therapy** (HRT) are significant in terms of stroke and myocardial infarction prevention, leading to a reduction in cardiovascular morbidity. HRT also leads to increased bone mineralization and a reduction in the incidence of hip fractures and other complications of osteoporosis. Other advantages include symptomatic relief of vasomotor flushing, mood improvement, prevention of urogenital and vaginal atrophy, and improvement in skin and muscle tone. Treatment must be carefully considered, however, and evidence of cholestatic hepatic dysfunction, known estrogen-dependent neoplasm (breast, ovary, uterus, cervix, vagina), history of thromboembolic disease, or undiagnosed vaginal bleeding are all contraindications to estrogen replacement therapy.

Estrogen replacement alone may cause endometrial hyperplasia and eventually cancer. Thus, progesterone is used in combination to offset the risks of unopposed estrogen. Either a combined continuous regimen (Premarin 0.625 mg every day/Provera 2.5 mg every day) or various combined sequential regimens can be used. The regimen of continuous progesterone is associated with more irregular breakthrough bleeding but may eventually lead to amenorrhea. Progesterone given periodically will result in regular withdrawal bleeding, which is more predictable but will not lead to amenorrhea.

Alternative Therapeutic Regimens

Alternative regimens for postmenopausal women who are unable to take hormone replacement therapy should be targeted toward treatment goals. Vasomotor flushes have been managed with behavioral therapy, herbal medications, and clonidine. Vaginal atrophy can be managed locally with lubricants and moisturizers.

The treatment for osteoporosis has been refined over the last few years and includes calcium/vitamin D supplements, bisphosphonates, calcitonin, and exercise. A bone density may be determined to follow bone resorption. From a cardiovascular standpoint, improvement in lifestyle and diet are key factors, as well as optimal blood pressure control to decrease morbidity and mortality.

Key Points

1. The mean age of menopause is 50.
2. Patients present with "hot flashes" and other symptoms consistent with decreased levels of estrogen. Diagnosis is made with elevated levels of FSH.
3. HRT with estrogen reduces morbidity and mortality from cardiovascular disease and bone demineralization.

Menopause: ↓estrogen, ↑FSH

HRT: 3x as many thromboembolic events & contraindicated in ♀ w/ this hx. (in HERS study).

CHAPTER 19

Amenorrhea

Amenorrhea, or the absence of menses, is described as either primary or secondary. **Primary** amenorrhea is the absence of menses in women who have not undergone menarche by the age of 16 or have not had menstruation by 4 years after thelarche. **Secondary** amenorrhea is the absence of menses for 3 menstrual cycles or a maximum of 6 months in women who have previously had normal menstruation. The pathophysiologic mechanisms underlying these two processes are quite different.

▶ PRIMARY AMENORRHEA

If menses has not occurred by the age of 16, the diagnosis of primary amenorrhea is made. In the United States, the prevalence of primary amenorrhea is 1 to 2%. The various causes of primary amenorrhea include congenital abnormalities, hormonal aberrations, chromosomal abnormalities, hypothalamic-pituitary disorders, and the variety of causes of secondary amenorrhea that may present before menarche. They can be considered in three categories: outflow tract obstruction, end-organ disorders, and central regulatory disorders (Table 19-1).

Outflow Tract Anomalies

Imperforate Hymen

The hymen sometimes forms a solid membrane across the introitus. If it is imperforate, it will not allow egress of menses. Over time, these patients present with pelvic or abdominal pain from the accumulation and subsequent dilation of the uterus by menstrual fluid. On physical examination they have a bulging membrane just inside the vagina, often with purple-red discoloration behind it consistent with hematocolpos.

Transverse Vaginal Septum

A transverse vaginal septum may result from failure to fuse the Müllerian-derived upper vagina and the urogenital sinus-derived lower vagina. Commonly found at the level of the midvagina, it is usually patent. However, in some cases it may be imperforate and cause primary amenorrhea. Diagnosis is made on careful examination of the female genital tract. Surgical therapy involves resection of the septum.

Vaginal Agenesis

Patients with **Rokitansky-Kuster-Hauser** (RKH) syndrome have Müllerian agenesis or dysgenesis. They may have complete vaginal agenesis and absence of a uterus or partial vaginal agenesis with a rudimentary uterus and distal vagina. This differs from **vaginal atresia** where the Müllerian system is developed, but the distal vagina is composed of fibrosed tissue. Diagnosis is made with physical examination that reveals no patent vagina, chromosomes that are 46,XX, and ovaries on ultrasound. With partial vaginal agenesis or vaginal atresia, a rectal examination may reveal a pelvic mass consistent with a uterus. The uterus can be visualized with ultrasound, computed tomography, or magnetic resonance imaging (MRI). Surgical therapy in either situation involves creating a vagina. In true vaginal atresia, the vaginoplasty may be connected with the upper genital tract.

Testicular Feminization

Testicular feminization results from a dysfunction or absence in the testosterone receptor that leads to a phenotypical female with 46,XY chromosomes. Because **Müllerian inhibiting factor** (MIF) was secreted, they have an absence of all Müllerian-derived structures. Usually estrogen is produced, and these patients develop breasts but present with primary amenorrhea. Similar to RKH syndrome, surgical therapy involves creating a vagina.

End-Organ Disorders

Ovarian Failure

Primary ovarian failure results in low levels of estradiol but elevated levels of gonadotropins termed **hypergonadotropic hypogonadism.** There are a variety of causes of primary ovarian failure (Table 19-2). **Savage's** syndrome is characterized by failure of the ovaries to respond to follicle-stimulating hormone (FSH) and luteinizing hormone (LH) secondary to a receptor defect. In **Turner's** syndrome (45,XO), the ovaries undergo such rapid atresia that by puberty there are no primordial oocytes. Defects in the enzymes involved in steroid biosynthesis, particularly 17-alpha-hydroxylase, can result in amenorrhea and absence of breast development because of lack of estradiol.

TABLE 19-1

Etiologies of Primary Amenorrhea

Outflow tract abnormalities
Imperforate hymen
Transverse vaginal septum
Vaginal agenesis
Vaginal atresia
Testicular feminization
Uterine agenesis with vaginal dysgenesis
Rokitansky-Kuster-Hauser syndrome
End-organ disorders
Ovarian agenesis
Gonadal agenesis 46,XX
Swyer's syndrome—gonadal agenesis 46,XY
Ovarian failure
Enzymatic defects leading to decreased steroid biosynthesis
Savage's syndrome—ovary fails to respond to FSH and LH
Turner's syndrome
Central disorders
Hypothalamic
Local tumor compression
Trauma
Tuberculosis
Sarcoidosis
Irradiation
Kallman's syndrome—congenital absence of GnRH
Pituitary
Damage from surgery or radiation therapy
Hemosiderosis deposition of iron in pituitary

TABLE 19-2

Causes of Primary Gonadal Failure (Hypergonadotropic Hypogonadism)

Idiopathic premature ovarian failure
Steroidogenic enzyme defects (primary amenorrhea)
Cholesterol side-chain cleavage
3β-ol-dehydrogenase
17-hydroxylase
17-desmolase
17-ketoreductase
Testicular regression syndrome
True hermaphroditism
Gonadal dysgenesis
Pure gonadal dysgenesis (Swyer's syndrome) (46,XX and 46,XY)
Turner's syndrome (45,XO)
Turner variants
Mixed gonadal dysgenesis
Ovarian resistance syndrome (Savage syndrome)
Autoimmune oophoritis
Postinfection (e.g., mumps)
Postoophorectomy (also wedge resections and bivalving)
Postirradiation
Postchemotherapy

DeCherney A, Pernoll M. Current obstetric & gynecologic diagnosis & treatment. Norwalk, CT: Appleton & Lange, 1994:1009.

Gonadal Agenesis with 46,XY Chromosomes

There are a variety of disorders that can lead to a 46,XY karyotype resulting in a female phenotype: absence of MIF, absence of testosterone, or absence of a response to testosterone. Gonadal agenesis in a genotypical male, **Swyer's syndrome,** results in a phenotypical picture similar to ovarian agenesis. Because the testes never develop, MIF is not released and these patients have both internal and external female genitalia. Without estrogen they will not develop breasts. If there is a defect in the enzymes **17-alpha-hydroxylase** or **17,20 desmolase,** which are involved in testicular steroid production, the patient will not produce testosterone. However, MIF will still be produced and hence there will be no female internal reproductive organs. They will otherwise be phenotypically female, usually without breast development. Patients with an absence or defect in the testosterone receptor develop **testicular feminization.**

Central Disorders

Hypothalamic Disorders

The pituitary will not release FSH and LH if the hypothalamus is unable to either produce gonadotropin-releasing hormone (GnRH), transport it to the pituitary, or release it in a pulsatile fashion. In this setting of hypogonadotropic hypogonadism, anovulation and amenorrhea result. Kallmann's syndrome involves a congenital absence of GnRH and is commonly associated with anosmia. GnRH transport may be disrupted with compression or destruction of the pituitary stalk or arcuate nucleus. This can result from tumor mass effect, trauma, sarcoidosis, tuberculosis, irradiation, or Hand-Schuller-Christian disease. There may be defects in GnRH pulsatility in the setting of anorexia nervosa, extreme stress, athletes, hyperprolactinemia, and constitutionally delayed puberty.

Pituitary Disorders

Primary defects of the pituitary are a rare cause of primary amenorrhea. Pituitary dysfunction is usually secondary to hypothalamic dysfunction. It may be caused by tumors, infiltration of the pituitary gland, or infarcts of the pituitary. Surgery or irradiation of pituitary tumors may lead to decreased or absence of LH and FSH. Hemosiderosis can result in iron deposition in the pituitary, leading to destruction of the gonadotrophs that produce FSH and LH.

Diagnosis

A patient who presents with primary amenorrhea can be worked up based on their phenotypic picture (Table 19-3 and Fig. 19-1). Lack of a uterus is seen in males because of the release of MIF by the testes and in females with Müllerian agenesis. Breast development is dependent on estradiol secretion by the ovaries. If a patient has neither a uterus nor breasts, they are generally 46,XY males with steroid synthesis defects or varying degrees of gonadal dysgenesis in which adequate MIF is produced by gonadal tissue but there is insufficient androgen synthesis.

TABLE 19-3

Diagnosis of Etiology of Primary Amenorrhea

	Uterus Absent	Uterus Present
Breasts absent	▲ Gonadal agenesis in 46,XY ▲ Enzyme deficiencies in testosterone synthesis	▲ Gonadal failure / agenesis in 46,XX ▲ Disruption of hypothalamic-pituitary axis
Breasts present	▲ Testicular feminization ▲ Müllerian agenesis or RKH	▲ Hypothalamic, pituitary, or ovarian pathogenesis similar to that of secondary amenorrhea ▲ Congenital abnormalities of the genital tract

If breasts are present but no uterus, the etiologies can include congenital absence of the uterus (Müllerian agenesis) in the female or testicular feminization in the male. In the latter case, estradiol from direct testicular secretion as well as peripheral conversion of testosterone and androstenedione leads to the development of breasts.

If the patient has a uterus but the absence of breast development, the differential includes hypergonadotropic hypogonadism as seen in gonadal dysgenesis in both sexes and defects in steroid pathways in 46,XX patients and hypogonadotropic hypogonadism, which is seen in central nervous system (CNS), hypothalamic, and pituitary dysfunction. A serum FSH level will differentiate between these two.

The workup for amenorrhea in phenotypic females with either absence of uterus or breasts must include karyotype analysis, followed by testosterone and FSH assays. Further biochemical and hormonal assays may be performed to elucidate specific enzyme defects. Patients with both a uterus and breasts present should be evaluated to determine whether there is a patent outflow tract from the uterus. If the vagina, cervix, and uterus are continuous, they can be evaluated as if presenting with secondary amenorrhea.

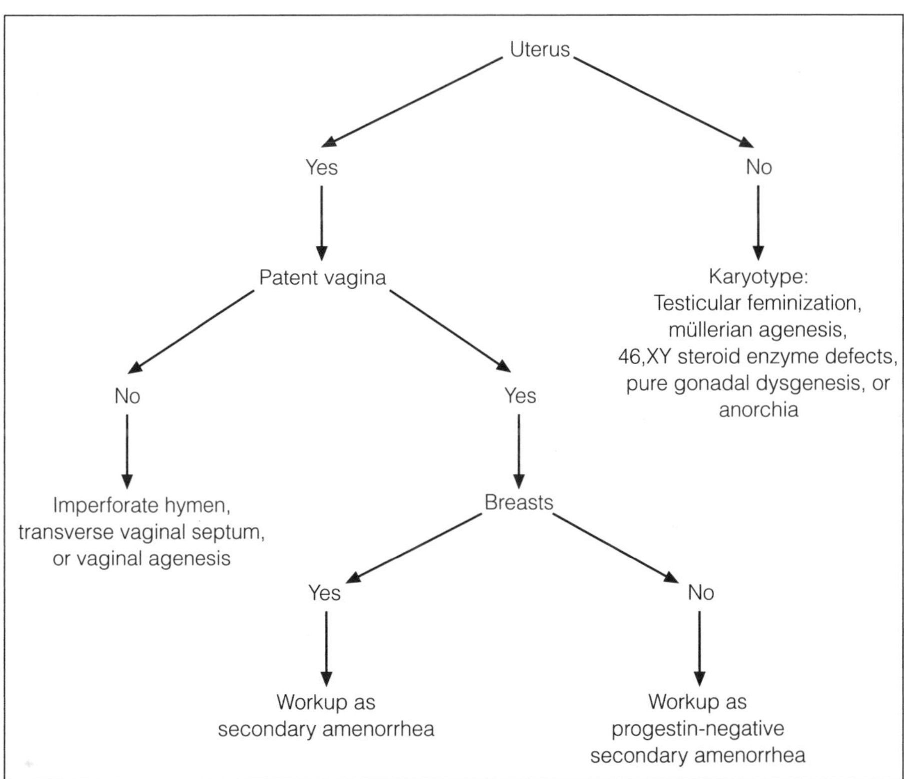

Figure 19-1 Workup for patients with primary amenorrhea.

Treatment

Patients with congenital abnormalities may be treated surgically with plastic procedures to allow egress of menses in those with a functional uterus or to create a functional vagina for sexual function. Patients with absent uterus and breasts can be treated with estrogen replacement to effect breast development and prevent osteoporosis. Patients with absent uterus but who have developed breasts may often require no medical therapy.

Patients with a uterus but without breast development with hypergonadotropic hypogonadism will often have irreversible ovarian failure. They will require estrogen replacement therapy. Patients with hypogonadotropic gonadism require further workup as patients with secondary amenorrhea.

Key Points

1. **Primary amenorrhea** is the absence of menarche by age 16.
2. Primary amenorrhea can be caused by congenital abnormalities of the genital tract, chromosomal abnormalities, enzyme or hormonal deficiencies, gonadal agenesis, ovarian failure, or disruption of the hypothalamic-pituitary axis.
3. The workup of primary amenorrhea is usually organized into four categories of patients using the categories of presence or absence of a uterus and the presence or absence of breast development.
4. In the absence of both uterus and breasts, karyotype will usually reveal 46,XY.
5. In the absence of a uterus and presence of breasts, karyotype will differentiate between Müllerian agenesis and testicular feminization.
6. In the absence of breasts and presence of a uterus, FSH will differentiate between hypergonadotropic and hypogonadotropic hypogonadism. Karyotype may be necessary to rule out gonadal agenesis in a 46,XY.
7. Patients with both a uterus and breasts should be evaluated as if presenting with secondary amenorrhea.

▶ SECONDARY AMENORRHEA

Secondary amenorrhea is the absence of menses for more than 6 months or for the equivalent of three menstrual cycles in a woman who previously had menstrual cycles. The leading cause of secondary amenorrhea is pregnancy. There are a variety of other causes due to anatomic and hormonal abnormalities.

Anatomic Abnormalities

Asherman's syndrome is the presence of intrauterine synechiae or adhesions usually secondary to intrauterine surgery or infection. The etiology of Asherman's syndrome includes dilatation and curettage, myomectomy, cesarean section, or endometritis. **Cervical stenosis** can present as secondary amenorrhea and dysmenorrhea. It is usually caused by scarring of the cervical os secondary to surgical or obstetric trauma.

Ovarian Dysfunction and Failure

Ovarian failure may result from ovarian surgery, infection, radiation, or chemotherapy. **Premature ovarian failure** (POF) is often idiopathic. Anytime menopause occurs without another etiology before the age of 40, it is considered POF. Before the age of 35, chromosomal analysis is usually done to rule out an obvious genetic basis for POF.

Polycystic ovarian disease as seen in **Stein-Leventhal** syndrome often leads to anovulation, oligomenorrhea, and amenorrhea. These patients are usually hirsute secondary to excess androgens and often obese. Increased androgens released from the ovaries and the adrenal cortex are converted peripherally in the adipose tissue into estrogens. This hyperestrogenic state leads to an increased LH-FSH ratio, atypical follicular development, anovulation, and increased androgen production. Once again the androgens are peripherally converted to estrogens, leading to a cyclical propagation of the disease.

Disruption of the Hypothalamic-Pituitary Axis

As in the hypothalamic and pituitary causes of primary amenorrhea disruption in the secretion and transport of GnRH, absence of pulsatility of GnRH or acquired pituitary lesions will all cause hypogonadotropic hypogonadism (Table 19-4). These patients are usually differentiated between those with galactorrhea and hyperprolactinemia and those without.

Hyperprolactinemia Associated Amenorrhea

Prolactin excess leads to amenorrhea and galactorrhea. Menstrual irregularities are secondary to interference with gonadotropin (FSH, LH) secretion, leading to hypogonadotropic hypogonadism. The etiologies and consequences of prolactin excess are numerous and should be understood in the approach to the patient with hyperprolactinemia. Prolactin release is inhibited by dopamine and stimulated by serotonin and thyrotropin-releasing hormone (TRH). Because of the constant suppression of prolactin release by hypothalamic release of dopamine, any disturbance in this process by a hypothalamic or pituitary lesion can lead to disinhibition of prolactin secretion.

Hyperprolactinemia has a variety of possible etiologies (Table 19-5). Primary hypothyroidism that leads to elevated thyroid stimulating hormone (TSH) and TRH can cause hyperprolactinemia. Medications that increase prolactin levels (by a hypothalamic pituitary effect) include dopamine antagonists (haldol, reglan, phenothiazines), tricyclic antidepressants, estrogen, mono amine oxidase (MAO) inhibitors, estrogen, and opiates. A prolactin-secreting pituitary adenoma will lead to elevated prolactin levels. The empty sella syndrome in which the subarachnoid membrane herniates into the sella turcica, causing it to enlarge and flatten, is another cause of hyperprolactinemia. Other conditions associated with high prolactin include pregnancy and breastfeeding.

Diagnosis

The approach to secondary amenorrhea always begins with a beta human chorionic gonadotropin assay to rule out pregnancy. TSH and prolactin levels should then be checked to rule out hypothyroidism and hyperprolactinemia, both of which can cause amenorrhea. If both are elevated, the hypothyroidism should be treated and the prolactin can be checked after thyroid studies have normalized to verify resolution.

If the prolactin level is elevated and TSH is normal, a workup for the other causes of prolactinemia should ensue (Fig. 19-2). In the diagnostic evaluation of the patient, a careful history should be taken, including a complete list of medications and clear documentation of the onset of symptoms. A thorough physical examination should include visual fields, cranial nerves, breast examination, and an attempt to express milk from the nipple. Consideration should be given for an MRI to rule out a hypothalamic or pituitary lesion.

If the prolactin level is normal, a progesterone challenge test (progesterone 200 mg intramuscularly or 10 mg orally for 5 to 7 days to mimic progesterone withdrawal) should be performed to assess the adequacy of

TABLE 19-4

Differential Diagnosis of Hypoestrogenic Amenorrhea (Hypogonadotropic Hypogonadism)

- Hypothalamic dysfunction
  - Kallmann's syndrome
  - Tumors of hypothalamus (craniopharyngioma)
  - Constitutional delay of puberty
  - Severe hypothalamic dysfunction
  - Anorexia nervosa
  - Severe weight loss
  - Severe stress
  - Exercise
- Pituitary disorder
  - Sheehans' syndrome
  - Panhypopituitarism
  - Isolated gonadotropin deficiency
  - Hemosiderosis (primarily from thalassemia major)

Reproduced by permission from DeCherney A, Pernoll M. Current obstetric and gynecologic diagnosis & treatment. Norwalk: Appleton & Lange, 1994:1013.

TABLE 19-5

Differential Diagnosis of Galactorrhea-Hyperprolactinemia

- Pituitary tumors secreting prolactin
  - Macroadenomas (> 10 mm)
  - Microadenomas (< 10 mm)
- Hypothyroidism
- Idiopathic hyperprolactinemia
- Drug-induced hyperprolactinemia
  - Dopamine antagonists
    - Phenothiazines
    - Thioxanthenes
    - Butyrophenone
    - Diphenylbutylpiperidine
    - Dibenzoxazepine
    - Dihydroindolone
    - Procainamide derivatives
  - Catecholamine-depleting agents
  - False transmitters (α-methyldopa)
- Interruption of normal hypothalamic-pituitary relationship
  - Pituitary stalk section
- Peripheral neural stimulation
  - Chest wall stimulation
    - Thoracotomy
    - Mastectomy
    - Thoracoplasty
    - Burns
    - Herpes zoster
    - Bronchogenic tumors
    - Bronchiectasis
    - Chronic bronchitis
  - Nipple stimulation
    - Stimulation of nipples
    - Chronic nipple irritation
  - Spinal cord lesion
    - Tabes dorsalis
    - Syringomyelia
  - CNS disease
    - Encephalitis
    - Craniopharyngioma
    - Pineal tumors
    - Hypothalamic tumors
    - Pseudotumor cerebri

Reproduced by permission from DeCherney A, Pernoll M. Current obstetric and gynecologic diagnosis & treatment. Norwalk: Appleton & Lange, 1994:1012.

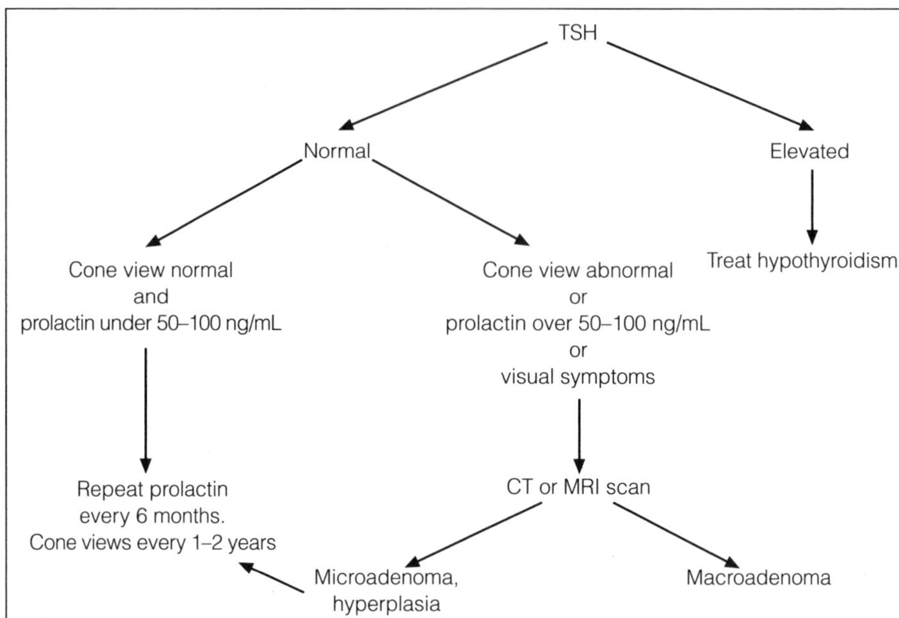

Figure 19-2 Workup for patients with amenorrhea-galactorrhea-hyperprolactinemia.

endogenous estrogen production. Subsequent withdrawal bleeding indicates estrogen presence, although amenorrhea is secondary to anovulation, which can be caused by a variety of endocrine disorders that alter pituitary/gonadal feedback such as polycystic ovaries, tumors of the ovary and adrenals, Cushing's syndrome, thyroid disorders, and adult-onset adrenal hyperplasia (Table 19-6).

Absence of withdrawal bleeding in response to progesterone alone must then be evaluated with estrogen and progesterone administration. If there is still no menstrual bleeding, an outflow tract disorder is suspected, such as Asherman's syndrome or cervical stenosis. If menstrual bleeding does occur in response to estrogen and progesterone administration, this suggests an intact and functional uterus without adequate endogenous hormone stimulation. Measurement of FSH and LH will help differentiate between a hypothalamic/pituitary disorder (low/normal FSH and LH levels) and ovarian failure (high FSH and LH levels) (Fig. 19-3).

Treatment

Patients with hypothyroidism are treated with thyroid hormone replacement. Those with pituitary macroadenomas are treated with surgical resection. Hyperprolactinemic patients without macroadenomas should be followed with serial prolactin levels and cone view radiographs to diagnose development of a macroadenoma.

Patients who respond to progesterone challenge should be withdrawn with progesterone on a regular basis to prevent endometrial hyperplasia. Oral contraceptive pills (OCPs) are useful in this setting and may be beneficial in the management of hirsutism. However, if the patient is a smoker over the age of 35, progesterone alone is indicated.

Patients who are hypoestrogenic should be treated with estrogen and progesterone for the effects on lipids, bone density, and genital atrophy. OCPs for

TABLE 19-6

Differential Diagnosis of Eugonadotropic Eugonadism (Progestin-Challenge Positive)

Mild hypothalamic dysfunction
- Emotional stress
- Psychologic disorder
- Weight loss
- Obesity
- Exercise-induced
- Idiopathic

Hirsutism-virilism
- Polycystic ovary syndrome (Stein-Leventhal syndrome)
- Ovarian tumor
- Adrenal tumor
- Cushing's syndrome
- Congenital and maturity-onset adrenal hyperplasia

Systemic disease
- Hypothyroidism
- Hyperthyroidism
- Addison's disease
- Cushing's syndrome
- Chronic renal failure
- Many others

Reproduced by permission from DeCherney A, Pernoll M. Current obstetric and gynecologic diagnosis & treatment. Norwalk: Appleton & Lange 1994:1013.

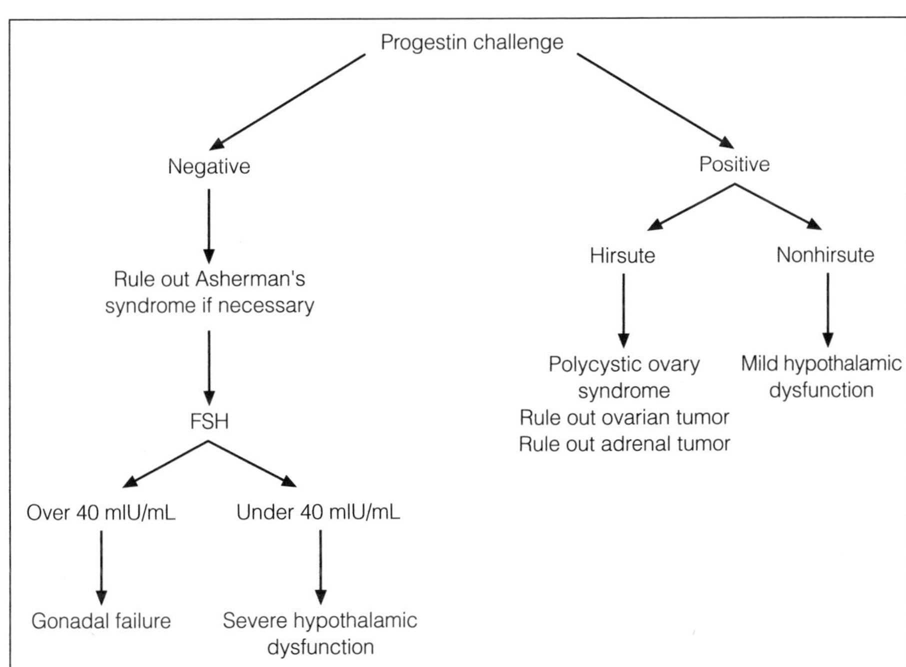

Figure 19-3 Workup for patients with secondary amenorrhea.

women under the age of 35 or those over 35 who are nonsmokers are often used. For other women, a regimen of 0.625 mg of conjugated estrogen cycled with 5 to 10 mg of medroxyprogesterone acetate is suitable. These patients should all received 1.2 g of elemental calcium supplementation per day.

Ovulation Induction

Ovulation induction with bromocriptine can be used in patients with hyperprolactinemia. If the cause of hyperprolactinemia is medication related, the medication should be discontinued or decreased.

Patients who respond to the progesterone challenge have evidence of estrogenation. Any specific cause of this amenorrheic state should be corrected. If menses do not resume, ovulation induction may be performed with clomiphene citrate, which acts as an antiestrogen to stimulate gonadotropin release. Those patients with elevated androgens may need combined therapy with clomiphene and corticosteroids.

Patients who do not respond to progesterone alone are presumed to have low esterogen levels; however, they will occasionally respond to clomiphene citrate as well. For patients who do not respond to clomiphene, human menopausal gonadotropin (hMG) can be used to stimulate ovulation. Careful monitoring with ultrasound and estradiol levels should be done in the setting of hMG ovulation induction because of the risk of ovarian hyperstimulation.

Key Points

1. Anatomic abnormalities including Asherman's syndrome and cervical stenosis may present with secondary amenorrhea. They will fail to respond to estrogen and progesterone withdrawal.
2. Hypothalamic-pituitary axis-related amenorrhea may be caused by hyperprolactinemia.
3. In the setting of normal prolactin levels, patients may be given a progesterone challenge to investigate whether the endometrium is estrogenized.
4. With progestin challenge failure the differential becomes hypergonadotropic or hypogonadotropic hypogonadism that can be differentiated by an FSH.
5. For patients not requiring fertility, it is important to treat the specific cause of amenorrhea and to ensure the hypoestrogenic patient receives replacement therapy.
6. For patients who wish fertility, ovulation induction may be carried out in most cases. Those with hyperprolactinemia will require bromocriptine, whereas patients with other forms of hypogonadism may respond to clomiphene and hMG.

CHAPTER 20

Abnormalities of the Menstrual Cycle

▶ DYSMENORRHEA

Dysmenorrhea is defined as pain and cramping during menstruation that interferes with the activities of daily living. Discomfort during menstruation ranges from mild discomfort to patients who are bedridden with pain. Dysmenorrhea is classified as primary, or idiopathic, and secondary.

Primary Dysmenorrhea

Primary dysmenorrhea usually presents before the age of 20 but after menarche. Although there is no obvious organic cause, women with dysmenorrhea have been documented to have higher tissue levels of prostaglandins. Additionally, there may be a psychological component involved for some patients that depends on attitudes toward menstruation learned from mothers, sisters, and friends.

Diagnosis

The diagnosis of primary dysmenorrhea is made on the basis of history and the absence of organic causes for the dysmenorrhea. Often, the pain of dysmenorrhea occurs with ovulatory cycles on the first or second day of menstruation. Associated symptoms include nausea, vomiting, and headache. On physical examination there are no obvious abnormalities with generalized tenderness throughout the pelvis.

Treatment

The treatment for primary dysmenorrhea is primarily medical with antiprostaglandin agents, nonsteroidal anti-inflammatory drugs (NSAIDs), and oral contraceptive pills (OCPs). The most commonly used NSAIDs include aspirin, ibuprofen, and naproxen. All are available over the counter; however, patients may need to be advised to take larger dosages than those recommended to achieve a tolerable comfort level. Patients should be advised to take the medications right at onset of symptoms.

OCPs should be used in those women who do not get relief from antiprostaglandin agents or who cannot tolerate them. Use of oral contraceptives usually prevents pain in even the most symptomatic patients. The mechanism of relief is either secondary to the cessation of ovulation or to an alteration of the endometrium, leading to decreased prostaglandin production. Most patients who have been cycled for a year will have reduction of symptoms if the OCPs are discontinued.

Surgical therapies including cervical dilatation and neurectomies have been used in the past but have little use in current management of true primary dysmenorrhea. Often, primary dysmenorrhea will decrease throughout a patient's 20s and early 30s. In addition, usually a pregnancy carried to viability will decrease the symptoms of primary dysmenorrhea.

Secondary Dysmenorrhea

Secondary dysmenorrhea implies that there is a cause of the symptoms of dysmenorrhea. The causes include endometriosis and adenomyosis (Chapter 13), fibroids, cervical stenosis, and pelvic adhesions. Because the first two causes are covered elsewhere, detailed management is referred to those particular chapters.

Cervical Stenosis

Cervical stenosis causes dysmenorrhea because of the obstruction of flow during menstruation. The stenosis can be congenital or secondary to scarring from infection, trauma, or surgery. Patients will often complain of scant menses associated with pain, which is relieved with increased menstrual flow. On physical examination there may be obvious scarring of the external os; often there is inability to pass a uterine sound through the cervical canal.

Treatment Dilatation of the cervix is the treatment for cervical stenosis. Either a surgical dilation can be performed or laminaria tents can be used. A dilatation is usually performed in an operating room. Progressively larger dilators are placed through the cervical canal until a curette may be placed through and use to clean the endometrial cavity. Laminaria may be placed in the office setting. Made from seaweed, they dilate over a period of 24 hours by absorbing water from the surrounding tissue.

Dilation will provide relief; however, patients will often develop recurrence of stenosis requiring multiple dilatations. Pregnancy with vaginal delivery often leads to a permanent cure.

Pelvic Adhesions

Patients with a history of pelvic infections including cervicitis, pelvic inflammatory disease, or tubo-ovarian abscess all may have symptoms of dysmenorrhea secondary to adhesion formation. Patients with other local inflammatory diseases (appendicitis, Crohn's disease) or prior pelvic surgery may also have adhesions leading to dysmenorrhea. Diagnosis is made via history of any of these problems in conjunction with laparoscopy revealing local adhesions. In some patients, the pelvic adhesions can be so extensive as to cement the uterus into a fixed position, which may be noted on pelvic examination.

Treatment These patients will occasionally respond to the antiprostaglandins prescribed for primary dysmenorrhea. For the more severe cases, which fail medical therapy, laparoscopy is indicated. At that time the diagnosis is made and the adhesions, if accessible, can be taken down. However, this surgery can lead to further adhesions and further problems with dysmenorrhea.

Key Points

1. Primary dysmenorrhea cannot be attributed to any organic cause.
2. Primary dysmenorrhea is treated with NSAIDs or OCPs.
3. Secondary dysmenorrhea needs to have the specific cause, usually fibroids, endometriosis, adenomyosis, cervical stenosis or pelvic adhesions, diagnosed and treated.

▶ PREMENSTRUAL SYNDROME

Premenstrual syndrome (PMS) is a constellation of symptoms that occur in the second half of the menstrual cycle including weight gain, edema, mood fluctuation, breast tenderness, and other depressive symptoms. Probably 90% of women suffer from some PMS symptoms and 5% of women are incapacitated at some point during the cycle.

Pathogenesis

The exact etiology of PMS has yet to be worked out. However, it is clear that it is likely to be due to both physiologic and psychological causes. Hypotheses include abnormalities in the estrogen/progesterone balance, disturbance of the renin-angiotensin-aldosterone pathway, excess prostaglandin production, and reduction of endogenous endorphins.

Treatment

There is often relief from NSAIDs, which supports the excess prostaglandin hypothesis. OCPs sometimes provide relief, supporting the idea that the symptoms are related to ovulation, low progesterone levels, or some imbalance in estrogen and progesterone. The idea that cyclic fluctuations in the steroid hormones affect PMS is supported by the fact that gonadotropin-releasing hormone agonists have been successful in treating symptoms in small trials. With severe edema, furosemide (Lasix) will offer some relief. Patients with incapacitating depressive symptoms of sleep disturbance, depressed mood, withdrawal from society, and lack of appetite may be helped by antidepressant medications.

Key Points

1. PMS is likely a multifactorial disease with physiologic and psychological components.
2. Though the cause is unknown, there are a variety of treatments that offer palliative treatment including NSAIDs and OCPs. These must often be tried as "hit or miss" therapies until one that is effective is found.

▶ ABNORMAL UTERINE BLEEDING

Abnormal uterine bleeding refers to any irregularity in the menstrual cycle from the norm. It can be too much bleeding with either heavy periods, frequent menses, or bleeding between periods or too little bleeding with light periods, infrequent periods, or complete absence of periods. Amenorrhea, complete absence of periods, is covered in Chapter 19.

Menorrhagia

Menorrhagia, or hypermenorrhea, is defined as heavy or prolonged menstrual bleeding. The average blood loss during a menstrual cycle is approximately 35 mL; menorrhagia is defined as bleeding greater than 80 mL in one menstrual cycle. Patients with menorrhagia will occasionally describe the blood as "pouring" out or "gushing" and may have blood clots with excessive flow. The diagnosis can be made by weighing the menstrual pads used in a cycle and calculating the volume of blood lost. Most gynecologists use a history of greater than 24 menstrual pads a day or soaking through a pad every hour as indicative of menorrhagia. A hematocrit and iron studies should be checked and contribute to the diagnosis. Bleeding from the cervix or vagina should be ruled out with speculum examination.

Menorrhagia can be caused by fibroids, adenomyosis, endometrial hyperplasia, endometrial polyps, endometrial or cervical cancer, dysfunctional uterine bleeding, primary bleeding disorders, or pregnancy complications.

Metrorrhagia

Metrorrhagia is characterized by bleeding between periods. It is usually less or equal to menses. If the bleeding is heavy (greater than 80 mL) and associated with heavy periods, it is described as menometrorrhagia. The usual causes include endometrial polyps, endometrial or cervical cancer, or complications of pregnancy. Occasionally, patients will have light spotting, which may be caused midcycle by ovulation.

Hypomenorrhea

Patients with hypomenorrhea have periods with unusually light flow. This is commonly caused by hypogonadotropic hypogonadism in anorexics and athletes. Atrophic endometrium in the setting of Asherman's syndrome, which is intrauterine adhesions or synechiae secondary to congenital effects or intrauterine trauma. Patients on OCPs or Depo-provera also have atrophic endometrium and will often have light menses. Outlet obstruction secondary to cervical stenosis or congenital abnormalities will also cause hypomenorrhea.

Polymenorrhea

Polymenorrhea, or frequent periods, can be confused with metrorrhagia. If all of the bleeding episodes are similar and there is less than 21 days between them, polymenorrhea should be considered. This is usually caused by anovulation.

Oligomenorrhea

Patients with periods greater than 35 days apart are described as having oligomenorrhea. The causes are similar to amenorrhea with disruption of the pituitary-gonadal axis by hypothalamic, pituitary or gonadal abnormalities, or systemic disease (Chapter 19). The most common cause of oligomenorrhea is pregnancy.

Evaluation

The workup of abnormal uterine bleeding includes a careful history and physical followed by diagnostic tests to determine the underlying etiology. The history should include timing of bleeding, quantity of bleeding, menstrual history with menarche and recent periods, and associated symptoms. It should also include a family history of bleeding disorders, particularly if menorrhagia presents at menarche.

On physical examination, vaginal and cervical causes of bleeding should be ruled out. The bimanual examination may reveal a uterus and adnexal masses consistent with fibroids, adenomyosis, or cancer. A Pap smear is used to screen for cervical cancer. An **endometrial biopsy** is used to screen for endometrial hyperplasia and cancer. Sometimes a polyp or submucous fibroid will be diagnosed in this fashion.

All patients should have a pregnancy test. A pelvic ultrasound can be used to examine the intrauterine cavity in a noninvasive manner. Endometrial polyps, fibroids, and extensive cancers may be seen with this modality. A sonohystogram or **hysterosalpingogram** may show intrauterine defects. **Hysteroscopy** gives direct visualization of the intrauterine cavity. A dilatation and curettage (D&C) provides tissue for diagnosis. The array of hormonal tests that can be performed are discussed with the workup of amenorrhea (Chapter 19).

Treatment

The treatment of abnormal uterine bleeding depends on the specific underlying etiology. A D&C may be therapeutic as well as diagnostic. Fibroids and polyps can be treated by removal. Cancer is diagnosed by biopsy and treated accordingly. Adenomyosis and the endocrinopathies will often respond to OCPs, as will dysfunctional uterine bleeding.

Key Points

1. The most common cause of oligomenorrhea and secondary amenorrhea is pregnancy.
2. Structural abnormalities including polyps, fibroids, adenomyosis, and cancer cause most of the menorrhagia, metrorrhagia, and menometrorrhagia except those related to pregnancy.

▶ DYSFUNCTIONAL UTERINE BLEEDING

If no pathologic cause of menorrhagia, metrorrhagia, or menometrorrhagia can be elucidated, the diagnosis of exclusion, dysfunctional uterine bleeding (DUB), is given. Most patients will be anovulatory, with disruption in the hypothalamic-pituitary-gonadal axis that leads to continuous estrogenic stimulation of the endometrium. The endometrium then sloughs off when it outgrows its blood supply rather than in any regular fashion. DUB usually occurs near menarche and menopause.

Diagnosis

Diagnosis is made by history and physical to rule out other causes of abnormal bleeding. A basal body temperature can be graphed daily to determine whether ovulation is occurring. An appropriate day 23 to 25 serum progesterone level also may indicate if a patient is ovulating. Endometrial sampling is the gold standard to determine whether ovulation is occurring. If there is concern about hemorrhage, a hematocrit and iron studies should be done.

Treatment

If patients are not hemorrhaging and are hemodynamically stable, OCPs are an effective means of regulating the menstrual cycle. They may also be cycled on progesterone alone. For patients with excessive blood loss, therapy to stop the bleeding should be initiated immediately. Conjugated estrogens given at 10 mg/day should control the bleeding within 24 to 48 hours. If this is not effective, the estrogens need to be increased. For hemodynamically unstable patients, intravenous estrogen can be used.

For patients with ovulatory DUB, NSAIDs have been shown to decrease menstrual blood loss by 20 to 50% and may be used alone or in conjunction with estrogen and progesterone therapy.

Patients who do not respond to medical therapy will require surgical intervention. D&C is the first treatment of choice, which may be diagnostic and occasionally therapeutic. Endometrial ablation with laser, electrocautery, or heated roller may be performed with the intent of causing Asherman's syndrome and decreased uterine bleeding. Hysterectomy is the definitive surgery but should be reserved for those cases refractory to all other treatment.

DUB is most likely to occur with the anovulatory cycles more common in adolescence and near menopause. In adolescence, the risk that there is a structural cause is small. However, any congenital possibilities and bleeding disorders should be eliminated. In the reproductive years, there is an increased risk of other etiologies ranging from structural to hormonal that need to be eliminated. During menopause, the risk for DUB increases as does the risk of other causes including cancer and fibroids. Thus, a careful workup of abnormal uterine bleeding must be performed before the diagnosis of DUB is given.

Key Points

1. DUB is a diagnosis of exclusion.
2. DUB is thought to be secondary to anovulation, thus more common near menarche and menopause.
3. Treatment includes initial medical therapy but may require surgical modalities for those patients who are not controlled with medical management.

► POSTMENOPAUSAL BLEEDING

Vaginal bleeding more than 12 months after menopause occurs is considered postmenopausal bleeding. Any bleeding after menopause is abnormal and should be investigated, because patients in this age group are much more likely to have cancer.

Bleeding in postmenopausal women can be due to nongynecologic etiologies, lower and upper genital tract sources, tumors, or exogenous hormonal stimulation. Nongynecologic causes include rectal bleeding from hemorrhoids, anal fissures, rectal prolapse, and lower gastrointestinal (GI) tumors. These can be identified by history and physical with anoscopy and occult blood screening. Further workup can include a barium enema or colonoscopy.

Vaginal atrophy is the most common source of lower genital tract bleeding. The thin vaginal mucosa is easily traumatized and therefore bleeds. Other causes of lower genital tract bleeding are lesions of the vulva, vagina, or exocervix.

Pathologic causes of postmenopausal bleeding from the upper genital tract include cervical cancer, endometrial hyperplasia, endometrial polyps, and endometrial cancer. Exogenous hormones are the most common cause of postmenopausal bleeding. However, bleeding that is abnormal with signs of menometrorrhagia should be worked up as abnormal postmenopausal bleeding.

Diagnosis

A careful history is important. Physical examination should include a careful inspection of the external anogenital region, the vagina, and cervix. A Pap smear should be performed as well as a digital rectal examination and occult blood screening.

Endometrial biopsy should be performed to rule out endometrial cancer if there is not an obvious nongynecologic or lower genital tract etiology. With heavy bleeding, a hematocrit should be obtained.

Hysteroscopy either in the office or operating room can further elucidate intrauterine structures such as an endometrial polyp. Ultrasound can identify polyps and is used to examine the thickness of the endometrial stripe. D&C is both diagnostic and therapeutic for some lesions of the uterus and cervix.

Treatment

If GI bleeding is suspected, referral to a gastroenterologist and colonoscopy is the routine management. Hemorrhoids and anal fissures should be referred to general surgeons for further management.

Lesions of the vulva and vagina should be biopsied. Lacerations of mucosa should be repaired. Atrophy should be treated with estrogen. Commonly, estrogen cream is used and may supplement hormone replacement therapy or be used alone.

Endometrial hyperplasia can be simple, complex, or atypical. Simple will progress to carcinoma in 1%, complex in 3%, and atypical in 15 to 20% of cases. Thus, therapy is different for each. Simple endometrial hyperplasia is often watched with repeated endometrial biopsies. Complex and atypical hyperplasia will often be treated with progestin therapy and can lead to reversal of lesions in greater than 85% of patients. Those without reversal or recurrence are treated surgically with hysterectomy.

Endometrial polyps may be removed by hysteroscopic resection or D&C. Endometrial cancer is usually treated by hysterectomy, which may or may not be done in conjunction with chemotherapy and radiation therapy.

Key Points

1. Postmenopausal bleeding should always be investigated to rule out cancer.
2. Causes of postmenopausal bleeding include tumors of the upper and lower genital tract, exogenous hormonal stimulation, vaginal atrophy, and nongynecologic sources.

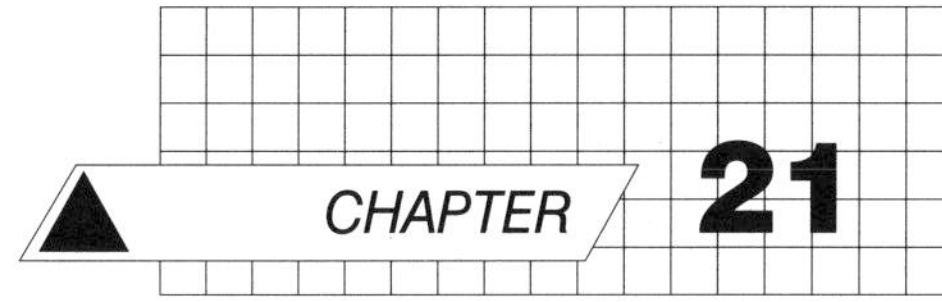

CHAPTER 21

Hirsutism and Virilism

Adults have two types of hair: vellus and terminal. Vellus hair is nonpigmented, soft, and covers the entire body. Terminal hairs, on the other hand, are pigmented and thick and cover the scalp, axilla, and pubic areas. Androgens are responsible for the conversion of vellus to terminal hairs at puberty, resulting in pubic and axillary hair. An abnormal increase in terminal hairs is due to androgen excess or increased **5α-reductase** activity, the enzyme that converts testosterone to the more potent dihydrotestosterone, which is believed to be the main stimulant of terminal hair development. **Hirsutism** refers to the increase in terminal hairs on the face, chest, back, lower abdomen, and inner thighs in a woman. The pubic hair is characterized by the development of a male escutcheon, which is diamond shaped as opposed to the triangular female escutcheon. **Virilization** refers to the development of male features, such as deepening of the voice, frontal balding, increased muscle mass, clitoromegaly, breast atrophy, and male body habitus.

The evaluation of hirsutism and virilism in the female patient is complex and requires understanding pituitary, adrenal, and ovarian function with detailed attention to the pathways of glucocorticoid, mineralocorticoid, androgen, and estrogen synthesis.

▶ NORMAL ANDROGEN SYNTHESIS

The adrenal gland can be divided into two components: the adrenal cortex, which is responsible for glucocorticoid, mineralocorticoid, and androgen synthesis, and the adrenal medulla, which is involved in catecholamine synthesis. The adrenal cortex is composed of three layers. An outer **zona glomerulosa** layer produces aldosterone and is regulated primarily by the renin-angiotensin system. Because this zone lacks **17α-hydroxylase,** cortisol and androgens are not synthesized. In contrast, the inner layers, the **zona fasciculata** and the **zona reticularis,** produce both cortisol and androgens but not aldosterone because they lack the enzyme **aldosterone synthase.** These two inner zones are highly regulated by adrenal corticotrophic hormone (ACTH).

Cholesterol is converted to pregnenolone by hydroxylation and side-chain cleavage, an enzymatically mediated process regulated by ACTH. Pregnenolone is then converted to progesterone and eventually aldosterone, cortisol, or shunted over to the production of sex steriods (Fig. 21-1).

In the adrenal glands, androgens are synthesized from the precursor **17α-hydroxypregnenolone,** which is converted to **dehydroepiandrosterone** (DHEA) and its sulfate (DHEAS), androstenedione, and finally to testosterone. DHEA and DHEAS are the most common adrenal androgens, whereas only small amounts of the others are secreted.

In the ovaries, the theca cells are stimulated by luteinizing hormone (LH) to produce androstenedione and testosterone. Both androstenedione and testosterone are then aromatized to estrone and estradiol, respectively, by the granulosa cells in response to follicle-stimulating hormone (FSH). Therefore, elevations in the ratio of LH to FSH may lead to elevated levels of androgens.

Pathologic Production of Androgens

Elevation of androgens can be primarily due to adrenal disorders or ovarian disorders. Because synthesis of steroid hormones in the adrenal cortex is stimulated by ACTH at a nondifferentiated step, elevated ACTH levels will increase all of the steroid hormones, including the androgens. If there are enzymatic defects, the precursor proximal to the defect accumulates and is shunted to another pathway. Thus, enzymatic blockade of either cortisol or aldosterone synthesis can lead to an increased androgen production. Because DHEAS is derived almost entirely from the adrenal glands, its elevation is used as a marker for adrenal androgen production.

In the ovary, any increase in LH or the LH to FSH ratio appears to lead to excess androgen production. Furthermore, there are tumors of both the adrenal gland and the ovary that can lead to excess androgens. Regardless of the source, elevated androgens lead to hirsutism and possibly virilism.

▶ ADRENAL DISORDERS

The adrenal disorders leading to virilization in a woman can be divided into two categories: nonneoplastic

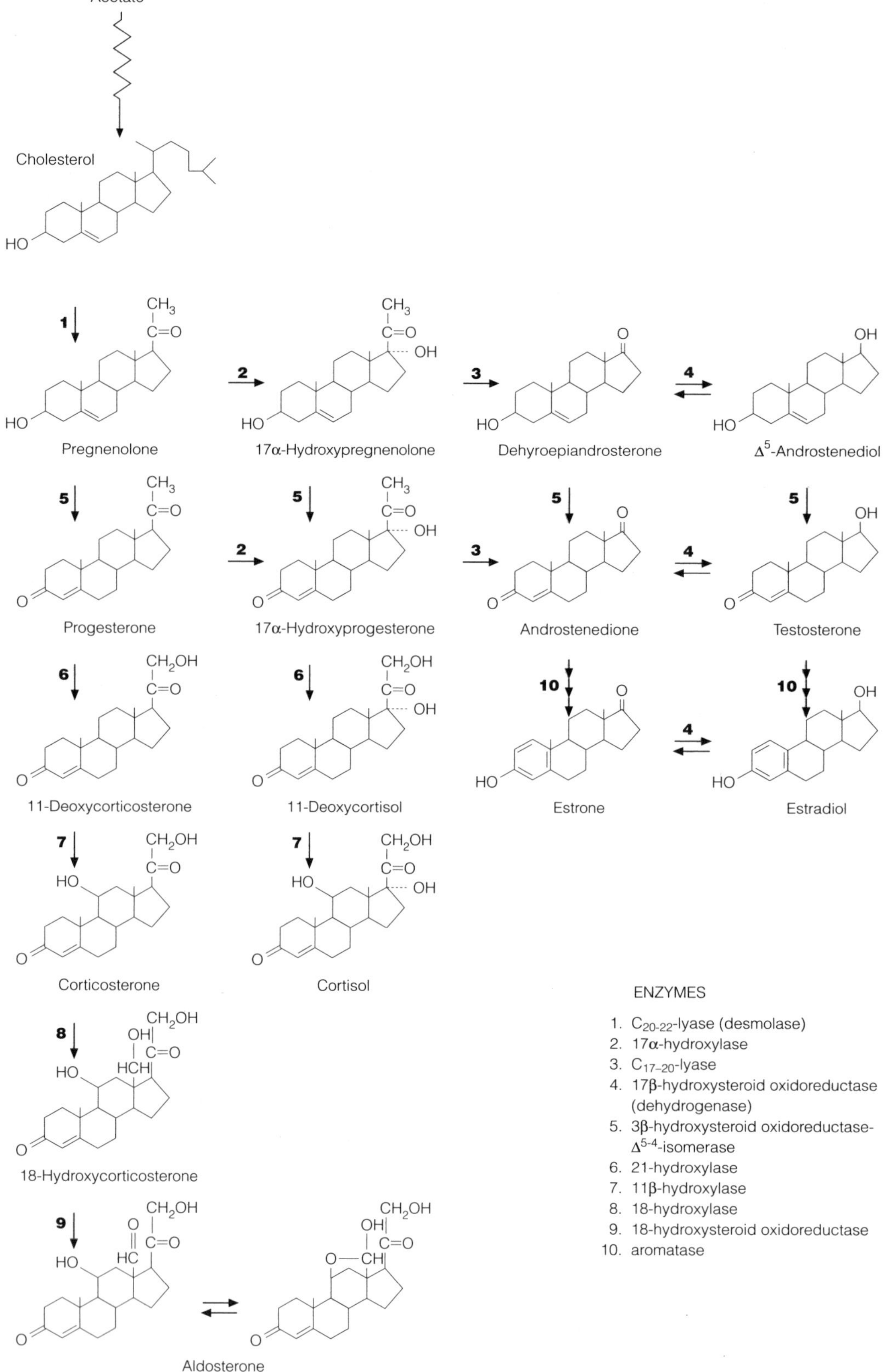

Figure 21-1 Biosynthesis of androgens, estrogens, and corticosteroids.

and neoplastic etiologies. Androgen-producing adrenal tumors may be either adenomas or carcinomas. Adrenal adenomas typically present with glucocorticoid excess and virilizing symptoms are rare. Carcinomas, on the other hand, can be more rapidly progressive and lead to marked elevations in glucocorticoid, mineralocorticoid, and androgen steroids.

Cushing's Syndrome

Cushing's syndrome is characterized by excess production of cortisol. Because the intermediates in production are androgens, there will be a concomitant hyperandrogenic state. Cushing's syndrome may be caused by pituitary adenomas, ectopic sources of ACTH, and tumors of the adrenal gland. **Cushing's disease** is caused by pituitary adenomas that hypersecrete ACTH. Paraneoplastic syndromes, such as nonpituitary ACTH-secreting tumors, will also lead to increased ACTH levels. Adrenal gland tumors usually have decreased levels of ACTH secondary to the negative feedback from the increased levels of adrenal steroid hormones. All three of these situations lead to the glucocorticoid excess characteristic of Cushing's disease, as well as hirsutism, acne, and menstrual irregularities related to adrenal androgen production.

Congenital Adrenal Hyperplasia

Congenital adrenal hyperplasia (CAH) refers to a constellation of enzyme deficiencies involved in steroidogenesis. The most common disorder is **21α-hydroxylase** deficiency. As seen in Figure 2-1, an enzymatic block at this step will lead to the accumulation of **17α-hydroxyprogesterone**, which is then shunted to the androgen pathway. These individuals do not synthesize cortisol or mineralocorticoids and thus present with salt-wasting and adrenal insufficiency at birth. Female infants will have ambiguous genitalia due to androgen excess. In more milder or "adult-onset" forms, the degree of deficiency can vary, and often the only presenting sign is mild virilization and menstrual irregularities.

The other types of CAH that can be associated with virilization include **11β-hydroxylase** and **3β-hydroxysteroid dehydrogenase** (3β-HSD) deficiencies. Patients with 11β-hydroxylase deficiency will present with similar symptoms of androgen excess as accumulated precursors are shunted to androstenedione and testosterone production pathways. Patients with 3β-HSD actually accumulate DHEA, because they are unable to convert either pregnenolone to progesterone or DHEA down the androgen synthesis pathway. DHEA and its sulfate, DHEAS, both have mild androgenic effects. Importantly, because the defect is also present in gonadal steroidogenesis, males have feminization and females have hirsutism and virilization. All patients have impaired cortisol synthesis and varying degrees of either mineralocorticoid excess or deficiency, depending on the location of the enzymatic block.

▶ FUNCTIONAL OVARIAN DISORDERS

The ovarian disorders leading to virilization can also be divided into the same categories: nonneoplastic and neoplastic etiologies. Nonneoplastic lesions include polycystic ovaries, theca lutein cysts, stromal hyperplasia, and stromal hyperthecosis. Neoplastic lesions vary and often present with rapid onset of virilization.

Nonneoplastic Ovarian Disorders

Polycystic Ovarian Syndrome

Polycystic ovarian syndrome (PCOS), known previously as the Stein-Leventhal syndrome, is a common disorder affecting up to 4% of reproductive age women and presents with a constellation of features that include hirsutism, virilization, anovulation, amenorrhea, and obesity. There is also an increased incidence of diabetes in this population. The cause of androgen excess appears to be related to excess LH stimulation leading to cystic changes in the ovaries and increased ovarian androgen secretion. Typically, the LH-FSH ratio is greater than 2:1. What actually causes the elevation in LH levels is not clear, although it appears that any number of factors can be involved in this cycle including obesity, insulin resistance, and excessive adrenal androgen production.

Theca Lutein Cysts

The **theca cells** of the ovary are stimulated by LH to produce androstenedione and testosterone. These androgens are normally shunted to the **granulosa cells** for aromatization to estrone and estradiol. Theca lutein cysts produce an excess amount of androgens that are secreted into the circulation. These cysts may be present in either normal pregnancy or molar pregnancy. The ovaries will be enlarged, and patients will present with hirsutism and occasionally virilization. Diagnosis is made by ovarian biopsy.

Stromal Hyperplasia and Hyperthecosis

Stromal hyperplasia is common between the ages of 50 and 70 and can present with hirsutism. The ovaries are uniformly enlarged. Stromal hyperthecosis is characterized by foci of luteinization within the hyperplastic stroma. It is more likely than simple hyperplasia to result in virilization as the luteinized cells continue to produce ovarian androgens. The ovaries typically appear enlarged and "fleshy," with the more florid cases seen in younger patients.

Neoplastic Ovarian Disorders

Functional Ovarian Tumors

Functional ovarian tumors that can produce varying amounts of androgen include the sex-cord mesenchymal tumors, **Sertoli-Leydig cell tumors** (arrhenoblastoma) and **granulosa-theca cell tumors, hilar (Leydig) cell tumors,** and germ cell tumors (gonadoblastomas). Sertoli-Leydig cell tumors usually occur in young women and make up less than 1% of all ovarian neoplasms. Hilar cell tumors are even more rare than Sertoli-Leydig cell tumors and are usually in postmenopausal women. These tumors may secrete androgens and present with hirsutism and virilism.

In pregnancy, there may be a luteoma of pregnancy, which is a benign tumor that grows in response to human chorionic gonadotropin. This tumor can result in high levels of testosterone and androstenedione and virilization in 25% of mothers. There will also be virilization of 65% of female fetuses. These findings should resolve in the postpartum period.

Nonfunctional Ovarian Tumors

Androgen excess can also occur in the setting of nonfunctional ovarian tumors (e.g., a cystadenoma or Krukenberg's tumor). Although these tumors do not secrete androgens themselves, they stimulate proliferation in the adjacent ovarian stroma that in turn may lead to increased androgen production.

▶ DRUGS AND EXOGENOUS HORMONES

There are a variety of drugs that can affect the circulating levels of sex hormone binding globulin (SHBG). SHBG is one of the major proteins that binds circulating testosterone, leaving a small proportion of "free" testosterone to interact at the cellular level. Androgens and corticosteroids decrease SHBG, leaving a greater percentage of free testosterone circulating. Patients engaged in the use of anabolic steroids will often present with hirsutism and virilization. In addition, there are several drugs that will cause hirsutism without using androgenic pathways. These include minoxidil, phenytoin, diazoxide, and cyclosporin.

Idiopathic Hirsutism

In the absence of adrenal or ovarian pathology or any exogenous source of androgens, hirsutism that occurs is considered idiopathic. Patients may actually have occult androgen production, but many of these patients will have normal circulating androgen levels. There may be an increase in peripheral androgen production at the level of the skin and hair follicles.

Clinical Manifestations

A detailed history including time of onset, progression, and symptoms of virilization/hirsutism should be obtained, as well as a pubertal, menstrual, and reproductive history. Because various medications can affect androgen levels by impacting SHBG or possess intrinsic androgenic activity, a detailed drug history should be obtained. A family history is also important to look for genetic disorders such as CAH.

Physical Examination On physical examination, the hair pattern should be noted, with attention to facial, chest, back, abdominal, and inner thigh hair, as well as the presence of frontal balding. The body habitus and presence or absence of female contours should be described. Breast examination will reveal atrophic changes, and a careful pelvic examination should include inspection of the escutcheon (pattern of pubic hair) and clitoris and palpation for ovarian masses. Cushingoid features should be ruled out and inspection for acanthosis nigricans (velvety, thickened hyperpigmentation) in the axilla and nape of neck should be done, as this dermatologic finding is often associated with polycystic ovaries.

Diagnostic Evaluation Laboratory evaluation should include testosterone, androstenedione, and DHEAS, a compound normally exclusive to the adrenal gland. An elevation in either testosterone or androstenedione confirms androgen excess and a concomitant elevation in DHEAS suggests an adrenal source. If an adrenal source is suspected, an abdominal computed tomography (CT) should be performed to rule out an adrenal tumor, as well as further tests to rule out Cushing's syndrome or CAH.

If the DHEAS is normal or minimally elevated an ovarian source should be considered and a pelvic ultrasound of CT should be performed to rule out an ovarian neoplasm. An elevation in the LH/FSH ratio greater than 3 is suggestive of PCOS. Rapid onset of virilization and testosterone levels greater than 200 ng/dL is suspicious for an ovarian neoplasm.

At times the source of androgen excess is not readily evident and further diagnostic tests such as abdominal magnetic resonance imaging and selective venous sampling need to be done for localization. In the hirsute woman with normal testosterone and androstenedione, a free testosterone should also be checked. If testosterone is also normal, an assay for 5α-reductase activity is performed to determine whether increased peripheral enzymatic activity is responsible for the development of hirsutism.

Treatment

Adrenal nonneoplastic androgen suppression can be achieved with glucocorticoid administration, such as prednisone 5 mg qhs. Antiandrogens such as spironolactone have been helpful as well, but are temporizing at best. In the setting of ovarian or adrenal tumors, the underlying disorder should be treated. Often surgical intervention is required.

In general, ovarian nonneoplastic androgen production can be suppressed with oral contraceptives, which will suppress LH and FSH as well as increase SHBG. Progestin therapy alone may help patients with contraindications to estrogen use. The progesterone decreases levels of LH and thus androgen production; furthermore, the catabolism of testosterone is increased resulting in decreased levels. Gonadotropin-releasing hormone agonists can also be used to suppress LH and FSH. However, this leads to a hypoestrogenic state and requires concomitant estrogen replacement.

Patients using exogenous androgens or other drugs leading to increased androgens or hair growth should be advised to discontinue use. For patients with idiopathic hirsutism or contraindications to hormonal use, waxing, depilatories, and electrolysis will often provide cosmetic improvement.

► KEY POINTS

1. Hirsutism is excess hair growth with a male pattern on the face, back, ears, chest, and abdomen, usually in response to excess androgens.
2. Virilism is a constellation of symptoms including hirsutism, deepening of the voice, frontal balding, clitoromegaly, and increased musculature.
3. Primary causes of hirsutism and virilization include PCOS, ovarian tumors, adrenal tumors, CAH, and Cushing's syndrome.
4. Diagnosis is made by history and physical, serum assays for testosterone and DHEAS, and imaging studies.
5. Treatment involves either primary treatment for the underlying cause; hormonal therapy with OCPs, GnRH, or progestins; and cosmetic treatment of hirsutism.

CHAPTER 22

Contraception and Sterilization

In weighing the risks and benefits of contraception methods, couples must keep in mind that no contraceptive or sterilization method is 100% effective. Table 22-1 shows relative failure rates or the number of women likely to become pregnant within the first year of using the method. **Theoretical efficacy rate** refers to the efficacy of contraception when used exactly as instructed. **Actual efficacy rate** refers to efficacy when used in "real life," assuming variations in the consistency of usage.

TABLE 22-1

Failure Rates for Various Contraceptive Methods

	Percent of Women with Pregnancy	
Method	Lowest Expected	Typical
No method	85.0	85.0
Combination pill	0.1	3.0
Progestin only	0.5	3.0
IUDs		3.0
Progesterone IUD	2.0	<2.0
Copper T 380A	0.8	<1.0
Norplant	0.2	0.2
Female sterilization	0.2	0.4
Male sterilization	0.1	0.15
Depo-Provera	0.3	0.3
Spermicides	3.0	21.0
Periodic abstinence		20.0
Calendar	9.0	
Ovulation method	3.0	
Symptothermal	2.0	
Postovulation	1.0	
Withdrawal	4.0	18.0
Cervical cap	6.0	18.0
Sponge		
Parous women	9.0	28.0
Nulliparous women	6.0	18.0
Diaphragm and spermicides	6.0	18.0
Condom	2.0	12.0

Reproduced with permission from Speroff L, Darney P. A clinical guide for contraception, 2nd ed. Baltimore: Williams and Wilkins, 1996:136.

▶ NATURAL METHODS

The methods of contraception covered in this section, periodic abstinence, coitus interruptus, and lactational amenorrhea, are **physiology-based methods** that use neither chemical nor mechanical barriers to contraception. Many couples, for deeply held religious or philosophic reasons, prefer these methods to other forms of contraception. However, these are the **least effective methods** of contraception and should not be used if pregnancy prevention is a high priority.

Periodic Abstinence

Method of Action

Periodic abstinence (the rhythm method) is a physiologic form of contraception that emphasizes **fertility awareness** and **abstinence** shortly before and after the estimated ovulation period. This method requires instruction on the physiology of menstruation and conception and on methods of determining ovulation. These **ovulation assessment** methods may include the use of basal body temperature (Fig. 22-1), menstrual cycle tracking, cervical mucus evaluation, and documentation of any premenstrual or ovulatory symptoms.

Effectiveness

The average effectiveness of periodic abstinence is relatively low (55 to 80%) compared with other forms of pregnancy prevention.

Advantages/Disadvantages

Periodic abstinence uses neither chemical nor mechanical barriers to conception and is, therefore, the method of choice for many couples for philosophic and/or religious reasons. However, this method requires a very motivated couple willing to learn reproductive physiology, to predict ovulation, and to abstain from intercourse. Periodic abstinence is relatively unreliable compared with the more traditional methods of contraception. This low reliability may require prolonged periods of abstinence, making it less desirable for some couples.

Coitus Interruptus

Method of Action

Coitus interruptus, or withdrawal of the penis from the vagina before ejaculation, is one of the oldest methods

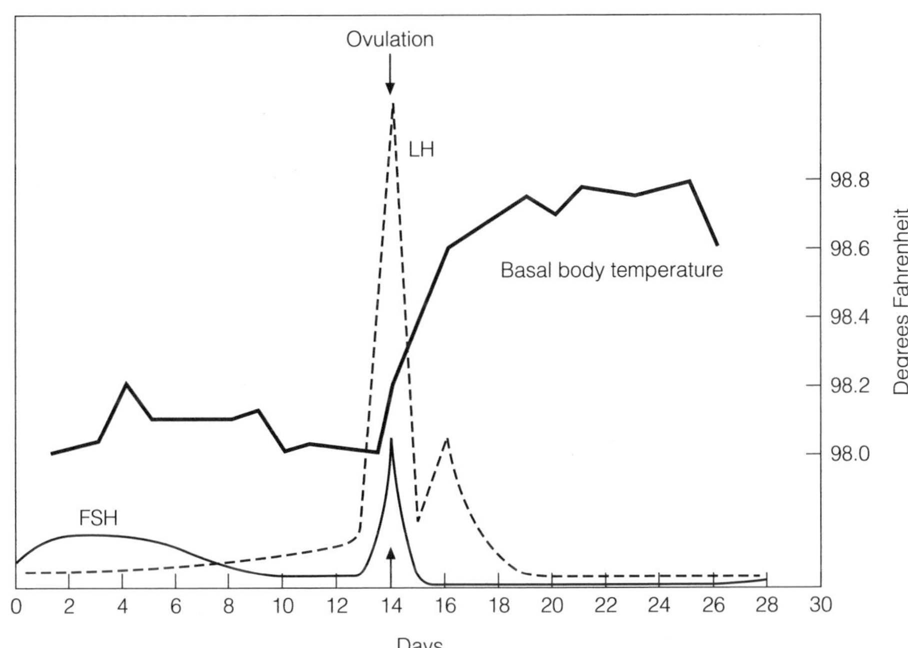

Figure 22-1 The relationship between ovulation and basal body temperature.

of contraception. With this method, the semen is deposited outside of the female reproductive tract with the intent of preventing fertilization.

Effectiveness

The failure rate for coitus interruptus is quite high (15 to 25%) compared with other forms of contraception. Failures can be attributed to the escape of semen into the vagina before orgasm or the deposition of semen near the introitus after intracrural intercourse.

Advantages/Disadvantages

The primary disadvantage of coitus interruptus is the high failure rate and the need for sufficient self-control to withdraw the penis before ejaculation.

Lactational Amenorrhea

Method of Action

After delivery, the restoration of ovulation is delayed because of a nursing-induced hypothalamic **suppression of ovulation**. Continuation of nursing has long been a widespread method of contraception for many couples.

Effectiveness

The duration of ovulatory suppression during nursing is highly variable. In fact, 50% of lactating mothers will begin to ovulate between 6 and 12 months after delivery, even while nursing. As a result, 15 to 55% of lactating mothers become pregnant even while nursing.

The effectiveness of lactational amenorrhea as a method of contraception can be enhanced by following certain principles. First, breastfeeding should be the only form of nutrition for the infant. Second, this method of contraception should be used only as long as the woman is experiencing amenorrhea, and even then, it should only be used for a **maximum of 6 months** after delivery. Following these guidelines, lactational amenorrhea as a method of contraception can have a failure rate as low as 2%.

Advantages/Disadvantages

Lactational amenorrhea has no effect on nursing. However, the efficacy rate is so low that it is an unacceptable and unreliable means of contraception.

Key Points

1. Natural family planning methods are the most ineffective methods of contraception and should not be used if pregnancy prevention is a high priority.
2. These methods rely on physiology to prevent pregnancy and require highly motivated users.
3. Periodic abstinence relies on accurate prediction of ovulation and abstinence from intercourse during periods of maximal fertility.
4. The length of lactational amenorrhea varies from woman to woman; therefore, this method should be used for a maximum of 6 months after delivery.

▶ BARRIER METHODS AND SPERMICIDES

These contraceptive methods work by preventing sperm from entering the endometrial cavity, fallopian tubes, and peritoneal cavity. Figure 22-2 shows the various forms of barrier and chemical contraceptives, including condoms, diaphragm, sponge, and spermicides.

Male Condoms

Method of Action

Condoms are latex sheaths placed over the erect penis before ejaculation. They prevent the ejaculate from being released into the reproductive tract of the woman.

Effectiveness

When properly used, the condom can be 98% effective in preventing conception. The actual efficacy rate in the population is 85 to 90%. To maximize effectiveness, it is important to leave a well at the tip of the condom to collect the ejaculate and to avoid leakage of semen as the penis is withdrawn.

Side Effects

Some individuals may experience an occasional hypersensitivity to the rubber, lubricant, or spermicide in condoms.

Advantages/Disadvantages

Condoms are widely available for a moderate cost and carry the added benefit of preventing the transmission of many **sexually transmitted infections.** They are the only method of contraception that offers protection against human immunodeficiency virus (HIV). Drawbacks of the condom include coital interruption and possible decreased male sensation.

Figure 22-2 Barrier and chemical methods of contraception.

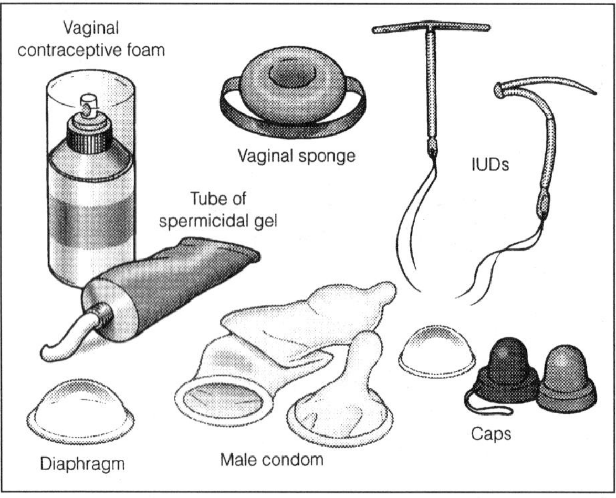

Female Condoms

Method of Action

The female condom or **Reality Vaginal Pouch** is a pouch made of polyurethane that has a flexible ring at each end. One ring fits into the depth of the vagina, and the other stays outside the vagina near the introitus (Fig. 22-3).

Effectiveness

Initial studies show that the failure rate of the female condom is 15 to 20%, somewhat higher than the male condom. However, these were short-term studies that may not reflect the failure rate with long-term usage.

Advantages/Disadvantages

Female condoms protect against many sexually transmitted infections while also placing the control of contraception with the female partner. Major drawbacks include their cost and their overall bulkiness. The overall acceptability rating is somewhat higher for the male partner (75 to 80%) than for the female partner (65 to 70%).

Figure 22-3 Placement of the female condom.

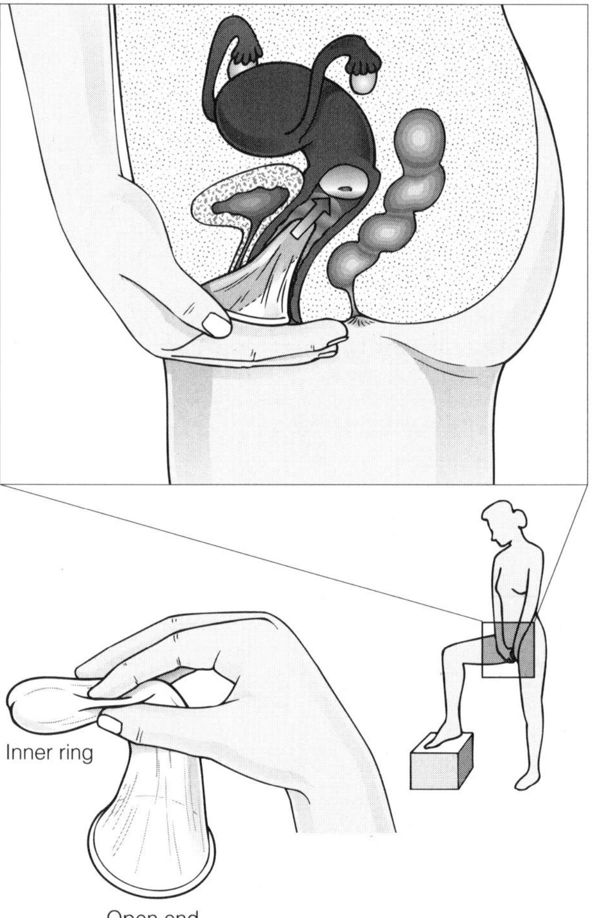

Diaphragm

Method of Action

The vaginal diaphragm is a domed sheet of rubber or latex stretched over a thin coiled rim. Spermicidal jelly is placed on the rim and on either side of the diaphragm, and it is placed into the vagina so that it covers the cervix (Fig. 22-4). The diaphragm and spermicide should be placed in the vagina before intercourse and left in place for **6 to 8 hours after intercourse.** If further intercourse is to take place before the diaphragm is removed, additional spermicide should be placed in the vagina without removing the diaphragm.

Effectiveness

The theoretic effectiveness of the diaphragm approaches 94%. The actual effectiveness rate of the diaphragm with spermicide is 80 to 85%.

Side Effects

Possible side effects include bladder irritation, which can lead to cystitis. If the diaphragm is left in place too long, colonization by *Staphylococcus aureus* may lead to the development of **toxic shock syndrome**. Some women also experience a hypersensitivity to the rubber or spermicide.

Figure 22-4 Placement of the vaginal diaphragm.

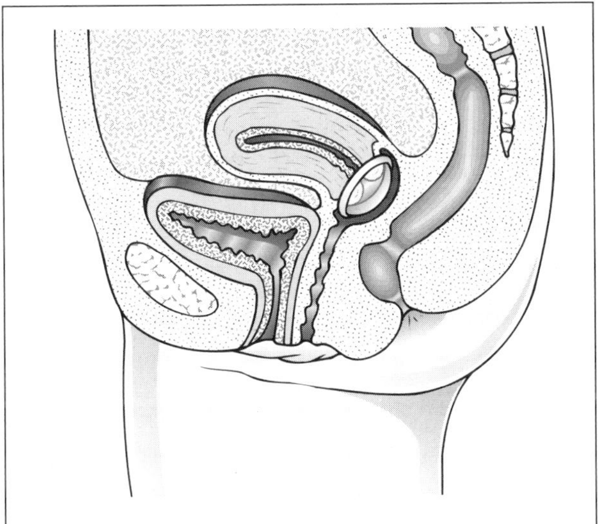

Advantages/Disadvantages

The diaphragm must be fitted and prescribed by a physician and costs significantly more than over-the-counter methods of contraception. The diaphragm should be replaced every 5 years or when the patient gains or loses more than 10 pounds. Women who are not comfortable with inserting the diaphragm or who cannot be properly fitted due to pelvic relaxation defects are poor candidates for the diaphragm.

Cervical Cap

Method of Action

The cervical cap is a small, soft, rubber cap that fits directly over the cervix (Fig. 22-5). It is held in place by suction and acts as a barrier to sperm. The cap must be fitted by a physician and must be used with a spermicidal jelly. Because of the variability in cervix size, proper fit and usage of the cap is essential to its effectiveness. Although it is widely used in Britain and Europe, the cervical cap is not widely available in the United States.

Figure 22-5 Placement of the cervical cap.

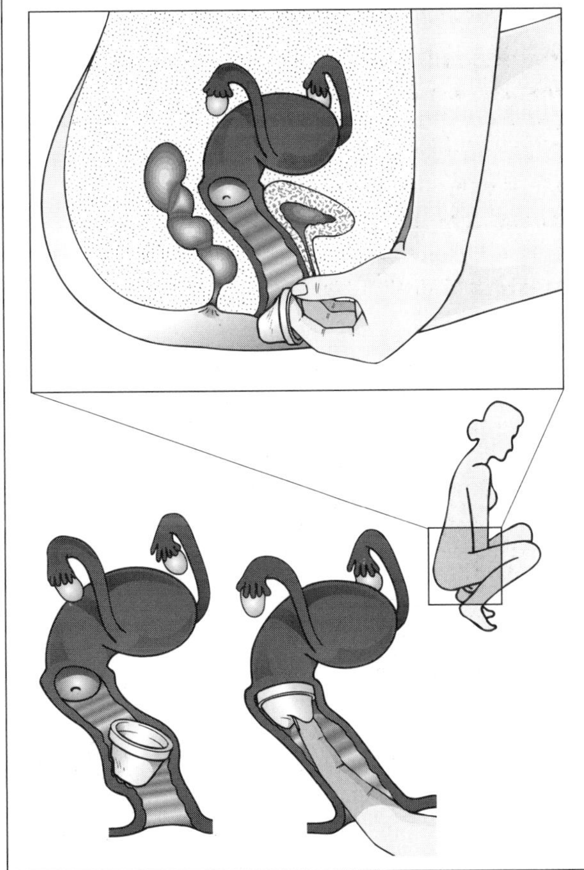

Effectiveness

The actual efficacy rate of the cervical cap is 80 to 85%, similar to the vaginal diaphragm. **Dislodgment** is the most common cause of failure.

Advantages/Disadvantages

One advantage of the cervical cap is that it can be left in place for 1 to 2 days. However, a foul discharge often develops after the first day. Also, many women have a difficult time mastering the placement and removal techniques for the cervical cap; as a result, the **continuation rate is low** (30 to 50%).

Contraceptive Sponge

Method of Action

The vaginal contraceptive sponge, or **Today sponge**, is a soft, polyurethane sponge embedded with the spermicide **nonoxynol-9**. The sponge is wetted before use to stimulate release of the spermicide and then it is placed high in the vagina over the cervix to act as both a chemical and physical barrier to sperm entry. The spermicide is **effective for 24 hours**. An elastic band on the sponge facilitates its removal. Production of the Today sponge in the United States ended in 1995.

Effectiveness

The efficacy of the Today sponge is similar to the vaginal diaphragm (80 to 85%). Pregnancy rates tend to be higher in parous women. This is thought to be due to dislodgment during intercourse.

Side Effects

Like the diaphragm, if the contraceptive sponge is left in place for extended periods, it may also pose the risk of **toxic shock syndrome**.

Advantages/Disadvantages

The contraceptive sponge can be purchased over the counter at a relatively low price. The failure rates are higher than some other methods of contraception.

Spermicides

Method of Action

Spermicidal agents come in a variety of forms, including creams, jellies, vaginal suppositories, foams, and vaginal contraceptive film. The most widely used spermicides are **nonoxynol-9 and octoxynol-9**. These agents both disrupt the cell membranes of spermatozoa and act as a mechanical barrier to the cervical canal. In general, spermicides should be placed in the vagina at least 30 minutes before intercourse to allow for dispersion throughout the vagina. Spermicides may be used alone or in conjunction with condoms, cervical caps, or diaphragms.

Effectiveness

When properly and consistently used, spermicides can have an effectiveness rate as high as 97%. However, in actual usage, the efficacy of spermicides when used alone is only 75 to 80%.

Side Effects

Occasionally, spermicides can irritate the vaginal mucosa and external genitalia.

Advantages/Disadvantages

Spermicidal agents are widely available in a variety of forms and are relatively inexpensive. Spermicides that contain nonoxynol-9 protect against **sexually transmitted infections**, including gonorrhea, syphilis, candida, trichomonas, and HIV.

Key Points

1. Condoms, diaphragms, cervical caps, and the sponge act as mechanical barriers between sperm and egg. Spermicides have both a barrier and spermicidal effect.
2. Condoms and spermicides containing nonoxynol-9 provide prophylaxis against sexually transmitted infections.
3. Diaphragms and cervical caps must be prescribed by a physician and are more expensive than other methods.
4. Chemical methods come in a variety of over-the-counter forms at minimal cost.
5. Efficacy for these methods is 75 to 80%, but variability in user technique can significantly lower efficacy.
6. Efficacy rates are greatly improved when using both barrier and spermicidal methods together.

▶ INTRAUTERINE DEVICES

Intrauterine devices (IUDs) have been used to prevent pregnancy since the 1800s. In the 1960s and 1970s, IUDs became extremely popular in the United States. However, legal problems stemming from pelvic infections caused by one particular IUD, the Dalkon shield, resulted in consumer fear and limited availability of all IUDs. Currently, only two IUDs are available in the United States: the copper **Paraguard** and the **Progestasert**. Despite this, with nearly 100 million users worldwide, the IUD is one of the most widely used methods of reversible contraception in the world (Fig. 22-6).

The IUD is especially indicated for women in whom oral contraceptives are contraindicated, those who are low risk for sexually transmitted infections,

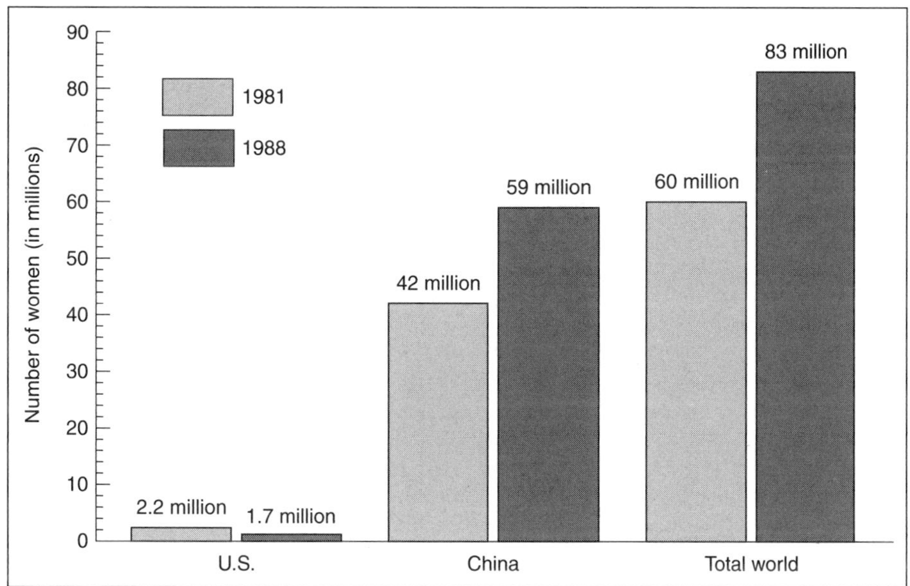

Figure 22-6 Use of IUD in the United States and the world.

and monogamous multigravid women. Absolute and relative contraindications for IUD use are shown in Table 22-2.

Method of Action

Intrauterine uterine devices made of plastic and/or metal are introduced into the endometrial cavity using a cervical cannula (Fig. 22-7). IUDs have one or two strings that extend through the cervix where it can be checked to detect expulsion or migration. The strings also facilitate removal of the device by the physician.

The mechanism of action for the IUD is not completely understood, but they are thought to elicit a sterile **spermicidal inflammatory response.** IUDs are also thought to inhibit implantation and alter tubal mobility. This foreign body reaction caused by IUDs is augmented by the addition of progesterone (Progestasert) or copper (Paraguard) to the device. IUDs do not affect ovulation nor do they act as abortifacients.

TABLE 22-2

Contraindications for IUD Use

Absolute contraindications
- Current pregnancy
- Undiagnosed abnormal vaginal bleeding
- Suspected gynecologic malignancy
- Acute cervical, uterine, or salpingeal infection
- Past salpingitis

Relative contraindications
- Nulliparity or desire for future child bearing
- Prior ectopic pregnancy
- History of sexually transmitted infections
- Multiple sexual partners
- Moderate or severe dysmenorrhea
- Congenital malformation of the uterus

Adapted from Speroff L, Darney P. A clinical guide for contraception. 2nd ed. Baltimore: Williams and Wilkins, 1996:195.

Effectiveness

The efficacy for IUDs is very high with a failure rate of less than 2% per year with prolonged use. During the first year of use, however, the failure rate is near 3% (thought to be due to unrecognized expulsions). IUDs also have a 10% expulsion rate and a 5 to 15% removal rate, mainly for pain and bleeding.

Side Effects

Although extremely safe, uncommon side effects and complications of intrauterine conception devices can be potentially severe and dangerous. These include pelvic infections, pain and bleeding, pregnancy, expulsion, and perforation.

Women who use IUDs appear to be at increased risk for **insertion-related salpingo-oophoritis.** This increased risk is now believed to be due to contamination of the endometrial cavity at the time of insertion. Otherwise, pelvic infection is rarely seen beyond the first 20 days after insertion. Prophylactic antibiotics (Doxycycline or azithromycin) at the time of insertion provide protection against insertion-related infections.

Intermenstrual **bleeding**, menorrhagia, and menstrual **pain** may occur in as many as 20% of women who use IUDs, particularly in nulliparous women. These are the primary reasons for discontinuation of IUD use.

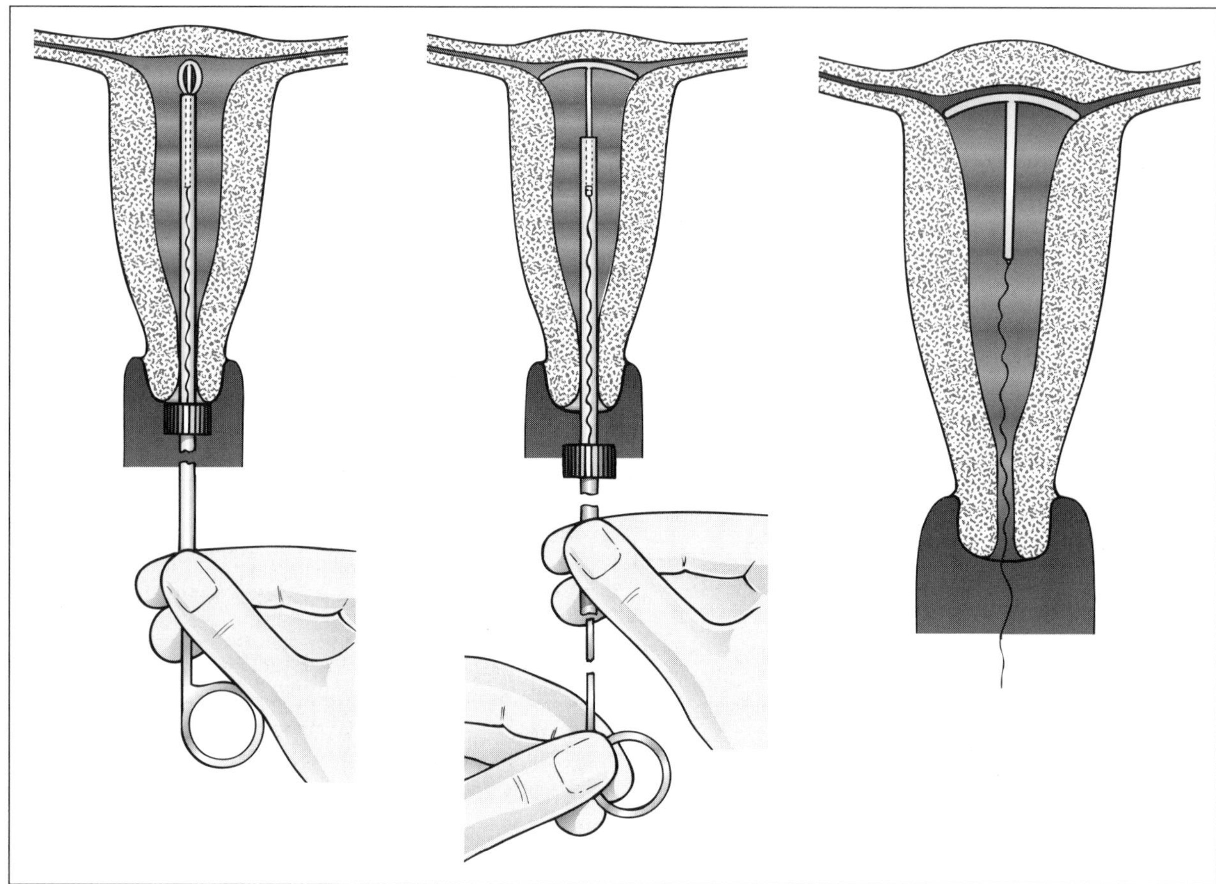

Figure 22-7 Placement of an intrauterine device.

The **spontaneous abortion** rate is increased to 40 to 50% for women who become pregnant with an IUD in place. Given this, if intrauterine pregnancy occurs while an IUD is in place, the device should be removed by gentle traction on the string. The risk of life-threatening, spontaneous septic abortion has only been seen with the Dalkon Shield. The IUD is not associated with an increased risk of congenital abnormalities.

Five percent of women with IUDs will experience an **expulsion** of the device usually with associated cramping or bleeding. The incidence is higher during the first year of use and in younger women with lower parity. **Perforation** of the uterine wall by an IUD is relatively rare, occurring in 1 of every 5,000 IUD users.

Advantages/Disadvantages

The IUD must be prescribed, inserted, and removed by a physician. However, once in place, the user must do little other than periodic follow-ups to check for expulsion and infection. The Progestasert must be replaced annually, whereas the lifespan of the Paraguard is 8 years. The IUD carries the added benefit of providing **protection against ectopic pregnancy** while in situ. Although this decreased risk of ectopic pregnancy is not as low as that found with oral contraceptives, use of an IUD lowers a woman's risk by 50% compared with noncontraceptive users.

Key Points

1. IUDs are less well tolerated by nulliparous women but are ideal for the monogamous multiparous women in whom the pill is contraindicated.
2. The primary mechanism of action is a sterile spermicidal inflammatory response. Other mechanisms include inhibition of implantation and alteration in tubal motility.
3. The failure rates for IUD use are very low ($<2\%$) with prolonged use but higher in first year of use.
4. Potentially serious side effects include insertion-related salpingitis, spontaneous abortion, and uterine perforation. The IUD provides protection against ectopic pregnancy while in situ.

▶ HORMONAL METHODS

Hormonal contraceptives are the most commonly used reversible means of preventing pregnancy in the United States.

Oral Contraception Pill

Method of Action

Oral contraceptive pills (OCPs) are composed of progesterone alone or a combination of progesterone and estrogen. Over 150 million women worldwide, including one third of sexually active women in the United States, use oral contraceptives. Oral contraceptives place the body in a **"pseudopregnancy"** state by interfering with the pulsatile release of follicle-stimulating hormone (FSH) and luteinizing hormone (LH) from the anterior pituitary. This **suppresses ovulation** and prevents pregnancy from occurring. Figure 22-8 illustrates the serum levels of FSH and LH during the normal menstrual cycle, and Figure 22-9 shows FSH and LH levels during a cycle on the combination pill. Because the FSH and LH surges do not occur, follicle growth, recruitment, and ovulation do not occur.

Secondary mechanisms of action for OCPs include changing the **cervical mucus** to render it less penetrable by sperm and changing the **endometrium** to make it unsuitable for implantation.

Monophasic (Fixed Combination) Pills Combination pills contain a fixed dose of estrogen and a fixed dose of progestin in each tablet. Nearly 30 different combinations of estrogen and progestins are available in the United States. In general, the selection of a particular pill for each patient depends on the individual side effects and risk factors for each patient.

Figure 22-8 Serum levels of FSH and LH during the normal menstrual cycle.

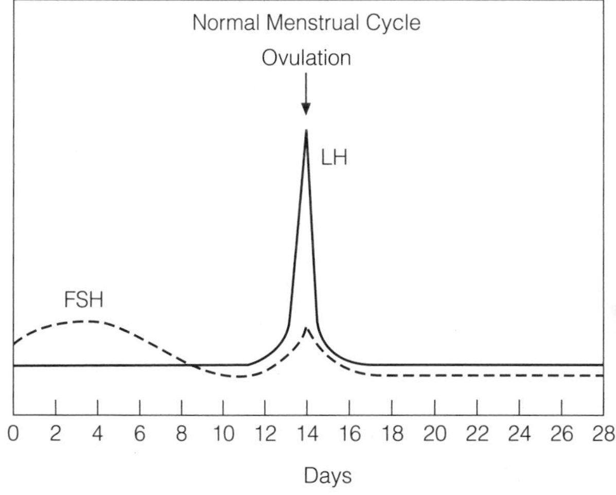

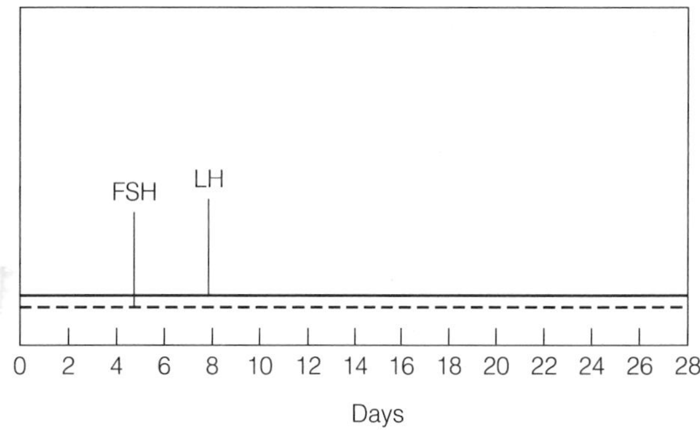

Figure 22-9 Serum levels of FSH and LH while taking monophasic oral contraceptive pills.

The combination pill is taken for the first 21 days out of a 28-day monthly cycle. During the last 7 days of the cycle, a placebo pill or no pill is taken. Bleeding should begin within 3 to 5 days of completion of the 21-day regimen.

Multiphasic (Dose Varying) Pills Multiphasic oral contraceptives differ from monophasic only in that they vary the dosage of progestin each week during these 21 days. The advantage of the multiphasic dosing is that they may provide a lower level of estrogen and progestin overall but are still highly effective at preventing pregnancy.

Progestin-Only Pills (The Minipill) Progestin-only pills are taken every day of the cycle to deliver a small daily dose of progestin. It is thought that the cervical mucus becomes less permeable to sperm and the endometrium becomes less appropriate for implantation. Progestin-only pills are generally **not as effective** (failure rate is 3 to 7%) as combination or multiphasic regimens and are also associated with irregular ovulatory cycles, breakthrough bleeding, and ectopic pregnancy. However, because they contain no estrogen, progestin-only pills are ideal for nursing mothers and patients for whom estrogens are contraindicated.

Effectiveness

OCPs are remarkably effective in preventing pregnancy. In fact, the theoretic failure rate for the first year of use is less than 1%. However, the actual failure rate is closer to 3%. Nausea, breakthrough bleeding, and the need to take the pill every day are often cited as reasons for discontinuing the pill.

Several medications interact with oral contraceptives and reduce the effectiveness of the pill. Conversely, oral contraceptives can also reduce the efficacy of many medications (Table 22-3).

TABLE 22-3
Interactions of Oral Contraceptives with Other Medications

Medications That Reduce the Efficacy of Oral Contraceptives	Medications Whose Efficacies are Reduced by Oral Contraceptives
Penicillins	Folates
Tetracycline	Anticoagulants
Rifampin	Insulin
Ibuprophen	Methyldopa
Phenytoin	Hypoglycemics
Barbiturates	Phenothiazides
Sulfonamides	Tricyclic antidepressants

TABLE 22-4
Complications Associated with Oral Contraceptives

Cardiovascular
- Thromboembolism*
- Pulmonary embolism*
- Cerebrovascular accident*
- Myocardial infarction*
- Hypertension*

Other complications
- Benign hepatic tumors
- Increase in gallbladder disease

*These complications occur mainly in smokers.

Adapted with permission from Hacker N, Moore JG. Essentials of obstetrics and gynecology. Philadelphia: WB Saunders, 1992:456.

Side Effects

Table 22-4 lists some of the cardiovascular, neoplastic, and biliary complications associated with oral contraceptive use.

Oral contraceptives with estrogen doses over 50 μg can increase coagulability, leading to higher rates of myocardial infarction, stroke, thromboembolism, and pulmonary embolism in women using these pills. The progestins in oral contraceptives have been found to raise low-density lipoproteins while lowering high-density lipoproteins in pill users smoking more than 1 pack per day. For these reasons, oral contraceptives are contraindicated in women over the age of 35 who smoke cigarettes. The advent of new progestins and lower estrogen doses has led to pill formulations that are essentially neutral in terms of cardiovascular effect. However, oral contraceptive use is still contraindicated in women over the age of 35 who smoke.

Neoplastic complications of oral contraceptive use are rare. The impact of the long-term oral contraceptive use on breast cancer has been studied extensively over the past decade with no conclusive findings. There is, however, an increased incidence of gallbladder disease and benign hepatic tumors associated with oral contraceptive use.

Table 22-5 illustrates both the absolute and relative contraindications to oral contraceptive use.

Advantages/Disadvantages

The major advantages of the pill include its extremely high efficacy rates and the noncontraceptive health benefits, including a reduced incidence of ovarian cancer, endometrial cancer, ectopic pregnancy, pelvic inflammatory disease, and benign breast disease (Table 22-6). Nearly 50,000 women avoid hospitalizations; of these, 10,000 avoid hospitalization for life-threatening

TABLE 22-5
Absolute and Relative Contraindications to Oral Contraceptives

Absolute Contraindications	Relative Contraindications	Other Relative Contraindications
Venous thrombosis	Uterine fibroids	An/oligo-ovulation
Pulmonary embolism	Lactation	Depression
Coronary vascular disease	Diabetes mellitus	Hyperlipidemia
Cerebrovascular accident	Sickle cell disease	Acne
Breast/endometrial CA	Hypertension	Severe varicose veins
Melanoma	Age 35+ and smoking	Severe headaches (especially vascular)
Hepatic tumor	Age 40+ and high risk for vascular disease	
Abnormal liver function		

Reproduced by permission from Hacker N, Moore JG. Essentials of obstetrics and gynecology. Philadelphia: WB Saunders, 1992:460.

TABLE 22-6
Noncontraceptive Health Benefits of Oral Contraceptives

Decreases life-threatening diseases
- Ovarian cancer
- Endometrial cancer
- Ectopic pregnancy
- Anemia
- Pelvic inflammatory disease

Alleviates quality-of-life problems
- Iron deficiency anemia
- Dysmenorrhea
- Functional ovarian cysts
- Benign breast disease
- Osteoporosis

Adapted from Hacker N, Moore JG. Essentials of obstetrics and gynecology. Philadelphia: WB Saunders, 1992:458.

illnesses due to the protection afforded them by oral contraceptives. Disadvantages include cardiovascular complications, increased gallbladder disease, increased incidence of benign hepatic tumors, and the need to take a medication every day.

Norplant

Method of Action

Norplant was approved for marketing in the United States in 1990. It is a "sustained release" system composed of six flexible silastic rods, each containing 36 mg of the progesterone **levonorgestrel**. The rods are placed in the subcutaneous tissue of the upper arm (Fig. 22-10) and progesterone is slowly released over a period of 5 years.

The progestin in Norplant circulates at levels one fourth to one tenth of the level obtained with oral contraceptives. Norplant acts by suppressing ovulation, thickening the cervical mucus to inhibit sperm penetration, and making the endometrium unsuitable for implantation.

Effectiveness

The efficacy of Norplant is extremely high, with a failure rate of 0.2%.

Side Effects

Because Norplant contains low levels of progestin and does not contain estrogen, it is not associated with any serious side effects. The sustained progestin release, however, does cause some bothersome side effects, including irregular vaginal bleeding, headaches, weight change, and mood changes. There are no long-term health sequelae associated with the use of Norplant. In contrast to Depo-Provera (see below), discontinuation of Norplant is not associated with any significant delay in the restoration of fertility.

Advantages/Disadvantages

The major advantages of Norplant are that it is a highly effective, long-term, reversible contraception method that does not have the adverse effects of estrogen. Norplant is as effective as sterilization and IUDs and more effective than oral contraceptives and barrier methods. Unlike injectable methods, Norplant is rapidly reversible. The major disadvantages are that it requires a physician to implant and remove the rods. The one-time cost of Norplant may be prohibitive for some women, but over the 5-year effectiveness period, the cost is equivalent to using oral contraceptives over the same period.

Depo-Provera

Method of Action

Although it was only approved for contraceptive use in the United States in 1992, Depo-Provera (**medroxyprogesterone acetate**) has been used in other countries since the mid-1960s. Depo-Provera is injected intramuscularly in a vehicle that allows the slow release of progesterone over 3 months. Depo-Provera acts by suppressing ovulation, thickening the cervical mucus, and making the endometrium unsuitable for implantation.

Effectiveness

With a failure rate of only 0.3%, Depo-Provera is one of the most effective contraceptive methods available.

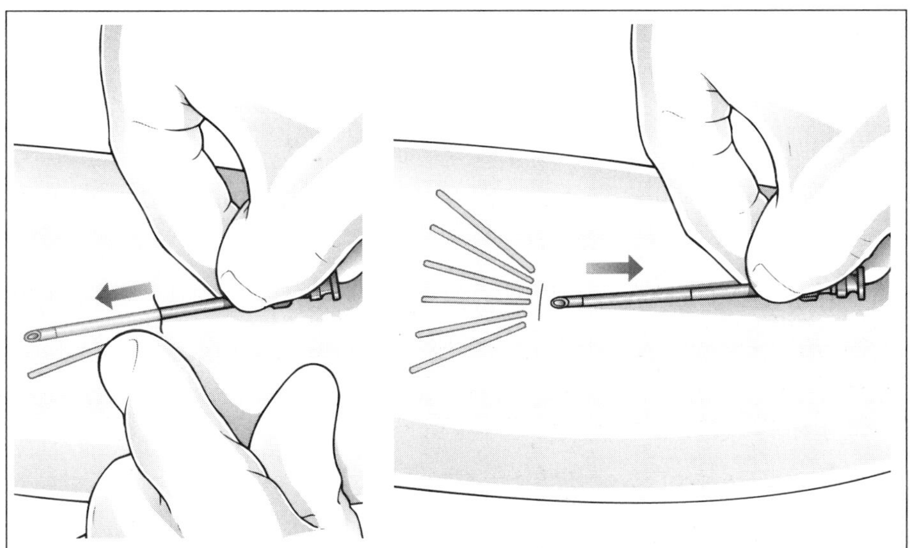

Figure 22-10 Norplant insertion.

Side Effects

The primary side effects experienced by Depo-Provera users include **irregular menstrual bleeding**, depression, weight gain, and breast tenderness. Over 70% of patients experience spotting and irregular menses during the first year of use. This is the primary reason for discontinuing Depo-Provera.

Advantages/Disadvantages

The primary advantages of Depo-Provera are that it is highly effective, long-lived, and acts independent of intercourse and only requires injections every 3 months. Irregular bleeding, weight gain, and mood changes are the major disadvantages. After discontinuation of Depo-Provera injections, many women experience a significant delay in the return of regular ovulation. Within 18 months, however, fertility rates return to normal levels.

Key Points

1. Hormonal contraceptives have extremely low failure rates.
2. Oral contraceptives prevent pregnancy by interfering with FSH and LH to suppress ovulation, alter cervical mucus, and cause atrophic changes in the endometrium.
3. Serious complications from OCP use occur mainly in smokers, including pulmonary embolism, stroke, deep venous thrombosis, heart attack, and hypertension.
4. Benefits of OCPs include protection from ovarian and endometrial cancer and reduction in ectopic pregnancy, pelvic inflammatory disease, osteoporosis, and benign breast disease.
5. Both Norplant and Depo-Provera use progestins to suppress ovulation, thicken the cervical mucus, and make the endometrium unsuitable for implantation. Norplant provides up to 5 years of protection and Depo-Provera provides 3 months of protection.
6. The side effects of Norplant include irregular bleeding, weight gain, and headaches. Primary side effects of Depo-Provera include irregular bleeding, weight gain, and depression.
7. Depo-Provera, *unlike* Norplant, is associated with significant delay in restoration of ovulation after discontinuation.

▶ SURGICAL STERILIZATION

The rate of surgical sterilization as a method of contraception has increased dramatically over the past three decades. Approximately 30% of reproductive-age couples in the Unites States and Great Britain choose female sterilization for contraceptive purposes. A similar number of men seek vasectomies each year. The rate of sterilization is higher in women who are married, divorced, over 30, or African-American.

Careful counseling and informed consent on the permanent nature of the procedure, operative risks, chance of failure, and possible side effects should be obtained before performing any sterilization procedure. Sterilization is ideal in stable monogamous relationships where no additional children are desired.

Tubal Sterilization

Method of Action

Tubal sterilization prevents pregnancy by surgically occluding both fallopian tubes to prevent the ovum and sperm from uniting. There are a number of methods by which tubal occlusion can be accomplished, including banding (Fig. 22-11), clipping (Fig. 22-12), and coagulating and/or ligating the fallopian tubes. These procedures are performed under general anesthesia. The most commonly used method, the Pomeroy tubal ligation, is shown in Figure 22-13.

Effectiveness

Tubal occlusion has a failure rate of < 1%.

Figure 22-11 Tubal occlusion with the Falope Ring.

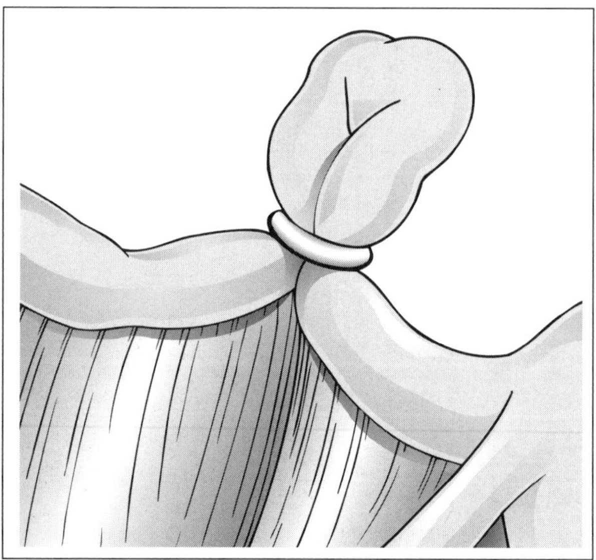

Figure 22-12 Tubal occlusion with the Hulka Clip.

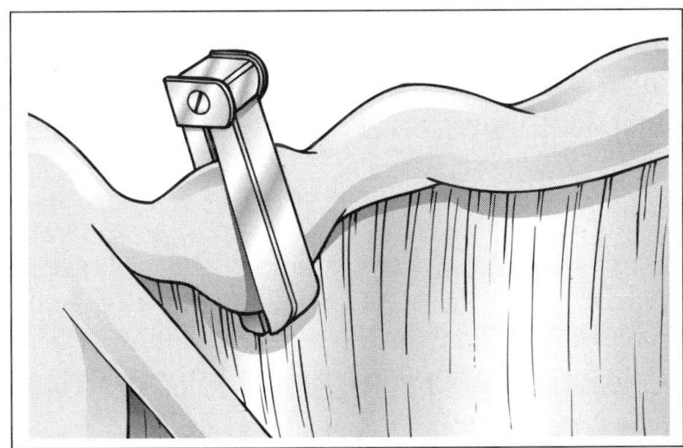

Side Effects

There are **no side effects** of tubal sterilization. Some women report pain and menstrual disturbances (post-tubal ligation syndrome) after the procedure. In most of these women, these symptoms are due to discontinuation of oral contraceptives that results in their baseline heavier periods and dysmenorrhea.

Advantages/Disadvantages

Tubal ligation offers the advantage of permanent effective contraception without continual expense, effort, or motivation. The mortality rate of bilateral tubal ligation is 4 women per 100,000. One in 15,000 women who undergo tubal sterilization will have an ectopic pregnancy at some point after the procedure. However, nearly 1,000 maternal lives are saved due to

Figure 22-13 The Pomeroy method of tubal sterilization.

A

B

C

D

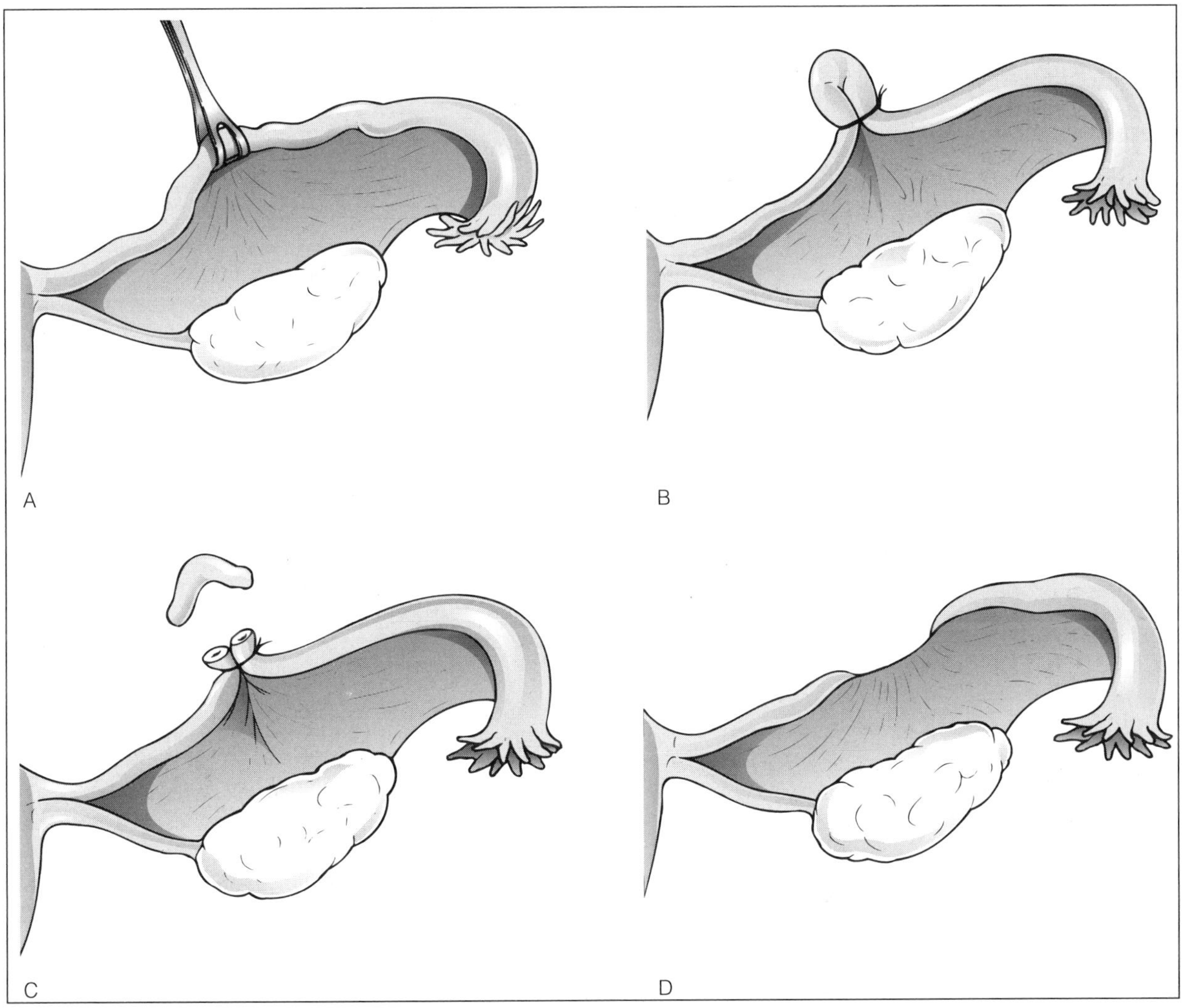

sterilization during the period from the time of sterilization to the end of the woman's reproductive period.

Studies estimate that only 1% of women seek reversal of tubal sterilization. The success of reversal varies from 41 to 84% depending on the method (Table 22-7). When pregnancy is desired after tubal ligation, in vitro fertilization offers a greater likelihood of pregnancy than does tubal microplasty.

TABLE 22-7

Success Rates of Tubal Occlusion Reversal by Method

Method of Tubal Sterilization	Success Rates for Reversal (%)
Clips	84
Bands	72
Pomeroy	50
Electrocauterization	41

Vasectomy

Methods of Action

Vasectomy is a simple and safe option for permanent sterilization involving ligation of the vas deferens. The procedure may be performed in a physician's office under local anesthesia through a small incision in the upper outer aspect of the scrotum (Fig. 22-14). Because sperm can remain viable in the proximal collecting system after vasectomy, patients should use another form of contraception for 4 to 6 weeks until azoospermia is confirmed by semen analysis.

Effectiveness

The failure rate for vasectomy is <1%. Many of these pregnancies are due to intercourse too soon after vasectomy rather than from recanalization.

Figure 22-14 (A–F) Sterilization by vasectomy.

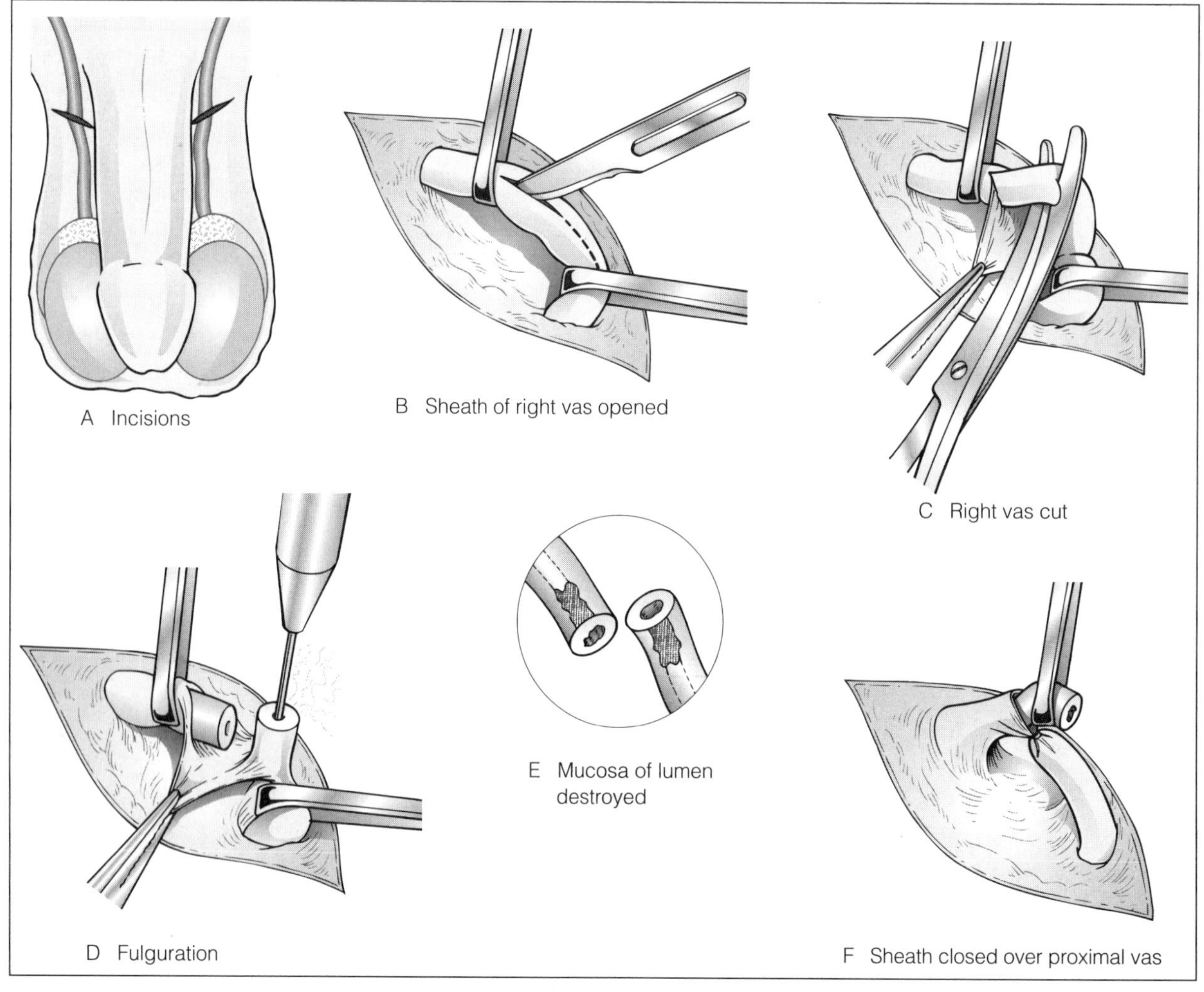

Side Effects

Complications after vasectomy are rare and usually involve slight bleeding, skin infection, and reactions to the sutures or local anesthesia. Fifty percent of patients will form **antisperm antibodies** after the procedure. However, there are no long-term side effects of vasectomy.

Advantages/Disadvantages

Vasectomy is a permanent highly effective form of contraception with few, if any, side effects. Vasectomy is generally safer and less expensive than tubal ligation. Vasectomy offers permanent sterility that may be a disadvantage for some couples. The success rate of vasal reanastomosis is 60 to 70%. Pregnancy rates after vasectomy reversal range from 18 to 60%.

Key Points

1. Surgical sterilization has increased dramatically in the past 30 years.
2. Both vasectomy and tubal occlusion are highly effective forms of permanent sterilization.
3. Tubal ligations are performed under general anesthesia with few, if any, side effects.
4. Reversal rates for tubal occlusion vary from 41 to 84% depending on the method used for sterilization.
5. Complications after vasectomy are rare and minimal.
6. The success rate of vasal reanastomosis is 60 to 70% with pregnancy rates from 18 to 60%.

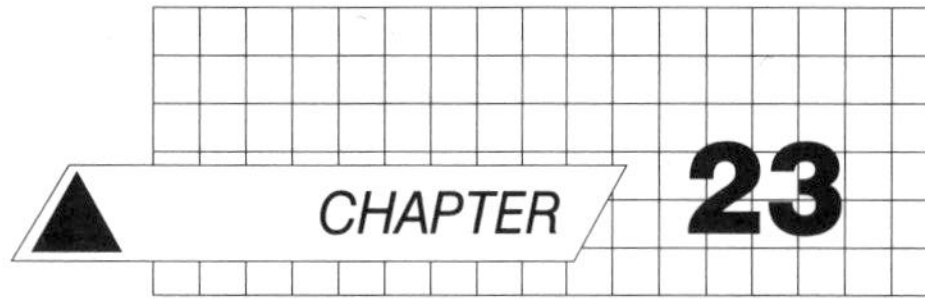

Therapeutic Abortion

It is estimated that 25% of all pregnancies worldwide end in induced abortion. Since its legalization in 1973, one legal abortion in the United States is performed for every four live births. Currently, about 1 million abortions are performed annually in the United States. One third of these procedures are performed on teenagers.

The abortion procedures used legally in the United States are both safe and effective. Risk of death from an abortion during the first 2 months of pregnancy is less than 1 per 100,000 procedures (Fig. 23-1). In fact, first trimester abortions have a lower mortality rate than using no birth control and giving birth. In general, however, maternal morbidity is lowest if legal abortion is performed before 8 weeks gestation (see Fig. 23-1). The major cause of abortion mortality is from general anesthesia.

There are many methods by which pregnancy terminations can be achieved. **Vaginal evacuation options** include suction curettage, dilatation and curettage, and dilatation and evacuation. The second option includes the **induction of labor** through intra-amniotic instillation of hypertonic saline, urea, or prostaglandins or by the use of prostaglandin suppositories. **Medical options** include the antiprogestin agent, RU-486, and the postcoital pill. In general, the technique to be used for termination is determined by the duration of the pregnancy. Table 23-1 shows the various options available for first versus second trimester abortions. Once the fetus has reached the stage of viability at about 24 weeks gestation, abortions are only allowed when necessary for the preservation of maternal life.

▶ FIRST TRIMESTER OPTIONS

Suction curettage, RU-486, and the postcoital pill are all methods of inducing abortion in the first trimester. Ninety percent of all abortions in the United States are achieved using suction curettage. The mortality incidence is 1 in 100,000 patients. In general, the risk of complications after suction curettage is directly proportional to the gestational age.

Suction Curettage

Methods of Action

Suction curettage (dilatation and vacuum aspiration) is both a safe and effective means of terminating a pregnancy at 12 weeks or less (Fig. 23-2). This procedure involves dilation of the cervix and removal of the products of conception using a suction cannula.

Effectiveness

When performed by a trained physician, the failure rate for suction curettage is extremely low.

Side Effects

Complications for suction curettage are rare and include infection (1%), excessive bleeding (2%), and uterine perforation (1%). There is no evidence that cervical dilatation for termination procedures leads to a higher incidence of cervical incompetence.

RU-486 (Mifepristone)

Methods of Action

RU-486, or mifepristone, is a synthetic hormone that binds to progesterone receptors to **block the effects of progesterone**. RU-486 is given orally in combination with a prostaglandin to stimulate abortion during the first half of the first trimester. The actual mechanism is unclear but it is thought to block the stimulatory effects of progesterone on endometrial growth.

Effectiveness

When given with a prostaglandin, the success rate of expulsion using RU-486 is over 90%. The efficacy rate for RU-486 declines significantly for pregnancies greater than 7 weeks gestation.

Side Effects

Side effects for RU-486 include incomplete abortion, failed abortion, and substantial uterine cramping.

Advantages/Disadvantages

RU-486 offers the advantages of being a highly effective noninvasive means of termination that can be achieved on an outpatient basis. The major disadvantage is that the woman must deal with the products of conception at home.

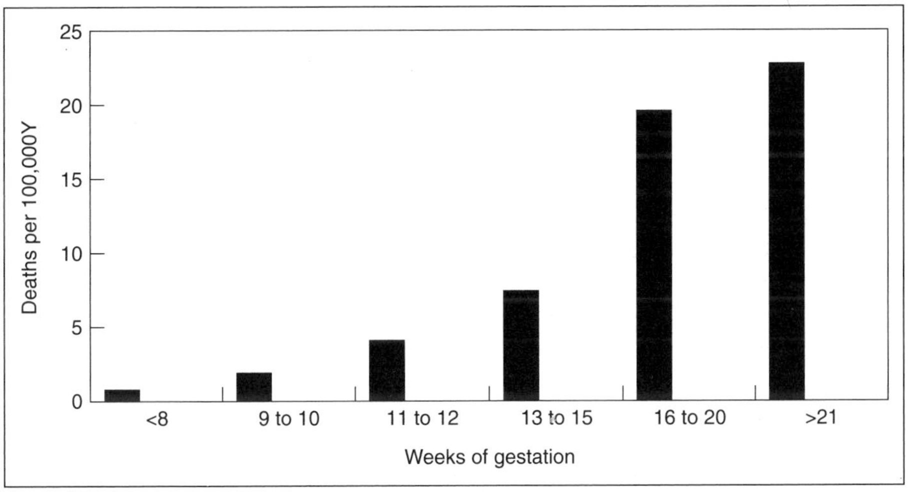

25
20
15
10
5
0
Deaths per 100,000Y
<8
9 to 10
11 to 12
13 to 15
16 to 20
>21
Weeks of gestation

Figure 23-1 The impact of gestational age on maternal mortality for legal abortions.

TABLE 23-1

Termination of Pregnancy Options by Gestational Age

First trimester terminations
Suction curettage
RU-486 (mifepristone)
Postcoital pill
Second trimester terminations
Intra-amniotic instillation
Intravaginal prostaglandins
Dilation and evacuation

Postcoital Pill

Methods of Action

The postcoital or "morning after" pill is a regimen of **high doses of estrogen** used to prevent pregnancy *after* intercourse has taken place. The mechanism of action varies widely depending on the point in the cycle in which the pill is given. Depending on when the pill is given in the cycle, it may act to suppress ovulation and to accelerate the ovum through the fallopian tube and endometrial cavity so that fertilization does not take place.

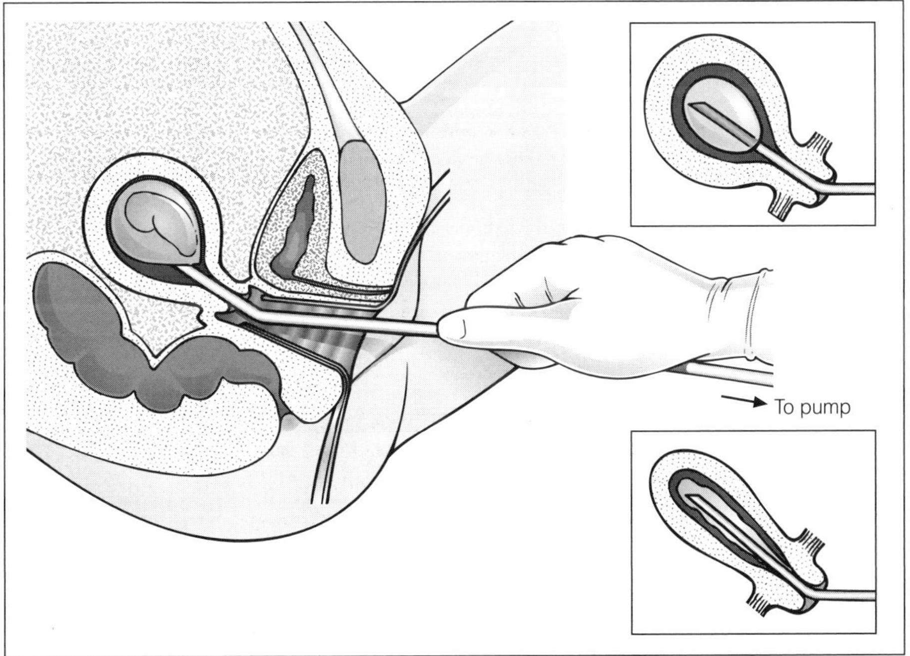

Figure 23-2 Suction of uterine cavity for termination of pregnancy.

Effectiveness

When taken within 72 hours of intercourse, the postcoital pill has a failure rate of 0 to 2.5%.

Side Effects

The primary side effects of postcoital estrogens include bloating, nausea, and vomiting during the drug regimen. The patient should also be advised that congenital malformations are possible if the pregnancy does occur.

Advantages/Disadvantages

The postcoital pill is extremely effective in preventing pregnancy. The major disadvantages include the short window of time when it can be used (within 72 hours of intercourse) and the possible teratogenic effects to the fetus in cases where a pregnancy ensues despite use of the postcoital pill.

Key Points

1. First trimester abortion options include suction curettage, RU-486 and the postcoital pill as very effective methods of termination.
2. Ninety percent of all abortions in the United States are achieved using suction curettage. Complications are rare including infection, bleeding, and perforation.
3. RU-486 is an abortifacient that blocks progesterone. It may be used in combination with a local prostaglandin. The mechanism of action is unclear but RU-486 is thought to cause asynchronization of the endometrium.
4. The postcoital pill contains high doses of estrogen given within 72 hours of intercourse to prevent pregnancy. The pill acts to suppress ovulation and to prevent fertilization or implantation.
5. Side effects of the postcoital pill are bloating, nausea, and vomiting. Estrogens can potentially cause congenital malformations if pregnancy does occur.

▶ SECOND TRIMESTER OPTIONS

Congenital abnormalities are the major reasons for second trimester abortions (12 to 24 weeks gestation). Termination of pregnancy options for the second trimester include intra-amniotic instillation agents, vaginal prostaglandins, and dilatation and evacuation (see Table 23-1). The upper limits of gestation at which these techniques can be legally performed varies from country to country. In the United States, these procedures, where permitted, may only be used up until the time of fetal viability (approximately 24 weeks), unless the mother's life is endangered. When a second trimester termination is necessary, **dilatation and evacuation** has been found to be safer than induction of labor procedures.

Induction of Labor

Method of Action

Labor can be induced to cause abortion by the instillation of agents into the amnion to stimulate uterine contractions and the expulsion of the fetus and placenta hours later (Table 23-2). The instillation substances include hypertonic saline, hyperosmolar urea, and prostaglandin F_{2alpha}. Induction of labor can also be achieved with prostaglandin E_2 suppositories placed in the vagina every 3 to 4 hours until labor begins.

Effectiveness

The success rates for second trimester abortions using induction of labor vary from 80 to 100% depending on the regimen used. The maternal mortality rate for second semester abortions using instillation agents or vaginal prostaglandins is comparable with that of term delivery.

Advantages/Disadvantages

The complication rate for abortion by induction of labor can be quite high (Table 23-3). Vaginal prostaglandins have a higher incidence of live births and significant gastrointestinal side effects, whereas instillation agents have a high rate of retained placenta (13 to 46%). Hypertonic saline may induce hyperosmotic coma, hypernatremia, and diffuse intravascular coagulation. As a result, urea and prostaglandin have largely replaced the use of hypertonic saline for amnioinfusion techniques.

TABLE 23-2

Injection-Abortion Intervals for Amniotic Infusion

Amnio-Infusion Agent	Injection-Abortion Interval (hr)
Hypertonic (20%) saline	<48
Prostaglandin F_{2alpha}	19–22
Hyperosmolar (59.7%) urea	16–17

TABLE 23-3

Complications Associated with Second Trimester Abortion by Induction of Labor

Complications	Side effects
Retained placenta	Nausea
Incomplete abortion	Vomiting
Hemorrhage	Diarrhea
Emotional stress	Fever

The disadvantages of induction of labor as a method of abortion include the high rate of complications and the profound emotional stress of abortion given that the patient is awake, the treatment-abortion intervals are lengthy, and the fetus is well formed at delivery. Intravaginal prostaglandins carry the added disadvantage of increased rates of live births.

Dilation and Evacuation

Method of Action

This method of termination is very similar to suction curettage but is reserved for second trimester terminations. It involves the gradual dilatation of the cervix using *Laminaria* tents or metal dilators followed by introduction of large suction cannulas into the uterus to extract the fetal tissue and placenta.

Advantages/Disadvantages

Complications from dilation and evacuation are uncommon but may include hemorrhage, perforation, infection, and retained tissues. As a method of second trimester abortion, dilation and evacuation offers the advantage of being performed on an outpatient basis without the need to undergo labor and delivery. Also, complications from dilation and evacuation occur at rates lower than those for intra-amniotic instillation or intravaginal prostaglandin abortions.

Key Points

1. During the second trimester, abortion may be achieved through induction of labor or dilation and evacuation. The mortality rate for these procedures is similar to a term delivery.
2. Induction of labor techniques includes instillation of saline, urea, or prostaglandins or use of intravaginal prostaglandin suppositories.
3. Complication rates are quite high for induction of labor (13 to 46%) and complications include retained placenta, hemorrhage, coagulopathy, infection, and cervical laceration. Intravaginal prostaglandins have an increased incidence of gastrointestinal side effects and live births.
4. Dilation and evacuation is similar to suction curettage and safer than induction of labor for second trimester abortion. Complications are uncommon but may include hemorrhage, infection, perforation, and retained tissue.

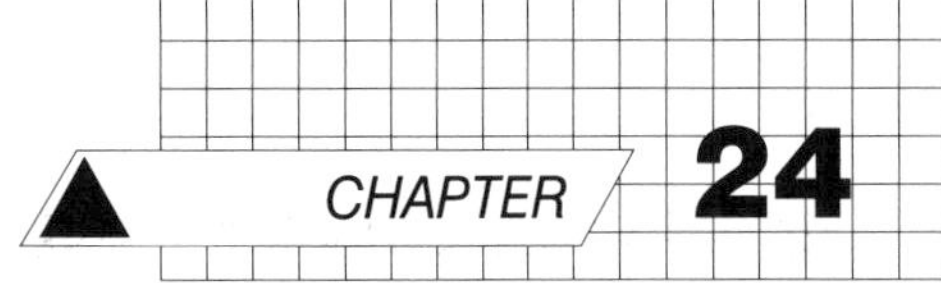

Infertility and Assisted Reproduction

▶ ETIOLOGY

Infertility is the inability to conceive after 1 year of unprotected intercourse. Although the overall incidence of infertility remained relatively unchanged between 1968 and 1992, the number of office visits to physicians by couples seeking infertility treatment nearly tripled, partially due to the availability of new treatment options for infertility. These treatments include ovulation induction, intrauterine insemination (IUI), in vitro fertilization (IVF), gamete intrafallopian transfer (GIFT), egg and sperm donation, and surrogacy.

Normally, 85 to 90% of couples are able to conceive within 18 months (Table 24-1). For the remaining 10 to 15% of couples who are incapable of conceiving on their own within that period, the factors contributing to infertility are varied and often multiple (20% of cases). Of couples who undergo evaluation for infertility, 40% of cases are attributed to male factors, 40% to female factors, and 20% have no identifiable cause (Table 24-2). Fortunately, modern technologies make it possible to identify the one or more possible causes for infertility in 80 to 90% of cases. In these cases, appropriate therapy will result in pregnancy in 50% of the time.

▶ MALE FACTOR INFERTILITY

Pathogenesis

There are multiple causes of male factor infertility (Table 24-3). Included among these are endocrine disorders, anatomic disorders, abnormal spermatogenesis, abnormal sperm motility, and sexual dysfunction.

TABLE 24-1

Average Conception Rates for All Couples

Percent of Couples		Length of Time Before Conception (mo)
20%	conceive within	1
60%	conceive within	6
75%	conceive within	9
80%	conceive within	12
90%	conceive within	18

Epidemiology

Male factor is the definitive cause or one of the contributing causes of infertility in 40% of cases (see Table 24-2).

Risk Factors

Men with occupational or environmental exposure to chemicals, radiation, or excessive heat are at increased risk for infertility as are those with a history of varicocele, mumps, hernia repair, pituitary tumor, anabolic steroid use, and impotence.

Clinical Manifestations

History

The physician should ask about previous pregnancies fathered by the patient, environmental exposures, and any history of sexually transmitted infections, mumps orchitis, hernia repair, or trauma to genitals.

Physical Examination

The physical examination should include a search for signs of testosterone deficiency and varicocele, identification of the urethral meatus, and measurement of testicular size.

Diagnostic Evaluation

A **semen analysis** is the primary investigative tool for male factor infertility. Sperm count, volume, motility, morphology, pH, and white blood cell count are analyzed.

The postcoital test examines the interaction between sperm and the cervical mucus. A healthy **sperm-mucus interaction** occurs when a large number of forwardly moving sperm are seen in a thin acellular mucus.

In the case of an abnormal semen analysis, an endocrine evaluation should include thyroid function tests, serum testosterone, prolactin, and follicle-stimulating hormone (FSH) (may identify parenchymal damage to testes).

Treatment

In general, the probability of conception can be enhanced by having intercourse every 2 days during ovulation with the female partner on bottom. The woman should lie on her back with her knees to her chest for at least 15 minutes after intercourse. Men should avoid the use of tight underwear, saunas and hot tubs, and unnecessary environmental exposures.

TABLE 24-2

Common Causes of Infertility and Basic Diagnostic Tools

Etiology	Incidence* (%)	Basic Investigative Tools
Male factor	40	Semen analysis Postcoital test
Ovulatory factor	15–20	Basal body temperature Serum progesterone Endometrial biopsy
Peritoneal factors	40	Laparoscopy
Uterine-tubal factor	30	Hysterosalpingogram Laparoscopy ± hysteroscopy
Cervical factors	5–10	Postcoital test

*Multiple factors are identified in 20% of cases.

Adapted from Hacker N, Moore JG. Essentials of obstetrics and gynecology. Philadelphia: WB Saunders 1992:553.

TABLE 24-3

Common Causes of Male Factor Infertility

Endocrine disorders
- Hypothalamic dysfunction (Kallman's)
- Pituitary failure (tumor, radiation, surgery)
- Hyperprolactinemia (drug, tumor)
- Exogenous androgens
- Thyroid disease
- Adrenal hyperplasia

Abnormal spermatogenesis
- Mumps orchitis
- Chemical/radiation/heat exposure
- Varicocele
- Cryptorchidism

Abnormal motility
- Varicocele
- Antisperm antibodies
- Kartagener's syndrome
- Idiopathic

Sexual dysfunction
- Retrograde ejaculation
- Impotence
- Decreased libido

Adapted from DeCherney A, Pernoll M. Current obstetric & gynecologic diagnosis and treatment. Norwalk, CT: Appleton and Lange, 1994:998.

Low semen volume is most often treated by using washed sperm for intrauterine insemination.

Treatment of low density or motility depends on the causal agent. Hypothalamic-pituitary failure can be treated with injections of human menopausal gonadotropins (hMGs) and varicoceles can be repaired by ligation. Intracytoplasmic sperm injection (ICSI) is another option for patients with low sperm density or impaired motility.

When no cause can be found, IUI or IVF may be attempted. In refractory cases, artificial insemination with donor sperm is highly effective.

Key Points

Male factor infertility

1. Is responsible for 40% of all infertility cases;
2. May be idiopathic or due to improper coital practices or abnormalities in sperm volume, density, or mobility;
3. Is diagnosed by semen analysis, a postcoital test, and endocrine evaluation;
4. Is treated when the causal agent is determined; beyond this, ICSI, IUI with washed sperm, IVF, and IVF with donor sperm may be effective.

▶ FEMALE FACTOR INFERTILITY

Forty percent of infertility is attributed to female factors. These factors can be subdivided into ovulatory factors and anatomic abnormalities. Ovulatory factors can impair folliculogenesis, ovulation, and endometrial development, thus preventing fertilization and implantation. Congenital and acquired **anatomic abnormalities** cause infertility by posing a mechanical barrier between sperm and oocyte.

Ovulatory Factors

Pathogenesis

Endocrine abnormalities at various points along the hypothalamic-pituitary-ovarian axis can contribute to female factor infertility (Table 24-4). Hypothalamic-pituitary insufficiency, hyperprolactinemia, polycystic ovarian disease, luteal phase defects, and premature ovarian failure are just a few of the endocrinologic causes of female factor infertility.

Epidemiology

Ovulatory factors are responsible for infertility in 15 to 20% of cases (see Table 24-2).

Clinical Manifestations

History The medical history should include a thorough menstrual history and inquiries about spontaneous abortions, endometriosis, galactorrhea, weight changes, or hot flushes.

Physical Examination Special effort should be made to look for hirsutism; obesity; and signs of virilism, hypothyroidism, premature ovarian failure, and insulin resistance.

TABLE 24-4
Causes of Ovulatory Factor Infertility

Central defects
Pituitary insufficiency (trauma, tumor, congenital)
Hypothalamic insufficiency
Hyperprolactinemia (drug, tumor, empty sella)
Polycystic ovarian disease (chronic hyperandrogenemic anovulation)
Luteal phase defects
Peripheral defects
Gonadal dysgenesis
Premature ovarian failure
Ovarian tumor
Ovarian resistance
Metabolic disease
Thyroid disease
Liver disease
Obesity
Androgen excess (adrenal, neoplastic)

From DeCherney A, Pernoll M. Current obstetric & gynecologic diagnosis and treatment. Norwalk, CT: Appleton and Lange, 1994:998.

Diagnostic Evaluation

The primary tests for the evaluation of ovulatory factor infertility look for **evidence of ovulation** by tracking the menstrual cycle, measuring the basal body temperature, monitoring the cervical mucus, measuring the midluteal progesterone, and documenting any premenstrual or ovulatory symptoms. An **endometrial biopsy** can be used to evaluate the morphology of the glands and stroma of the endometrium to determine the adequacy of progesterone's affects on the endometrial lining. This is also the most accurate method to time ovulation and to look for luteal phase defects. Finally, **endocrine evaluation** may include measurement of FSH, luteinizing hormone (LH), prolactin, thyroid function tests, and thyroid antibodies.

Treatment

The underlying etiology of ovulatory dysfunction should be identified and corrected. Regular ovulation can be restored in 90% of fertility cases due to endocrine factors. For uncorrectable cases, ovulation induction with fertility drugs can be used. Of note, there is no treatment for premature ovarian failure. Patients with this diagnosis should be offered the option of egg donation, embryo donation, surrogacy, and adoption.

Key Points

Ovulatory factor infertility

1. Is caused by pituitary and hypothalamic insufficiency, polycystic ovarian disease, luteal phase defects, hyperprolactinemia, and premature ovarian failure;
2. Is primarily diagnosed by evaluation of ovulation, endometrial biopsy, and endocrine tests;
3. Is treated contingent upon the nature of the defect; diagnosis should be made before a treatment plan is instigated.

Anatomic Causes of Infertility

Pathogenesis

Anatomic causes of infertility include conditions resulting in mechanical barriers of the cervix, uterus, fallopian tubes, ovaries, and adjacent pelvic structures (Table 24-5). Cervical factors and uterine abnormalities are relatively rare causes of infertility. The primary anatomic factors are tubal occlusion and endometriosis. **Tubal occlusion** typically results from prior salpingitis, use of intrauterine device (IUD), or endometriosis. **Endometriosis** may interfere with tubal mobility, cause tubal obstruction, or result in pelvic adhesions that contribute to infertility by holding the fallopian tube away from the ovary or trapping the released oocyte.

Epidemiology

Cervical factor accounts for 5 to 10% of infertility cases, uterine and tubal factors account for 30%, and peritoneal factors account for 40% of infertility cases (see Table 24-2).

Risk Factors

Diethylstilbestrol (DES) exposure in utero, previous cervical surgery, and cervicitis are risk factors for

TABLE 24-5
Anatomic Causes of Infertility

Anomalies of the cervix
DES exposure in utero
Müllerian duct abnormality
Cervical stenosis
Surgical treatment (cryotherapy, conization)
Cervicitis or chronic inflammation
Hostile cervical mucus
Abnormalities of the uterine cavity
Congenital malformations
Submucosal leiomyoma
Intrauterine synechiae (Asherman's syndrome)
Tubal occlusion
Pelvic inflammatory disease
IUD use
Tubal ligation
Endometriosis
Peritoneal factors
Endometriosis
Pelvic adhesions

cervical causes of infertility. Risk factors for uterine and tubal infertility include prior history of pelvic inflammatory disease or IUD use, endometriosis, adenomyosis, or adnexal surgery. Endometriosis and prior pelvic surgery are the primary risk factors for pelvic factor infertility.

Clinical Manifestations

History Information about prior IUD use, salpingitis, endometriosis, adenomyosis, or tubal sterilization should be elicited as should a history of ectopic pregnancy, adnexal surgery, cryotherapy, conization, or in utero DES exposure.

Physical Examination Special attention should be taken to evaluate the adnexa and to look for leiomyoma and any signs of current or prior pelvic infection. Cervical cultures should also be collected.

Diagnostic Evaluation

The primary investigative tools for anatomic abnormalities of the female reproductive tract are **hysterosalpingogram** and **laparoscopy**. These studies may be supplemented by transvaginal ultrasound and hysteroscopy as indicated. Cervical mucous studies and a postcoital test may be used to evaluate the quality of the cervical mucus.

Treatment

Intrauterine insemination appears to be most effective treatment for cervical factor infertility. Pregnancy rates have been as high as 20 to 30% after three cycles. In cases that are refractory to other treatments, patients should be offered IVF, GIFT, or zygote intrafallopian tube transfer (ZIFT).

Uterine synechiae can be treated with surgical ligation of adhesions via operative hysteroscopy, insertion of an IUD, or estrogen therapy. Most surgeons reserve myomectomy for treatment after recurrent abortion or when submucosal **fibroids** have been identified.

Microsurgical tuboplasty has proven to be effective for **tubal occlusion** due to prior infection or from prior tubal ligation. However, because it is more effective, most couples undergo IVF rather than attempt tuboplasty.

Endometriosis can be treated medically with Danazol (Table 24-6), gonadotropin-releasing hormone analogues, oral medroxyprogesterone (Provera), or continuous oral contraceptives or surgically by ligation periadnexal adhesions during laparoscopy or laparotomy. Pregnancy rates after treatment often depend on the extent of the disease.

Key Points

1. Tubal occlusion and endometriosis are the most common causes of anatomic factor infertility.
2. Pelvic examination, hysterosalpingogram, and laparoscopy are the primary investigative tools for these disorders. These are augmented by cervical mucous studies, postcoital tests, and hysteroscopy as indicated.
3. Tubal occlusion may be repaired with microsurgical tuboplasty, but most couples opt for IVF. Endometriosis may be treated medically or the implants and pelvic adhesions can be ligated during laparoscopy.

▶ UNEXPLAINED INFERTILITY

Pathogenesis

Five to 10% of couples who complete an initial assessment find no cause for their infertility. When the initial infertility evaluation reveals no cause for infertility, the problem often involves abnormalities in **sperm transport**, the presence of **antisperm antibodies**, or problems with penetration and fertilization of the egg. When problems in sperm transport, motility, or functional capacity are identified, IVF or GIFT may be used for treatment. If this fails, the use of donor sperm may offer an opportunity for pregnancy.

TABLE 24-6

Drugs Used in the Treatment of Infertility and in Assisted Reproductive Technologies

Commercial Name	Generic Name	Mechanism
Clomid/ Serophene	Clomiphene citrate	Antiestrogen, stimulates follicular development for ovulation induction
Pergonal	Human gonadotropins	Purified FSH/LH, stimulates follicular development during ovulation induction
Danocrine	Danazol	Androgen derivative, decreases FSH and LH used to treat endometriosis
hCG	Human chorionic gonadotropin	Triggers ovulation
Lutrepulse	Pulsatile GnRH	Stimulates release of FSH/LH from pituitary
Lupron	Leuprolide acetate	GnRH agonist, decreases estrogen levels, shrinks fibroids, causes regression of endometriosis

When no cause for infertility is identified after in-depth testing, studies show that most therapies have no higher success rates than no treatment at all. Although some patients with unexplained infertility may undergo three to six cycles of Pergonal stimulation with IUI before trying IVF or GIFT, many opt for no treatment. The eventual pregnancy rate for couples with unexplained infertility who receive no treatment approaches 60% over 3 to 5 years. Other options include use of donor sperm, surrogacy, adoption, or acceptance of childless infertility.

Key Points

In unexplained infertility,

1. Between 5 and 10% of couples find no explanation for infertility after their initial assessment;
2. Further studies should look for problems with sperm transport, ability to penetrate and fertilize the egg, and antisperm antibodies; IVF can be used to treat these patients;
3. Most therapies for couples have not been shown to have higher success rates than no treatment;
4. If no cause for infertility is identified after a second evaluation, no treatment will result in pregnancy up to 60% of the time over 3 to 5 years.

▶ ASSISTED REPRODUCTIVE TECHNOLOGIES

Since their conception, the treatment of infertility with assisted reproductive technologies has progressed rapidly and now includes not only "fertility drugs" (Pergonal, Metrodin, and Clomid), which stimulate multiple follicular development, but also technologies that combine ovulation induction agents with IUI, IVF, GIFT, or ZIFT.

Ovulation Induction

Method of Action

Clomifene citrate (Clomid) is an **antiestrogen** that stimulates increased production of FSH through feedback upregulation of FSH from the pituitary (see Table 24-6). This leads to follicular maturation and ovulation. Clomid is generally given orally during days 5 through 10 of the follicular phase of the menstrual cycle. Clomid is used for ovulation induction in women with anovulation, normal prolactin, and normal FSH.

If a woman fails to respond to Clomid, ovulation induction can be attempted with **Pergonal** (see Table 24-6), a purified preparation of **FSH and LH** from the urine of postmenopausal women. Pergonal is a human menopausal gonadotropin (hMG) that acts to stimulate follicular maturation directly. Pergonal is administered through intramuscular injection during the follicular phase of the menstrual cycle. Pergonal is useful in women who are unsuccessful with Clomid, who have hypothalamic or pituitary insufficiency, or unexplained infertility.

Both Clomid and Pergonal cause **multiple follicular development**. Once ovulation occurs, fertilization may be attempted by intercourse or IUI where washed sperm are placed directly into the uterine cavity. After ovulation induction, the oocytes may also be aspirated for fertilization via IVF, GIFT, or ZIFT.

Effectiveness

Clomid is successful in inducing ovulation in 70% of correctly selected patients. While 60% of patients achieve ovulation, if pregnancy does not occur after 3 to 6 cycles of Clomid, more aggressive therapies are needed. Pergonal has a 85 to 90% success rate of induction but also carries a much higher risk of **ovarian hyperstimulation and multiple gestation pregnancy**.

Side Effects and Complications

The side effects of Clomid, including hot flashes, emotional lability, depression, and visual changes, are mostly mild and disappear after discontinuation of the medication. Multiple gestation pregnancy occur in 8% of Clomid-induced pregnancies. The major complications of ovulation induction with Pergonal include ovarian hyperstimulation (1 to 3%) and multiple gestation pregnancy (20%).

Advanced Reproductive Techniques (IVF, GIFT, ZIFT)

Method of Action

Assisted reproductive technologies have advanced the treatment of infertility by allowing physicians to successfully bypass the normal mechanisms of gamete transportation and fertilization. In conjunction with ovulation induction, multiple oocytes may be harvested from the ovary using ultrasound or laparoscopic guidance. During IVF and ZIFT, the oocytes are allowed to mature briefly in vitro before washed sperm are added. Fertilization is verified 14 to 18 hours later by the presence of two pronuclei. In the case of IVF, the conceptuses are then placed into the uterus using a catheter, making IVF a relatively noninvasive procedure compared with ZIFT and GIFT. In the case of ZIFT, the zygotes are placed directly into the fallopian tubes via laparoscopy. When GIFT is being attempted, mature eggs are laparoscopically placed into the healthy fallopian tube along with washed sperm.

Effectiveness

The success rate of these advanced reproductive technologies varies from center to center. On average, with IVF, a successful outcome is achieved 18 to 22% per cycle. GIFT and ZIFT have slightly higher success rates of 22 to 28% per cycle in properly selected couples.

Key Points

1. Clomid is an antiestrogen that promotes follicular maturation and ovulation by increasing FSH levels.
2. Pergonal is a preparation of FSH and LH that stimulates follicular maturation for patients who have failed Clomid, or those with hypothalamic or pituitary insufficiency, or unexplained infertility.
3. The primary complications of fertility drugs include ovarian hyperstimulation and multiple gestation pregnancy.
4. IVF, GIFT, and ZIFT may be used to bypass the normal mechanisms or gamete transport with fertilization success rates of 18 to 28%.

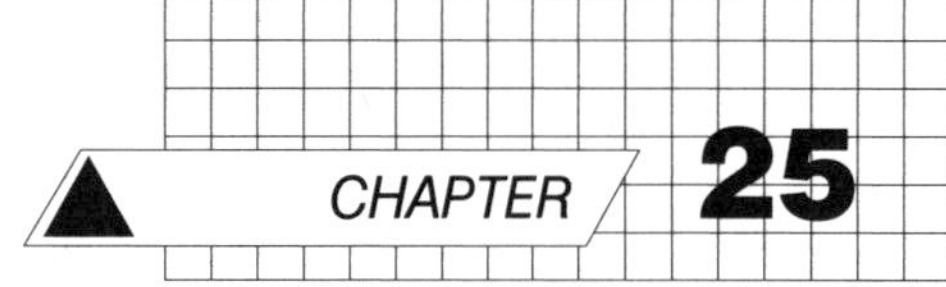

CHAPTER 25 Neoplastic Disease of the Vulva and Vagina

▶ PREINVASIVE NEOPLASTIC DISEASE OF THE VULVA

Anytime a pruritic area of the vulva does not respond to topical antifungals and creams, further workup with biopsy should be performed. If there are no obvious lesions, colposcopy may be performed. Diagnosis is then often made pathologically. Histologically, Paget's disease, intraepithelial neoplasia, and melanoma of the vulva can all be quite similar (Table 25-1). Diagnosis is then made by immunohistochemical staining.

Extramammary Paget's Disease

In the vulva, Paget's disease is an intraepithelial neoplasia of the skin overlying this region. In addition, about 20% of patients with Paget's disease will have adenocarcinoma underlying the outward changes. When this occurs, metastasis is common. Without the adenocarcinoma, Paget's disease can be treated locally without concern for metastases.

Diagnosis

The lesions of Paget's disease are consistent with chronic inflammatory changes. Commonly, there is a long-standing pruritus that accompanies velvety-red lesions of the skin that eventually became eczematous and scar into white plaques. The lesions may be focal on the labia, perineum, or perianal region or may encompass the entire region. The disease is most common in patients over the age of 60, and the symptoms of vulvar pruritus and vulvodynia can precede diagnosis for years. Absolute diagnosis is made with vulvar biopsy.

Therapy

Wide local excision of this intraepithelial lesion should be curative. Because microscopic Paget's disease often extends beyond the obvious gross lesions, wide margins should be taken and excised segments checked in pathology for clean margins. It is also important to rule out underlying adenocarcinoma with pathology. Finally, even with clean margins, Paget's disease has a high recurrence rate and often may need multiple local excisions. Without nodal metastases, the disease is commonly cured with local excision; however, with spread to nodes, the disease is likely to be fatal.

TABLE 25-1
Diagnostic Tests for Vulvar Disease

Disease	Carcino-embryonic Antigen	S-100 Antigen	Melanoma Antigen
Paget's	Positive	Negative	Negative
VIN	Negative	Positive	Negative
Melanoma	Negative	Negative	Positive

Key Points

1. Paget's disease is an intraepithelial neoplasia; however, it is associated with adenocarcinoma 20% of the time.
2. The lesions are often velvety-red in appearance.
3. Diagnosis is made by biopsy.
4. Treatment is with wide local excision; there is a high recurrence rate and close follow-up of patients is important.

▶ PREINVASIVE DISEASE OF THE VULVA

Premalignant disease of the vulva, or vulvar intraepithelial neoplasia (VIN) has a peak incidence in postmenopausal women in their late 50s and early 60s, although lesions can be seen in many patients under the age of 35. As the incidence of cervical dysplasia has been rising in younger women, so has VIN. This concomitant rise is not surprising because both cervical and vulvar neoplastic disease is correlated with HPV infection; 80 to 90% of VIN lesions will have DNA fragments from HPV. These lesions have also been associated with condylomata. The disease differs in younger and older patients. Younger women will have multifocal lesions that become invasive and more aggressive rapidly, whereas older women tend to have single lesions that are slow to become invasive.

Diagnosis

Patients will commonly present with complaints of vulvar pruritus or vulvodynia. Often times they will have been seen several times and diagnosed with candidiasis but will have no relief of symptoms with antifungal treatments. On physical examination there may be a variety of lesions that can be diffuse or focal, raised or flat, white, red, brown, or black. Extensive colposcopy of the entire vulvar region will often reveal multiple suspicious lesions that can be biopsied. The diagnosis is then made by pathologic specimen (Fig. 25-1).

Treatment

It is assumed that VIN will progress to invasive vulvar cancer if not treated. If all of the biopsies taken reveal VIN without any evidence for invasiveness, then wide local excision is commonly used. Often times, split-thickness skin grafts are used to replace the excised lesions, known as "skinning." More recently, laser vaporization has been used to eradicate the lesions; this results in less scar tissue and decreased healing times but provides no pathologic specimen so should only be used when nothing more extensive is suspected. These therapies are curative for VIN, but close follow-up is required. Patients should be followed up with colposcopy every 3 months until disease free for 2 years, when examinations are reduced to every 6 months.

Figure 25-1 Vulvar intraepithelial neoplasia.

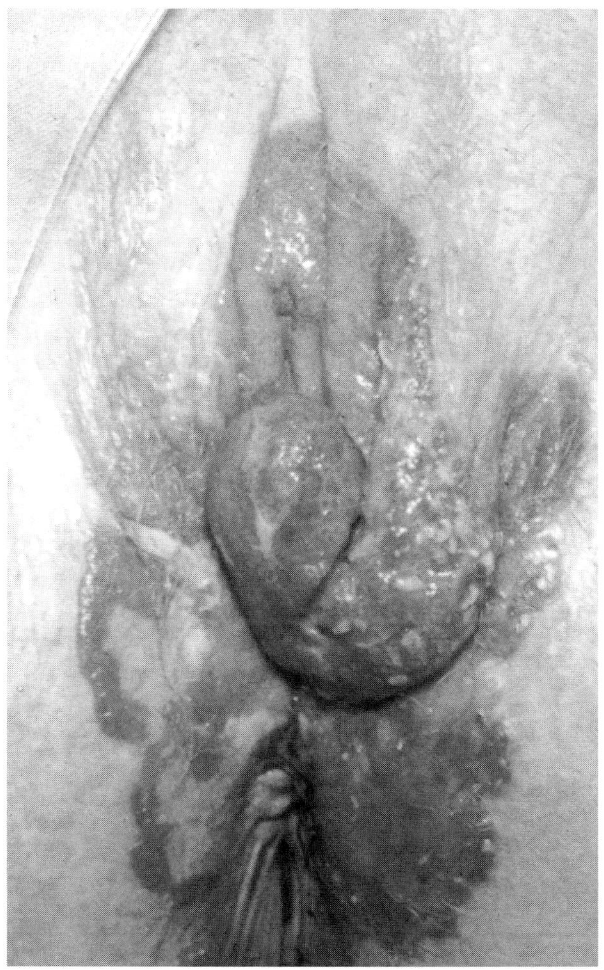

Key Points

1. Presenting symptoms are vulvar pruritus and vulvodynia, nonrefractory to treatment with antifungals.
2. The lesions are quite varied and are difficult to differentiate on the basis of physical examination; thus, diagnosis is made strictly by biopsy.
3. These lesions are thought to be premalignant.
4. Treatments include wide local excision or laser vaporization of tissue.

► CANCER OF THE VULVA

Epidemiology

Vulvar cancer accounts for only 5% of gynecologic malignancies. It is more common in the elderly and the poor. It has a peak incidence in patients in their 60s. Associated conditions include diabetes, hypertension, obesity, the vulvar dystrophies, and any granulomatous pelvic infection.

Diagnosis

Patients present with long histories of vulvar pruritus and vulvodynia. They will also present with vulvar bleeding or a vulvar mass. They will often have focal lesions that are simply inflamed and erythematous in early cancers and heaped up or ulcerated as the lesions progress. Final diagnosis is made by pathologic examination of a biopsy specimen.

There are a variety of possible vulvar cancers, the most common being the epidermoid cancer, which occurs in 85 to 90% of cases. This lesion ranges in appearance from a cauliflower-like mass to a hard indurated ulcer. The other types of vulvar cancers include malignant melanoma (5 to 10%), basal cell carcinoma (2 to 3%), and sarcomas (< 1%) including leiomyosarcomas and fibrous histiocytomas.

Staging

Staging of vulvar carcinoma is done with International Federation of Gynecologists and Obstetricians (FIGO) staging criteria using tumor size and invasiveness, nodal involvement, and distant metastases (Table 25-2). Thus, without doing a lymphadenectomy, it is impossible to definitively stage someone. Staging may be approximated by a thorough examination for palpable lymph nodes, although 25% of those with positive nodes will have none on physical examination.

TABLE 25-2

International Federation of Gynecology and Obstetrics (FIGO) Staging for Vulvar Cancer

FIGO Stage	TNM*	Clinical/Pathologic Findings
Stage 0	T_{is}	Carcinoma in situ, intraepithelial carcinoma
Stage I	$T_1N_0M_0$	Lesions 2 cm or less in size confined to the vulva or perineum. No nodal metastasis.
Stage IA		Lesions 2 cm or less in size confined to the vulva or perineum and with stromal invasion no greater than 1.0 mm.† No nodal metastasis.
Stage IB		Lesions 2 cm or less in size confined to the vulva or perineum and with stromal invasion greater than 1.0 mm. No nodal metastasis.
Stage II	$T_2N_0M_0$	Tumor confined to the vulva and/or perineum, >2 cm in greatest dimension, nodes are not palpable
Stage III	$T_3N_0M_0$	Tumor of any size with
	$T_3N_1M_0$	1. Adjacent spread to the lower urethra or the anus
	$T_1N_1M_0$	2. Unilateral regional lymph node metastasis
	$T_2N_1M_0$	
Stage IVA	$T_1N_2M_0$	Tumor invades any of the following:
	$T_2N_2M_0$	Upper urethra, bladder mucosa, rectal mucosa, pelvic bone, or bilateral regional node metastasis
	$T_3N_2M_0$	
	T_4 any N M_0	
Stage IVB	Any T, any N M_1	Any distant metastasis including pelvic lymph nodes

*TNM classification

T: Primary Tumor

T_x Primary tumor cannot be assessed

T_0 No evidence of primary tumor

T_{is} Carcinoma in situ (preinvasive carcinoma)

T_1 Tumor confined to the vulva and/or perineum 2 cm or less in greatest dimension

T_2 Tumor confined to the vulva and/or perineum more than 2 cm in greatest dimension

T_3 Tumor involves any of the following: lower urethra, vagina, anus

T_4 Tumor involves any of the following: bladder mucosa, rectal mucosa, upper urethra, pelvic bone

N: Regional Lymph Nodes

Regional lymph nodes are the femoral and inguinal nodes

N_x Regional lymph nodes cannot be assessed

N_0 No lymph node metastasis

N_1 Unilateral regional lymph node metastasis

N_2 Bilateral regional lymph node metastasis

M: Distant Metastasis

M_x Presence of distant metastasis cannot be assessed

M_0 No distant metastasis

M_1 Distant metastasis (pelvic lymph node metastasis is M_1)

†The depth of invasion is defined as the measurement of the tumor from the epithelial-stromal junction of the adjacent most superficial dermal papilla to the deepest point of invasion.

From American College of Obstetricians and Gynecologists. Prolog: gynecologic oncology and surgery. 3rd ed. Washington DC: 196:184.

Treatment and Prognosis

For a primary occurrence of vulvar epidermoid carcinoma, wide local excision with regional lymphadenectomy is the treatment of choice. Stage I disease rarely has positive contralateral lymph nodes, thus ipsilateral lymphadenectomy is sufficient. Most stage II and III disease can be treated with separate inguinal incisions for resection of lymph nodes. Stage IV disease and advanced stage III disease may require radical vulvectomy with en bloc lymphadenectomy.

If lymphadenectomy reveals metastatic disease, pelvic radiation is used as adjunct therapy. In patients in whom extensive surgery is contraindicated, the procedure may be confined to vulvectomy. In these patients, preoperative radiation therapy with and without chemotherapy has been used to reduce tumor burden. For recurrence, secondary excision or radiation therapy can be used.

The 5-year survival rate for all patients after surgical treatment of invasive epidermoid carcinoma is approximately 75%. In patients with metastases to local lymph nodes, 5-year survival rates are 90 to 95% for one positive lymph node, 75 to 80% for two positive lymph nodes, and less than 15% for three or more positive lymph nodes.

Melanoma of the vulva can be treated similarly to squamous cell carcinoma, except lymphadenectomy is rarely performed. Once the melanoma has metastasized, the mortality rate is near 100%; thus, these patients will not benefit from further surgery to document the spread of the disease. Basal cell carcinoma can be treated with wide local excision. These lesions rarely metastasize to the lymph nodes; thus, lymphadenectomy is not required.

Key Points

1. Vulvar cancer often presents with similar symptoms and lesions to VIN.
2. Diagnosis is made by biopsy.
3. Most treatment includes wide excision and regional lymphadenectomy; radiation therapy is used to reduce tumor burden and for recurrence.
4. Five-year survival rates are excellent for two or less positive nodes, but for three or more positive nodes it drops to 15%.

▶ PREINVASIVE DISEASE OF THE VAGINA

Vaginal intraepithelial neoplasia (VAIN) is similar to its counterparts of the vulva and cervix. It is designated I, II, or III depending on its thickness, and carcinoma in situ of the vagina is VAIN III. It is also associated with condylomas and history of infection with HPV. The peak incidence is patients in their mid to late 40s, younger than patients with VIN and older than patients with CIN.

Diagnosis

Patients with VAIN are usually asymptomatic and are usually diagnosed on Pap smear. Patients who have undergone hysterectomy should continue to have annual Pap smears to screen for VAIN. In the setting of a positive Pap, colposcopy should follow, and often suspicious lesions will be diagnosed with acetic acid application. These lesions should then be biopsied to give a final pathologic diagnosis.

Treatment

For focal lesions, local resection is curative. If lesions are found on both the cervix and extend into the upper third of the vagina, they can be removed with hysterectomy. If invasive disease has been ruled out with extensive biopsies, the lesions can be vaporized with CO_2 laser or application of topical 5-FU. Many of these patients tend to have multifocal lesions of both the vulva and cervix as well and need close follow-up with colposcopy every 3 months until disease free for 2 years.

Key Points

1. VAIN lesions are often asymptomatic and usually only found with careful Pap smear screening; diagnosis is made by biopsy.
2. Local excision or vaporization are common therapies.
3. Patients need close follow-up with colposcopy to rule out recurrence.

▶ CANCER OF THE VAGINA

Epidemiology

Invasive cancer of the vagina has a peak incidence in women in their 50s (mean age of 55). This pertains primarily to the most common cancer of the vagina, which is epithelial. However, women who were exposed in utero to diethylstilbestrol (DES) have a propensity to develop clear cell adenocarcinoma of the vagina, which is not uncommonly found in these women under the age of 30.

Diagnosis

Many patients are asymptomatic with vaginal cancer. The most common presenting symptoms are that of increasing vaginal discharge, bleeding, and vaginal pruritus. As in VAIN, diagnosis is screened for with Pap smear, follow-up colposcopy, and pathologic diagnosis is made with biopsy of suspicious lesions.

Staging and Treatment

Invasive squamous cell carcinoma (SCC) of the vagina is often complicated by involvement with local structures such as the rectum or bladder. Stage I and II lesions of the upper third of the vagina are amenable to surgical resection, but those of the lower two thirds of the vagina and stage III and IV lesions are treated with radiation therapy alone (Table 25-3). Lesions that are invading into local structures may often require palliative surgical therapy, but this does not affect survival rates in any way. Adenocarcinoma of the vagina is treated similarly to SCC. However, a clear-cut therapy

TABLE 25-3

International Federation of Gynecology and Obstetrics Staging for Carcinoma of the Vagina

Stage	Clinical/Pathologic Findings
Stage 0	Carcinoma in situ, intraepithelial carcinoma
Stage I	The carcinoma is limited to the vaginal wall
Stage II	The carcinoma has involved the subvaginal tissue but has not extended to the pelvic wall
Stage III	The carcinoma has extended to the pelvic wall
Stage IV	The carcinoma has extended beyond the true pelvis or has clinically involved the mucosa of the bladder or rectum. Bullous edema as such does not permit a case to be allotted to stage IV.
Stage IVA	Spread of the growth to adjacent organs and/or direct extension beyond the true pelvis
Stage IVB	Spread to distant organs

From American College of Obstetricians and Gynecologists. Prolog: gynecologic oncology and surgery. 3rd ed. Washington DC: 1996:183.

for clear cell carcinoma has not been established, so they are often treated similarly with resection of earlier staged lesions and radiation for stage III and IV lesions or those involving the lower vagina.

Prognosis

The 5-year survival rate of SCC of the vagina is highly dependent on the clinical stage. State I and II lesions have a 5-year survival rate of 70 to 75%. Stage III has a 5-year survival rate of approximately 30%. Stage IV has few survivors.

Key Points

1. Vaginal cancer will often be asymptomatic, with the most common presenting symptoms being vaginal pruritus, discharge, or bleeding.
2. Diagnosis is made by biopsy.
3. Stage I and II lesions of the upper vagina can be treated with excision; all other lesions are treated with radiation therapy.

CHAPTER 26

Cervical Cancer

▶ NEOPLASTIC DISEASE OF THE CERVIX

In the United States, cervical cancer was the leading cause of death from malignancy in women at the turn of the century. Since the onset of the **Papanicolaou smear,** which gained widespread acceptance in the 1950s and 1960s, it has been easier to detect in earlier nonlethal stages. Although cervical cancer has decreased to the sixth leading cause of death from cancer in women, it still leads to about 5,000 deaths per year. Cervical cancer and the premalignant cervical dysplasia are correlated with onset of sexual activity at an early age, increasing number of sexual partners, while being notably decreased by celibacy. Thus, for years it was suspected that cervical cancer was caused by a sexually transmitted agent.

Human Papilloma Virus

Human papilloma virus (**HPV**) is now accepted as the primary causative agent in cervical cancer. DNA fragments of HPV have been found incorporated into the DNA of cells from invasive cervical cancer in over 90% of cases studied. Furthermore, male partners of patients with cervical cancer can often be found to have subclinical infections of HPV. Although subtypes 6 and 11 seem to predispose to cause condylomas, serotypes 16, 18, and 31 are correlated with cervical cancer.

Epidemiology

There are approximately 15,000 cases of cervical cancer diagnosed annually in the United States that lead to an estimated 4,600 deaths. Risk factors for cervical cancer and dysplasia include cigarette smoking, number of sexual partners, age of onset of sexual activity, and a history of sexually transmitted infections. Additionally, patients with human immunodeficiency virus infections are considered at risk for cervical neoplasia and invasive cervical cancer is considered an AIDS-defining illness.

Pap Smear

The Pap smear involves scraping cells from the external os of the cervix with a blunt spatula to gain cells from the transformation zone. Because the squamocolumnar junction may be in the endocervical canal, it is important to also sample the endocervical canal with a cytobrush. Current recommendations call for annual Pap smears in anyone who has started sexual activity. Pap smears may show findings consistent with normal cellular material, inflammatory changes, dysplasia, carcinoma in situ, or invasive carcinoma.

In 1988, The Bethesda System of reporting Pap smears was created. This system gives three categories of squamous cell abnormalities:

- Atypical squamous cells of undetermined significance (ASCUS)
- Squamous intraepithelial lesions (SIL) subdivided into low and high grade
- Squamous cell carcinoma

The cellular changes in ASCUS may represent benign inflammatory response to infection or trauma but may herald a preinvasive neoplastic lesion. In patients who are reliable, follow-up with repeat Pap smear in 4 to 6 months is indicated. If follow-up is a concern, the patient may proceed immediately to colposcopy where directed biopsies may be performed. Ten to 15% of ASCUS evaluations will have significant lesions on colposcopy, whereas 80 to 85% of these lesions will resolve on repeat Pap smears.

Cytologic changes consistent with HPV infection, mild cervical dysplasia, and cervical intraepithelial neoplasia (CIN I) all correspond to low-grade SIL. Moderate dysplasia (CIN II) and severe dysplasia (CIN III), known as carcinoma in situ, are described as high-grade SIL. Patients with SIL should proceed to colposcopy for further workup of their abnormal Pap smear.

Colposcopy

Cervical dysplasia is categorized as mild (CIN I), moderate (CIN II), or severe (CIN III) depending on the depth and involvement of the epithelium. To determine the severity of dysplasia or if there is invasive carcinoma, colposcopy can be performed and directed biopsies taken. The colposcope gives a magnified view of the cervix and, when stained with acetic acid, cervical lesions can be noted and biopsied. These specimens are sent to pathology where a more definitive diagnosis can be made. However, if the Pap smear is suspicious for CIN III and the biopsy shows CIN I, further biopsies should be done to rule out more advanced disease.

Key Points

1. Cervical cancer leads to 5,000 deaths per year and is the sixth leading cause of death from cancer in women.
2. The Pap smear should be performed annually in any woman with a history of sexual activity.
3. Cervical cancer is highly correlated with infection with HPV. The progression of the disease is from dysplasia to cervical intraepithelial neoplasia to invasive disease.
4. Abnormal Pap smears need to be followed up with repeat Pap smears or colposcopy which offers the ability to make directed biopsies of cervical lesions.

▶ CERVICAL INTRAEPITHELIAL NEOPLASIA

Cervical dysplasia is thought to be the precursor to cervical cancer. In the case of CIN I, approximately 30% of these lesions will resolve if followed. On average, it takes about 7 years before CIN I will become cervical cancer and about 4 years for CIN II. However, because of the severity of this disease and the rapidity of progression of an occasional lesion, often CIN is treated by surgical excision.

Treatment of CIN

When the diagnosis is made by biopsy of a CIN lesion, there are several treatments that may ensue. For small lesions confined to the exocervix with invasive disease ruled out, **cryotherapy** or **laser therapy** may be used to destroy the epithelial tissue without causing extensive damage to the cervix. If the lesion involves the endocervix surgical excision of the transformation zone and distal endocervical canal must ensue. The **loop electrosurgical excision procedure** (LEEP) or **surgical conization** (Fig. 26-1) can be performed to remove endocervical lesions. In general, the LEEP removes cervical tissue without causing as extensive damage to the stroma of the cervix, although scarring of the endocervical canal still ensues. The specimens of excisions should always be sent to pathology to ensure adequate margins surrounding the excised lesions.

Key Points

1. CIN may be treated by destruction of the lesion if confined to the exocervix with laser therapy or cryotherapy.
2. CIN involving the endocervix requires conization either surgically or with LEEP.
3. On average, CIN I will advance to cervical cancer in about 7 years.

▶ CERVICAL CANCER

Squamous cell carcinoma makes up about 90% of all cervical cancer. It can be subdivided into large cell keratinizing, large cell nonkeratinizing, and small cell. **Adenocarcinoma** makes up most of the remaining cervical cancers. One type of adenocarcinoma is clear cell carcinoma, which is correlated with in utero diethylstilbestrol (DES) exposure. Rarely, a malignancy of the cervix will be a sarcoma or lymphoma.

Diagnosis

Although the Pap smear has proven to be an excellent screening method for cervical cancer, patients still present with advanced stages of this disease. The classic presentation is with postcoital bleeding. Other signs and symptoms that will accompany cervical cancer include any abnormal vaginal bleeding, watery discharge, pelvic pain or pressure, and rectal or urinary tract symptoms. On speculum examination, one may see an exophytic lesion on the cervix or invading into the upper vagina. On bimanual examination, a mass within the cervix may be palpated as well as invasive lesions into the upper vagina, cul de sac, or adnexa.

If a lesion is seen it should be biopsied. If the Pap smear is abnormal, the cervix should be biopsied. If the physical examination is abnormal, ultrasound or computed tomography may be performed to confirm these findings, but for a pathologic diagnosis, tissue still needs to be obtained if there are lesions to biopsy.

Cervical cancer is clinically staged by the amount of metastatic involvement of other tissues (Table 26-1 and Fig. 26-2). **Stage I** is confined to the cervix. **Stage II** extends beyond the cervix but not to the pelvic sidewalls or the lower third of the vagina. **Stage III** extends to the pelvic sidewalls or lower third of the vagina. Extension beyond the pelvis, invasion into local structures including the bladder or rectum or distant metastases all give the diagnosis of **stage IV.**

Treatment

In the setting of **microinvasive carcinoma** (stage IA1 and IA2), a cone biopsy may be adequate therapy if there is a wish to maintain fertility. The pathologic specimen should have the depth of invasion less than 5 mm, the horizontal spread less than 7 mm, and there should be clean margins. The standard of care is

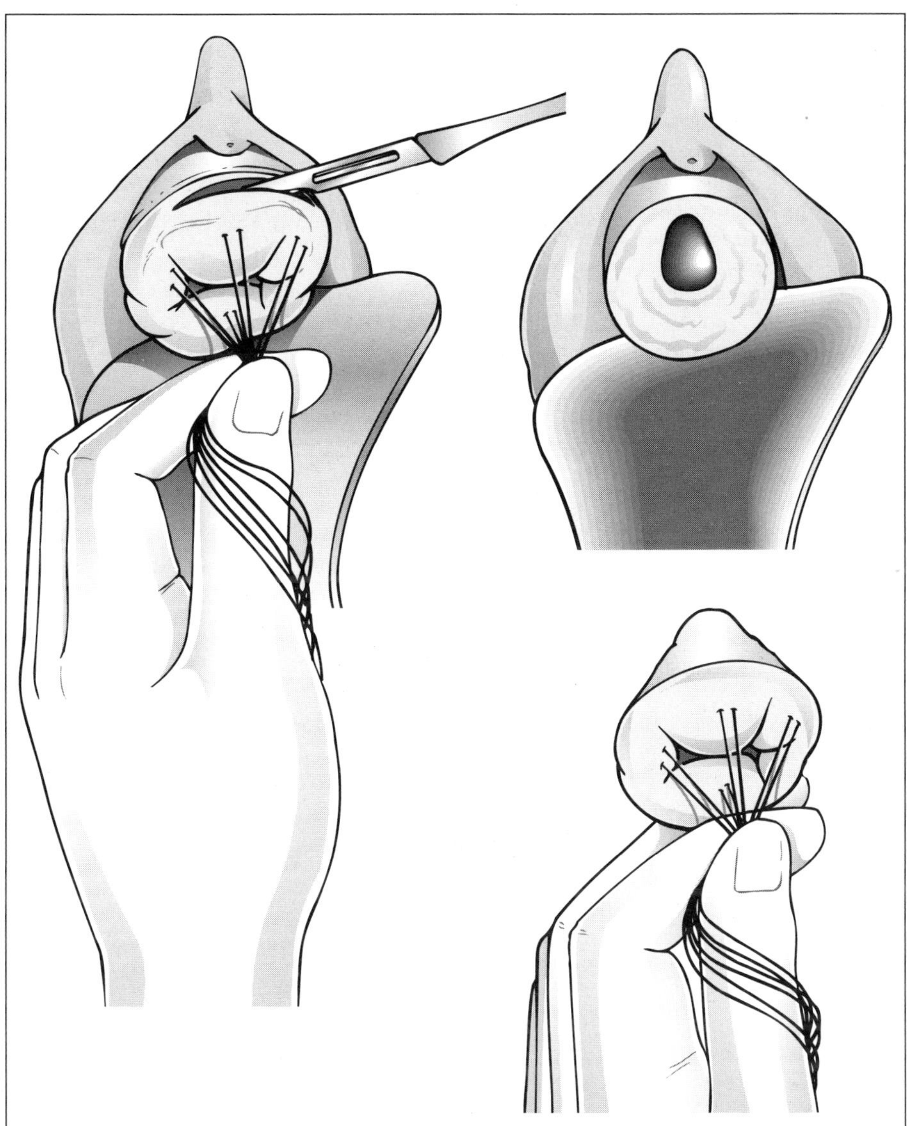

Figure 26-1 Conization of the cervix.

hysterectomy, which can be simple hysterectomy in the setting of stage IA1 disease and radical hysterectomy with stage IA2.

Surgical Therapy

In the treatment of **invasive cervical carcinoma**, radical hysterectomy only offers benefit in the setting of cancer that has not spread beyond the cervix, uterine corpus, and vagina. Approximately 40% of cervical cancer will be stage IB. This has an 85% cure rate regardless of whether radical hysterectomy or radiation therapy is used. Considerations of mode of treatment include the patient's ability to tolerate surgery and the length of treatment involved in radiation therapy. After treatment, patients need close follow-up for recurrence, although the benefit of secondary treatment for recurrent cancer is minimal.

Radiation Therapy

Radiation therapy can be used for curative and palliative purposes. Both external beam radiation and intracavitary radiation are used in the curative setting, whereas palliative radiation to control bleeding or for pain management may use either modality. In using the combination radiation therapy, the goals are eradication of local disease, prevention of metastatic disease, and to minimize irradiation of other local structures. Once the cancer has spread to the parametria or

TABLE 26-1

International Federation of Gynecology and Obstetrics Staging for Carcinoma of the Cervix Uteri

Stage	Clinical/Pathologic Findings
Stage 0	Carcinoma in situ, intraepithelial carcinoma
Stage I	The carcinoma is strictly confined to the cervix (extension to the corpus should be disregarded)
Stage IA	Invasive cancer identified only microscopically. All gross lesions even with superficial invasion are stage IB cancers. Invasion is limited to measured stromal invasion with maximum depth of 5.0 mm and no wider than 7.0 mm*
Stage IA1	Measured invasion of stroma no greater than 3.0 mm in depth and no wider than 7.0 mm
Stage IA2	Measured invasion of stroma greater than 3 mm and no greater than 5 mm and no wider than 7 mm
Stage IB	Clinical lesions confined to the cervix or preclinical lesions greater than stage IA
Stage IB1	Clinical lesions no greater than 4.0 cm in size
Stage IB2	Clinical lesions greater than 4 cm in size
Stage II	The carcinoma extends beyond the cervix but has not extended to the pelvic wall. The carcinoma involves the vagina but not as far as the lower third
Stage IIA	No obvious parametrial involvement
Stage IIB	Obvious parametrial involvement
Stage III	The carcinoma has extended to the pelvic wall. On rectal examination, there is no cancer-free space between the tumor and the pelvic wall The tumor involves the lower third of the vagina All cases with hydronephrosis or nonfunctioning kidney are included unless they are known to be due to other causes
Stage IIIA	No extension to the pelvic wall
Stage IIIB	Extension to the pelvic wall and/or hydronephrosis or nonfunctioning kidney
Stage IV	The carcinoma has extended beyond the true pelvis or has clinically involved the mucosa of the bladder or rectum. A bullous edema as such does not permit a case to be allotted to stage IV
Stage IVA	Spread of the growth to adjacent organs
Stage IVB	Spread to distant organs

*The depth of invasion should not be more than 5 mm taken from the base of the epithelium, either surface or glandular, from which it originates. Vascular space involvement, either venous or lymphatic, should not alter the staging.

From American College of Obstetricians and Gynecologists. Prolog: gynecologic oncology and surgery. 3rd ed. Washington DC: 1996:183.

beyond, the treatment is radiation therapy. This is actually relatively effective with 5-year survival rates close to 50% for stage IIIA disease.

Chemotherapy

Chemotherapeutic measures in cervical cancer have been only minimally effective. This may be in part that they are usually added to the treatment regimen after surgery and radiation have failed. Doxorubicin, bleomycin, and cisplatin are the most potent agents used to treat squamous cell cervical cancer. In addition to the minimal benefit predicted, all are quite toxic with serious side effects. There have been reports in the literature of response rates greater than 50%, but in multiple trials in the United States, remission rates range from 0 to 15%. Whether single agent treatment is given with cisplatin or multiple agents used, there appears to be little difference in the response rates.

Key Points

1. Early microinvasive disease, stage IA1 and IA2, can be treated with cone biopsy.
2. Stage IB lesions are equally responsive to surgery or radiation therapy with an 85% cure rate.
3. More advanced lesions, stage III or greater, require radiation therapy and occasionally chemotherapy may offer some help.

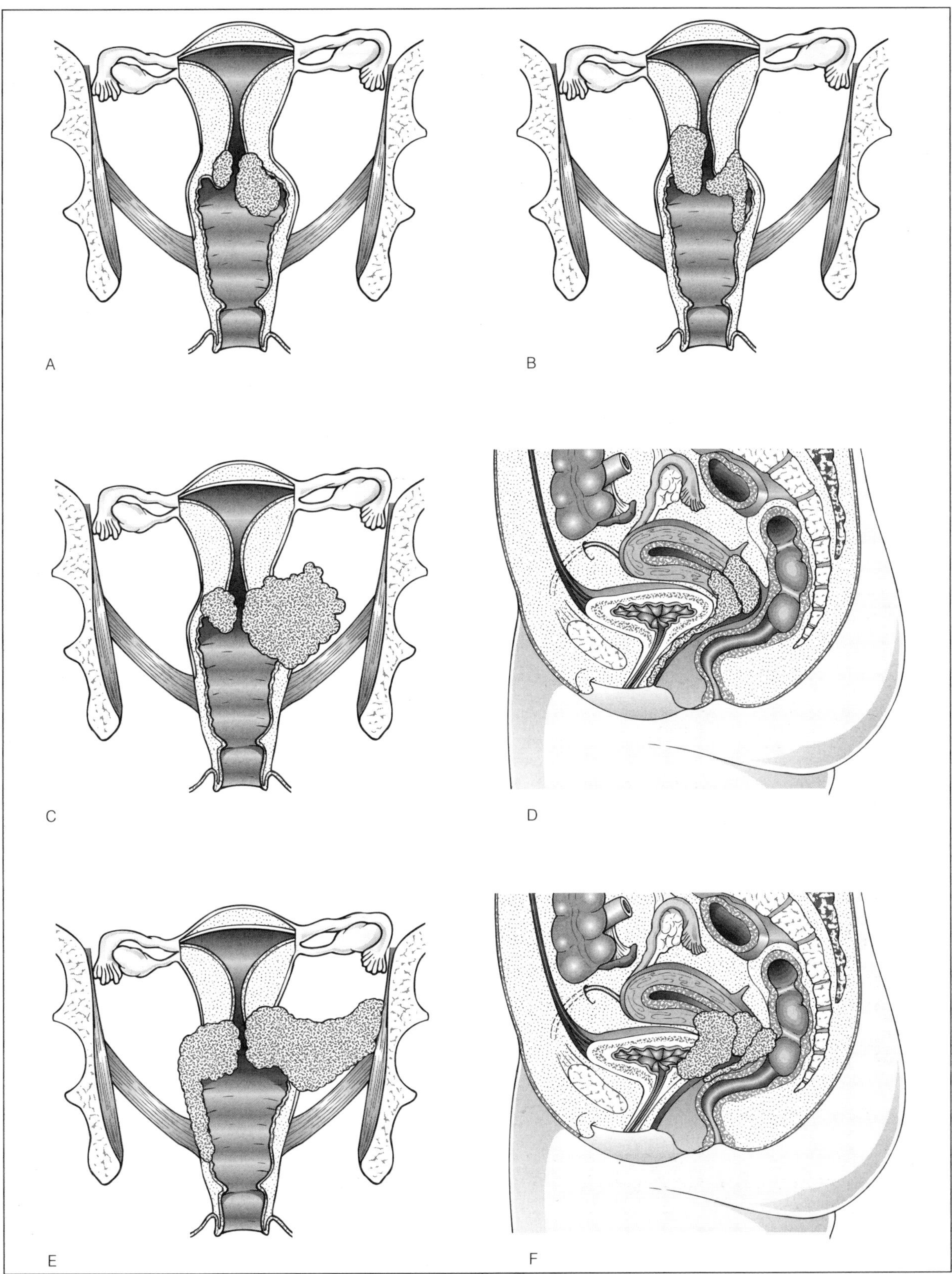

Figure 26-2 FIGO classification of carcinoma of the cervix. (A) Stage IB: carcinoma continued to the cervix, exophytic. (B) Stage IIA: carcinoma extends into the upper vagina or fornix. (C) Stage IIB: carcinoma extends into the parametrium but does not extend to pelvic wall. (D) Stage IIIA: carcinoma involves the anterior vaginal wall, extending to the lower one third. (E) Stage IIIB: the parametrium is infiltrated and the carcinoma extends to the pelvic wall. (F) Stage IVA: the bladder base or rectum is involved.

CHAPTER 27

Endometrial Cancer

▶ PATHOGENESIS

Endometrial carcinoma is known as an "**estrogen-dependent neoplasm**" because of the strong association between *atypical* endometrial hyperplasia and its progression to endometrial carcinoma in the setting of chronic exposure to **unopposed estrogen**. Between 20 and 30% of patients with atypical adenomatous hyperplasia progress to endometrial carcinoma if not treated.

Nearly 75% of cases of endometrial cancers are **adenocarcinomas**. Other types are adenosquamous carcinoma, clear cell carcinoma, squamous carcinoma, and papillary serous carcinoma. Invasive adenocarcinoma usually represents a proliferation of the glandular cells of the endometrium rather than stromal proliferation. The degree of abnormality in these glandular cells is used to determine the grade of the tumor.

Endometrial carcinoma has four primary routes of spread. The most common route is **direct extension** of tumor downward to the cervix or outward through the myometrium and serosa. When there is significant myometrial penetration, cells may spread through the lymphatic system via the pelvic and periaortic lymph nodes. Exfoliated cells may also be shed out through the fallopian tubes to the ovaries, parietal peritoneum, and omentum. Hematogenous spread occurs less frequently but can result in metastasis to the liver, lungs, and/or bone.

Histologic grade is the most important prognostic factor for endometrial carcinoma. Poorly differentiated tumors have a higher grade and a much poorer prognosis due to the likelihood of spread outside of the uterus. Depth of the **myometrial invasion** is the second most important prognostic factor. The prognosis is dramatically worsened when the cancer has invaded greater than one third of the thickness of the myometrium. The **histologic type** of carcinoma also effects prognosis. In general, adenosquamous (found in older women), clear cell squamous, and papillary serous carcinoma have worse prognoses than the much more common adenocarcinoma. Other important prognostic factors are pelvic node metastases, original tumor volume, extension to the cervix, adnexal metastases, and positive peritoneal washings.

▶ EPIDEMIOLOGY

Endometrial cancer is the **most common gynecologic malignancy** in the United States and the fourth most common malignancy in American women after breast, colorectal, and lung carcinoma. Over 70% of endometrial cancer cases occur before the age of 50, and the median age of diagnosis is 60 years. Most tumors are caught early when they are of low grade and low stage; therefore, the overall prognosis for the disease is good and overall mortality rates are declining.

▶ RISK FACTORS

Most women with endometrial cancer have a history of **unopposed estrogen exposure**, including obesity (>30 lbs overweight), nulliparity or low parity, chronic anovulation, menopause after age 50, or a history unopposed exogenous estrogen use. Other risk factors include diabetes mellitus, hypertension, cancer of the breast or ovary, and a family history of endometrial cancer.

Despite these known risk factors, no effective screening mechanism exists for endometrial carcinoma. Neither annual Pap smears nor endometrial biopsies have been shown to effectively screen asymptomatic patients.

▶ CLINICAL MANIFESTATIONS

History

The most common symptom of endometrial cancer is **postmenopausal bleeding**. Some form of abnormal vaginal bleeding occurs in 90% of patients with endometrial cancer. The premenopausal patient may report menorrhagia or metrorrhagia.

Physical Examination

The physical examination may reveal hypertension, obesity, or stigmata of diabetes. Care should be given to look for signs of metastatic disease including pleural effusion, ascites, hepatosplenomegaly, general lymphadenopathy, and abdominal masses.

Women with endometrial carcinoma typically have a **normal pelvic examination**. In more advanced stages of the disease, the cervical os may be patulous and the cervix may be firm and expanded. The uterus may be of normal size or enlarged and the adnexae should be carefully examined for extrauterine metastasis and coexistent ovarian carcinoma.

Differential Diagnosis

The differential diagnosis for postmenopausal bleeding is shown in Table 27-1. The older the patient, the more likely that malignancy is the cause of the bleeding.

▶ DIAGNOSTIC EVALUATION

The initial workup for endometrial carcinoma in a postmenopausal woman with vaginal bleeding should include a Pap smear, an endocervical curettage, and an endometrial biopsy. Although only 30 to 40% of patients with endometrial cancer will have an abnormal Pap smear, outpatient techniques of endometrial sampling have 90% accuracy. If the biopsy is negative, fractional dilatation and curettage and hysteroscopy should be performed. If bone pain is present, a chest radiograph and bone scan should also be performed.

▶ TREATMENT

The treatment of endometrial carcinoma is based on a surgical staging system by the International Federation of Gynecology and Obstetrics, which relies on pathologic confirmation of the extent of spread of the disease (Table 27-2).

The treatment plan for the various stages of endometrial cancer are summarized in Table 27-3. In general, treatment includes **surgical staging**, total abdominal hysterectomy, bilateral salpingo-oophorectomy (TAHBSO), and postoperative **radiation treatment**.

Hormonal therapy using high-dose progestins and antiestrogens is the first line of treatment for advanced disease and recurrent disease. Single-agent nonhormonal chemotherapy may be used in advanced or recurrent disease but has a low efficacy.

TABLE 27-1

Differential Diagnosis of Postmenopausal Bleeding

Diagnosis	No. of Cases
Exogenous estrogens	30
Atrophic vaginitis/endometritis	30
Endometrial cancer	**15**
Endometrial or cervical polyps	10
Endometrial hyperplasia	5
Miscellaneous*	10

*For example, cervical cancer, uterine sarcoma, urethral carbuncle, trauma.

Adapted from Hacker N, Moore JG. Essentials of obstetrics and gynecology. Philadelphia: WB Saunders Company, 1992:577.

TABLE 27-2

FIGO Surgical Staging of Endometrial Carcinoma (1988)

Stages		Extension of Disease
IA	G123	Tumor limited to endometrium
IB	G123	Invasion of <0.5 myometrium
IC	G123	Invasion of >0.5 myometrium
IIA	G123	Endocervical glandular involvement only
IIB	G123	Cervical stromal invasion
IIIA	G123	Tumor invades serosa and/or positive peritoneal cytology
IIIB	G123	Vaginal metastases
IIIC	G123	Metastases to pelvic and/or paraaortic lymph nodes
IVA	G123	Tumor invasion of bladder and/or bowel mucosa
IVB	G123	Distant metastases including intra-abdominal and/or inguinal lymph nodes

Reproduced with permission from American College of Obstetricians and Gynecologists. Prolog: gynecologic oncology and surgery. 3rd ed. Washington DC: 1996:182.

Because most endometrial cancers are **stage I at diagnosis**, the overall 5-year survival is 65%. The survival rates for the various stages of endometrial cancer are 73% for stage I, 56% for stage II, 32% for stage III, and 10% for stage IV.

▶ FOLLOW-UP

Seventy-five percent of recurrences of endometrial carcinoma will happen within the first 2 years after treatment and 85% by the end of the third year. Follow-up should occur every 3 months for 2 years, then twice a year for 3 years, and then annually. The first line of treatment for recurrent disease is hormonal therapy.

TABLE 27-3

Treatment of Endometrial Carcinoma

Stages I and II	Stages III and IV
Surgical staging	Surgical staging
Total abdominal hysterectomy	Total abdominal hysterectomy
Bilateral salpingo-oophorectomy	Bilateral salpingo-oophorectomy
Peritoneal washings	Peritoneal washing
Pelvic/aortic node sampling*	Pelvic/aortic node sampling*
Local or regional radiation	Local or regional radiation
	Hormonal therapy
	Chemotherapy

*The decision to perform a biopsy on the lymph nodes depends on the depth of myometrial invasion.

The use of estrogen replacement therapy in patients treated for endometrial carcinoma is controversial and is usually reserved for the patient treated for a well-differentiated minimally invasive disease that has not recurred for 5 years.

▶ KEY POINTS

Endometrial cancer

1. Is the most common gynecologic cancer and the fourth most common cancer in women;
2. Is an adenocarcinoma in over 75% of cases;
3. Is diagnosed at an average age of 60;
4. Is caused by prolonged exposure to exogenous or endogenous estrogen in the absence of progesterone;
5. Is more common in women using unopposed exogenous estrogen, obese and postmenopausal women, and women with chronic anovulation or late menopause;
6. Most often presents with abnormal vaginal bleeding and is diagnosed with a Pap smear, endocervical curettage, and endometrial biopsy;
7. Has no effective screening tools; fortunately, 75% of lesions are at stage I at the time of diagnosis;
8. Is treated by TAHBSO followed by radiation depending on the stage;
9. Has an overall 5-year survival rate of 65%;
10. Uses hormonal therapy (high-dose progestins) as the first line of treatment for recurrent disease (85% of recurrences happen in the first 3 years after treatment).

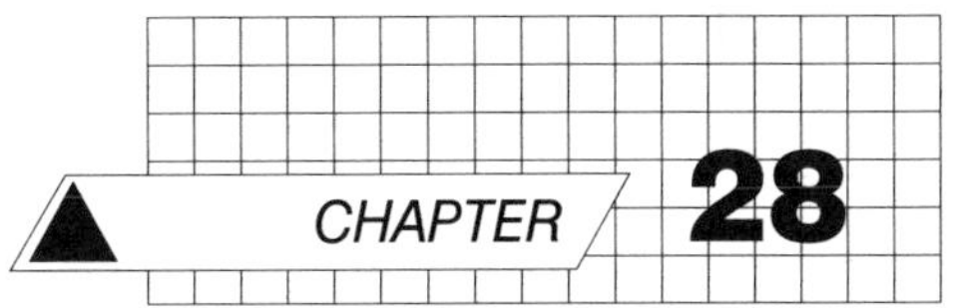

Ovarian and Fallopian Tube Tumors

There are many types of benign and malignant tumors of the ovaries (Table 28-1) each with their own characteristics (Table 28-2). Fortunately, 80% of ovarian tumors are benign. While fallopian tube carcinoma is extremely rare, ovarian cancer is the fifth most common cancer in women in the United States and the third most common cancer of the female genital tract, second only to endometrial and cervical cancer.

Although ovarian carcinoma comprises 25% of all gynecologic malignancies, it is responsible for nearly 50% of deaths from cancer of the female genital tract. This high mortality is due in part to the lack of effective screening tools for early diagnosis and partially to the spread by direct extension into the peritoneal cavity. Because the overall 5-year survival rate for women with ovarian carcinoma is only 25 to 30%, a high degree of suspicion and prompt diagnosis and intervention can be critical to survival.

▶ PATHOGENESIS

Tumors of the ovaries are derived from one of the three distinct components of the ovary: the surface coelomic epithelium, the ovarian stroma, or the germ cells (Fig. 28-1). Over 65% of all ovarian tumors and 90% of all ovarian cancers originate from **celomic epithelium** in the ovary capsule. About 5 to 10% of ovarian cancers are metastatic from other primary tumors in the body, usually from the gastrointestinal tract, breast, or endometrium, and are known as **Krukenberg tumors.**

Ovarian carcinoma is primarily spread by **direct exfoliation** of malignant cells from the ovaries. As a result, the sites of metastasis often follow the circulatory path of the peritoneal fluid, and the regional lymph nodes are often involved. Hematogenous spread is responsible for more rare and distant metastases to the lung and brain. In advanced disease, this pattern of spread and tumor mass is responsible for accumulation of ascites in the abdomen as well as the encasement of the bowel which can result in an intermittent bowel obstruction known as a carcinomatous ileus. In many cases, this progression results in a slow "starvation," cachexia, and death.

▶ ETIOLOGY

Although the cause of ovarian carcinoma is unclear, it is thought to result from malignant transformation of ovarian tissue after prolonged periods of chronic uninterrupted ovulation. Ovulation disrupts the germinal epithelium of the ovary and activates the cellular repair mechanism. When ovulation occurs for long periods of time without interruption, this mechanism is thought to provide the opportunity for somatic gene deletions and mutations. High dietary fat, mumps virus, and agents such as talc and asbestos have also been proposed as possible etiologic agents in the pathogenesis of ovarian carcinoma.

▶ RISK FACTORS

Women at the highest risk for ovarian cancer are those with a family history of the disease and those with a history of uninterrupted ovulation, including nulliparous women, and women with decreased fertility, delayed childbearing, or late onset menopause. Women with breast cancer also have a twofold increase in the incidence of ovarian cancer. Oral contraceptives have been found to have a modest protective effect against ovarian cancer. This is attributed to the suppression of ovulation by oral contraceptives.

▶ DIFFERENTIAL DIAGNOSIS

Patients with ovarian cancer are often **asymptomatic** until the disease has progressed to the advanced stages. Some patients may present with vague lower abdominal pain and abdominal enlargement. As the tumors progress, other symptoms may develop including gastrointestinal complaints, urinary frequency, dysuria, and pelvic pressure. Ascites may develop in later stages.

The primary finding on examination is a **solid fixed pelvic mass** that may extend into the upper abdomen and **ascites** (Table 28-3). **Pelvic ultrasound** is the primary diagnostic tool for investigating an adnexal mass (Table 28-4). These physical and radiographic findings help to distinguish between benign and malignant tumors. Other studies, including computed tomography and magnetic resonance imaging of the pelvis and abdomen, can be helpful in specific cases but do not play significant roles in the diagnosis

TABLE 28-1

Benign and Malignant Ovarian Tumors

Tumors of surface epithelium	Serous tumors Serous cystadenoma Borderline serous tumor Serous cystadenocarcinoma Adenofibroma and cystadenofibroma
	Mucinous tumors Mucinous cystadenoma Borderline mucinous tumor Mucinous cystadenocarcinoma
	Endometrioid carcinoma
	Clear cell adenocarcinoma
	Brenner tumor
	Undifferentiated carcinoma
Germ cell tumors	Teratoma Benign (mature, adult) Cystic teratoma (dermoid cyst) Solid teratoma Malignant (immature) Monodermal or specialized (e.g., carcinoid, struma ovarii)
	Dysgerminoma
	Endodermal sinus tumor
	Choriocarcinoma
	Others (embryonal carcinoma, polyembryoma, mixed germ cell tumors)
Sex cord–stromal tumors	Granulosa-theca cell tumors Granulosa cell tumor Thecoma Fibroma
	Sertoli-Leydig cell tumor (androblastoma)
	Gonadoblastoma
Unclassified tumors	
Metastatic tumors	

Reproduced with permission from Robbins S, Cotran R, Kumar V. Robbins pathologic basis of disease. Philadelphia: WB Saunders Company, 1991:1158.

of most ovarian cancers. Because malignant cells can be spread via direct exfoliation, paracentesis and cyst aspiration should be avoided. Once the diagnosis is made, studies are undertaken to look for **metastatic disease** and to distinguish between primary and secondary ovarian cancer.

Depending of the type of tumor, ovarian malignancies can be monitored using the **serum tumor markers** CA-125, alpha-fetoprotein (AFP), lactate dehydrogenase (LDH), and human chorionic gonadotropins (hCG).

TABLE 28-2

Frequency of the Major Ovarian Tumors

Type	Percentage of Malignant Ovarian Tumors	Percentage that Are Bilateral
Serous	40	
Benign (60%)		25
Borderline (15%)		30
Malignant (25%)		65
Mucinous	10	
Benign (80%)		5
Borderline (10%)		10
Malignant (10%)		20
Endometrioid carcinoma	20	40
Undifferentiated carcinoma	10	—
Clear cell carcinoma	6	40
Granuloma cell tumor	5	5
Teratoma		
Benign (96%)		15
Malignant (4%)	1	Rare
Metastatic	6	>50
Others	3	—

Reproduced with permission from Robbins S, Cotran R, Kumar V. Robbins pathologic basis of disease. Philadelphia: WB Saunders Company, 1991:1159.

▶ SURGICAL STAGING

Ovarian carcinoma is staged surgically (Table 28-5), including collecting ascites and peritoneal washings and sampling the regional lymph nodes. Nearly 75% of patients present with stage III or more advanced disease.

▶ EPITHELIAL TUMORS

Pathogenesis

Epithelial cell tumors of the ovaries are derived from the surface mesothelial cells of the ovary (see Fig. 28-1). The six primary types of epithelial tumors are serous, mucinous, endometroid, clear cell, Brenner's, and undifferentiated. The neoplasms in this group range in malignant potential from benign to borderline to frankly malignant.

Malignant epithelial tumors extend through the capsule of the ovary to seed the peritoneal cavity and rarely invade the underlying ovary. These are slow growing tumors that often remain undiagnosed until they are very large and at an advanced stage. Over 75% of patients have spread beyond the ovary at the time of diagnosis; thus, the **prognosis is very poor.**

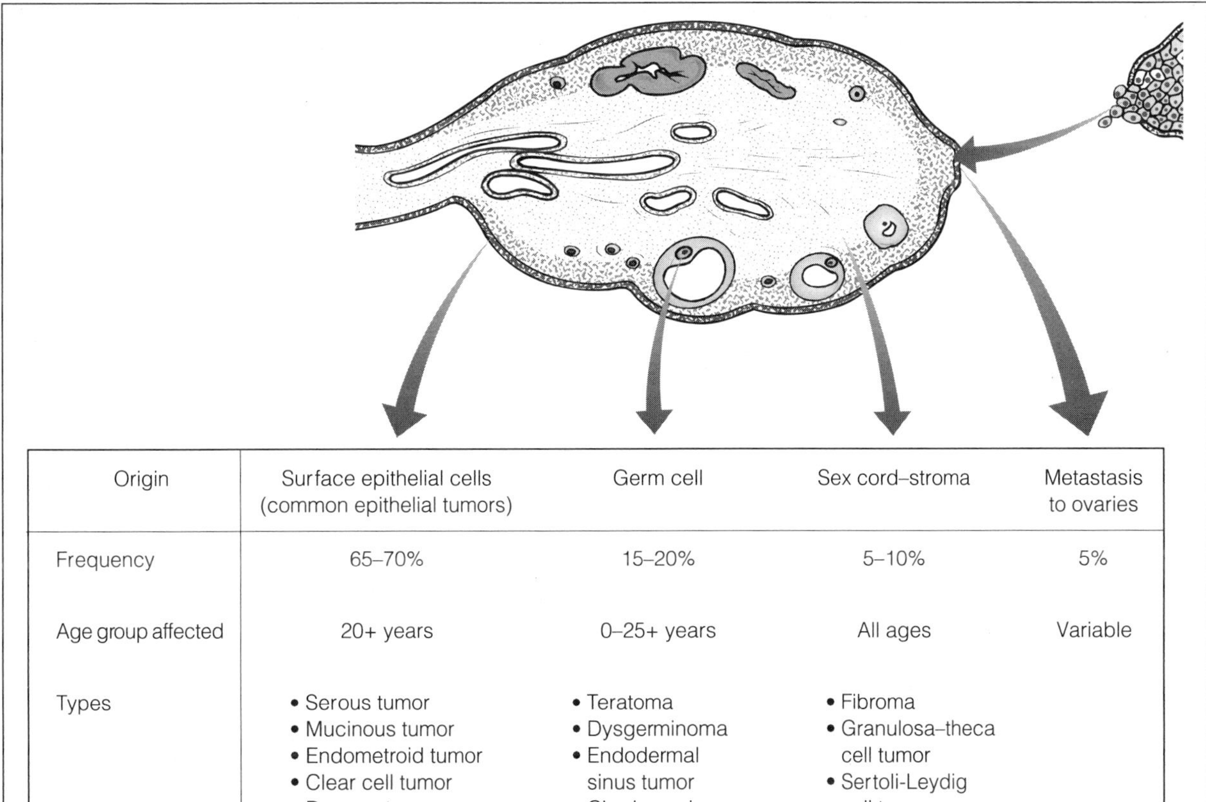

Origin	Surface epithelial cells (common epithelial tumors)	Germ cell	Sex cord–stroma	Metastasis to ovaries
Frequency	65–70%	15–20%	5–10%	5%
Age group affected	20+ years	0–25+ years	All ages	Variable
Types	• Serous tumor • Mucinous tumor • Endometroid tumor • Clear cell tumor • Brenner tumor • Undifferentiated	• Teratoma • Dysgerminoma • Endodermal sinus tumor • Choriocarcinoma	• Fibroma • Granulosa–theca cell tumor • Sertoli-Leydig cell tumor	

Figure 28-1 Classification of various ovarian neoplasms.

Epidemiology

Epithelial cell cancers account for 65 to 70% of all ovarian tumors and more than 90% of ovarian cancers. Epithelial tumors tend to occur during the sixth decade of life.

Clinical Manifestations

The serum tumor marker **CA-125** is elevated in 80% of epithelial cell cancers. Because CA-125 levels correlate with the progression and regression of these tumors, it has been useful in tracking the effect of treatment for epithelial ovarian carcinoma. Its value as a screening tool for the detection of ovarian cancer has not yet been established.

TABLE 28-3

Characteristics of Pelvic Mass on Physical Examination

	Benign	Malignant
Mobility	Mobile	Fixed
Consistency	Cystic	Solid or firm
Bilateral or unilateral	Unilateral	Bilateral
Cul de sac	Smooth	Nodular

Adapted from De Cherney A, Pernoll M. Current obstetric and gynecologic diagnosis and treatment. Norwalk: Appleton and Lange, 1994:960, Table 49-3.

TABLE 28-4

Radiographic Characteristics of Adnexal Masses

	Benign	Malignant
Size	<8 cm	>8 cm
Consistency	Cystic	Solid or cystic and solid
Septation	Unilocular	Multilocular
Bilateral or unilateral	Unilateral	Bilateral
Other	Calcification, esp teeth	Ascites

Adapted from De Cherney A, Pernoll M. Current obstetric and gynecologic diagnosis and treatment. Norwalk: Appleton and Lange, 1994:961, Table 49-4.

TABLE 28-5
Staging of Ovarian Carconima

Stage I. Growth limited to the ovaries
- Ia—one ovary involved
- Ib—both ovaries involved
- Ic—Ia or Ib and ovarian surface tumor, ruptured capsule, malignant ascites, or peritoneal cytology positive for malignant cells

Stage II. Extension of the neoplasm from the ovary to the pelvis
- IIa—extension to the uterus or fallopian tube
- IIb—extension to other pelvic tissues
- IIc—IIa or IIb and ovarian surface tumor, ruptured capsule, malignant ascites, or peritoneal cytology positive for malignant cells

Stage III. Disease extension to the abdominal cavity
- IIIa—abdominal peritoneal surfaces with microscopic metastases
- IIIb—tumor metastases <2 cm in size
- IIIc—tumor metastases >2 cm in size or metastatic disease in the pelvic, para-aortic or inguinal lymph nodes

Stage IV. Distant metastatic disease
- Malignant pleural effusion
- Pulmonary parenchymal metastases
- Liver or splenic parenchymal metastases (not surface implants)
- Metastases to the supraclavicular lymph nodes or skin

Reproduced with permission from American College of Obstetricians and Gynecologists. Prolog: gynecologic oncology and surgery. 3rd ed. Washington DC: 1996:181.

Treatment

Surgery is the mainstay of treatment for epithelial cell tumors, including total abdominal hysterectomy, bilateral salpingo-oophorectomy, omentectomy, and cytoreductive surgery.

Epithelial cell carcinoma is **very sensitive to cisplatin-based combination chemotherapeutic** agents and taxol. After chemotherapy, a "second look" laparotomy may be performed to evaluate the patient's response to treatment. Unfortunately, the tumors **frequently recur.** Radiation therapy plays a very limited role in the treatment of epithelial ovarian carcinoma.

The overall 5-year survival for patients with epithelial cell carcinoma is less than 20% (80 to 95% for stage I, 40 to 70% for stage II, 30% for stage III, and less than 10% for stage IV disease).

Key Points

1. Ninety percent of ovarian cancers are epithelial cell tumors derived from the coelomic epithelium of the surface of the ovary.
2. Epithelial ovarian tumors are slow-growing but aggressive tumors that may cause few symptoms until significantly advanced. Over 75% are diagnosed at stage III or higher.
3. These tumors typically occur in the sixth decade of life.
4. Treatment includes surgery (TAHBSO, omentectomy, debulking procedures) and platinum-based chemotherapy.
5. The 5-year survival for patients with epithelial cell carcinoma is less than 20%.

► GERM CELL TUMORS

Pathogenesis

Germ cell ovarian tumors are thought to arise from totipotential germ cells capable of differentiating into the three germ cell layers (Fig. 28-2). Ovarian germ cell

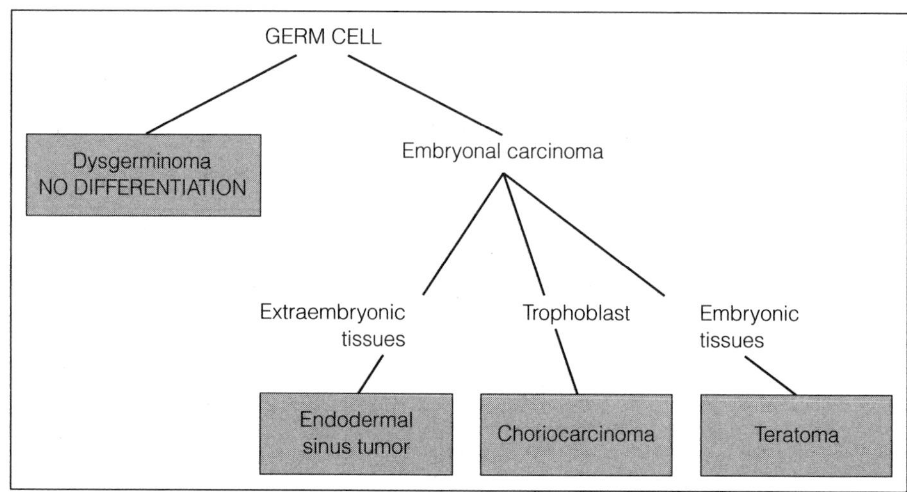

Figure 28-2 Histogenesis of tumors of germ cell origin.

tumors are very similar to germ cell tumors in the male. The most common types of germ cell cancers are **dygerminomas and immature teratomas.** Endodermal sinus (yolk sac) tumors, embryonal cell carcinoma, mixed germ cell tumors, and nongestational choriocarcinoma are less common. Many of these tumors produce **serum tumor markers** that can be used to assess response to therapy (Table 28-6).

In contrast to epithelial tumors, most germ cell tumors are in the **early stage** at the time of diagnosis. The prognosis for germ cell tumors, therefore, is much better than that of epithelial tumors. In most cases, these tumors are **considered curable.**

Epidemiology

Germ cell tumors make up 15 to 20% of all ovarian tumors. Although **95% are benign**, the remaining 5% of germ cell tumors are malignant and found primarily in children and young women. Germ cell tumors tend to occur during the second and third decades of life.

Clinical Manifestations

Patients with germ cell carcinoma present with **rapidly enlarging adnexal mass.** Functional germ cell tumors may produce hCG, AFP, LDH and/or CA-125 depending on the cell type (see Table 28-6).

Treatment

Because most germ cell tumors are diagnosed in the early stage and are rarely bilateral, surgery is typically limited to **removal of the involved ovary.** However, complete surgical staging should still be performed. Most cases of germ cell cancer is considered curable with **combination chemotherapy** (e.g., vinblastine, bleomycin, and cisplatin).

Radiation therapy is not a major component of treatment for germ cell tumors except in the case of dysgerminomas, which are exquisitely sensitive to whole abdominal radiation.

TABLE 28-6

Serum Tumor Markers for Germ Cell Neoplasia

Tumor	hCG	AFP	LDH	CA-125
Mixed germ cell tumor	+	+	+	+
Embryonal carcinoma	+	+	±	+
Endodermal sinus tumor	–	+	±	?
Dysgerminoma	±	–	+	+
Immature teratoma	–	±	±	+
Choriocarcinoma	+	–	±	?

Reproduced with permission from Frederickson H, Wilkins-Haug L. OB/GYN secrets. Philadelphia: Hanley and Belfus, Inc., 1991:119.

The 5-year survival rate is 85% for dysgerminomas, 70 to 80% for immature teratomas, and 60 to 70% for endodermal sinus tumors.

Key Points

Germ cell tumors

1. Arise from totipotential germ cells;
2. Are most commonly dysgerminomas and immature teratomas;
3. Produce serum tumor markers (AFP, LDH, CA-125, and/or hCG) that can be used to assess response to therapy;
4. Occur primarily in women under the age of 20 and present with a unilateral rapidly enlarging adnexal mass;
5. Are usually diagnosed at an early stage;
6. Are treated by combination chemotherapy and removal of the affected ovary; dysgerminomas are extremely sensitive to radiation therapy;
7. Have a good 5-year survival rate.

▶ SEX CORD–STROMAL TUMORS

Pathogenesis

These tumors originate from either the **sex cords** of the embryonic gonad (before the differentiation into male or female) or from the **ovarian stroma** (see Fig. 28-1). This group of tumors includes granulosa-theca cell tumors, Sertoli-Leydig cell tumors, and fibromas, and is characterized by **hormone production.** Ovarian stroma can develop into an ovary or a testes. As a result, ovarian granulosa-theca cell tumors resemble fetal ovaries and produce large amounts of estrogens, whereas ovarian Sertoli-Leydig cell tumors resemble fetal testes and produce testosterone and other androgens.

The ovarian fibroma is derived from mature fibroblasts and, unlike the other stromal cell neoplasms, is not a functioning tumor. Occasionally, fibromas are associated with ascites. The presence of ovarian tumor, ascites, and right hydrothorax is known as **Meigs' syndrome.**

Epidemiology

Stromal cell ovarian carcinoma is primary a disease of **older women.** It affects women in the fifth through eighth decades of life.

Clinical Manifestations

Granulosa-theca cell tumors often produce estrogen, which can cause feminization, precocious puberty, or postmenopausal bleeding. Sertoli-Leydig cell tumors produce androgenic compounds, which can cause virilizing effects including hirsutism, deepened voice, acne, and clitoromegaly.

Treatment

Because most occur in postmenopausal women, surgery for stromal cell tumors typically includes total abdominal hysterectomy and bilateral salpingo-oophorectomy. Chemotherapy is ineffective in treating stromal cell carcinoma. Even with aggressive treatment, the tumor typically recurs. Postoperative pelvic radiation is occasionally used in early stage disease.

The 5-year survival for patients with stromal carcinomas is 90% for stage I disease. However, these tumors are slow growing and recurrences can be detected 15 to 20 years after removal of the primary lesion.

Key Points

Sex cord–stromal tumors

1. Are derived from the sex cords of the embryonic gonad or from the ovarian stroma;
2. Are characterized by hormone production;
3. Are slow growing tumors that are often found only incidentally, usually in postmenopausal women in their sixth through eighth decades of life;
4. Are treated surgically, including TAHBSO, but recurrences can be detected 15 to 20 years later.

▶ CANCER OF THE FALLOPIAN TUBES

Pathogenesis

The cause of fallopian tube carcinoma is unknown. Most fallopian tube cancers are **adenocarcinomas** arising from the mucosa. Sarcomas and mixed tumors are less common. The disease progression of these tumors is similar to ovarian cancer, including wide **peritoneal spread** and ascites accumulation. The cancer is bilateral in 10 to 20% of cases and is often the result of metastasis from other primary tumors.

Epidemiology

Primary fallopian tube carcinoma is **extremely rare** and accounts for less than 0.5% of gynecologic malignancies. These tumors can occur at any age (18 to 80), but the mean age is 52.

Clinical Manifestations

The diagnosis of fallopian tube cancer is almost never made preoperatively. The disease is typically **asymptomatic** and is usually diagnosed during laparotomy for other indications. Some patients may report a history of vague lower abdominal pain and serous or bloody vaginal discharge.

Treatment

Treatment of these tumors include total abdominal hysterectomy, bilateral salpingo-oophorectomy, and omentectomy. Adjunctive chemotherapy includes cisplatin and cyclophosphamide. Whole-abdominal radiation is given for patients with completely resected disease. The prognosis for fallopian tube cancer is similar to ovarian cancer.

Key Points

Fallopian tube cancers

1. Are rare malignancies that can occur at any age;
2. Are usually adenocarcinomas arising from the mucosa or metastases from other primary tumors;
3. Are usually asymptomatic and rarely diagnosed preoperatively;
4. Are treated with TAHBSO and adjunctive chemotherapy;
5. Have a prognosis similar to ovarian cancer.

CHAPTER 29

Gestational Trophoblastic Disease

Gestational trophoblastic disease (GTD) is a diverse group of disorders resulting in the abnormal proliferation of trophoblastic (placental) tissue. GTD represents a spectrum of neoplasms that can be grouped into three major classifications (Table 29-1): molar pregnancies (80%), invasive moles (10 to 15%), and choriocarcinomas (2 to 5%). Each neoplasm shares the ability to produce **human chorionic gonadotropin** (hCG). This serves both as a tumor marker for diagnosing the disease and a tool for measuring the effects of treatment. Another distinguishing feature of GTD is its **extreme sensitivity to chemotherapy**. As a result, the cure rate for properly treated GTD is near 95%.

Molar pregnancies, also known as hydatidiform moles, make up the 80% of all GTD. Ninety percent of molar pregnancies are classified as complete moles, which are comprised of molar degeneration but have no associated fetus. Ten percent of molar pregnancies are classified as partial or incomplete moles, which are comprised of molar degeneration in association with an abnormal fetus. Ninety percent of molar pregnancies are benign. The remainder may progress to invasive moles or can give rise to choriocarcinoma.

The remaining 10% of patients with GTD are diagnosed with a malignant form of the disease. These include invasive moles and choriocarcinoma. Most patients with malignant GTD can be effectively cured with chemotherapy.

TABLE 29-1

Classification of Gestational Trophoblastic Disease

Benign GTD
- Molar pregnancy (80% of GTD)
  - Complete mole
  - Incomplete mole (partial mole)

Malignant GTD*
- Invasive mole (10 to 15% of GTD)
- Choriocarcinoma (2 to 5% of GTD)

*Malignant GTD may be divided into nonmetoplastic and metastatic with good prognosis or poor prognosis.

Adapted from Hacker N, Moore JG. Essentials of obstetrics and gynecology. Philadelphia: WB Saunders Company, 1992:628.

▶ KEY POINTS

Gestational trophoblastic disease

1. Can be classified as molar pregnancy (80%), invasive mole (10 to 15%), or choriocarcinoma (2 to 5%); all forms produce β-hCG and are very sensitive to chemotherapy;
2. Has a good prognosis.

▶ COMPLETE MOLAR PREGNANCIES

Pathogenesis

Although the cause of molar pregnancy is unknown, it is thought that **complete moles** result from the fertilization of an **empty ovum**, one whose nucleus is missing or nonfunctional, by a normal sperm (Fig. 29-1). All chromosomes, therefore, are paternally derived. The most common chromosomal pattern for complete moles is **46XX**. A complete mole is characterized by trophoblastic proliferation and the absence of fetal parts. Although most molar pregnancies are benign, complete moles have a higher **malignant potential** than do incomplete moles.

Epidemiology

The incidence of molar pregnancy is about 1 in 2,000 normal pregnancies among white women in the United States. The worldwide rate is highest among Asian women in the Far East where molar pregnancies occur in 1 in every 200 normal pregnancies.

Risk Factors

Gestational trophoblastic disease occurs most commonly in women under 20 or over 40 years of age. Higher incidences have also been found in geographic areas where the diet is low in beta-carotene and folic acid and in women with blood type group A who are married to men with blood type group O.

Clinical Manifestations

History

The most common presenting symptom of molar pregnancy is irregular or heavy **vaginal bleeding** during early pregnancy (97%). The bleeding is typically painless but may also be associated with uterine contractions. Table 29-2 shows other conditions associated with molar pregnancy in descending order of

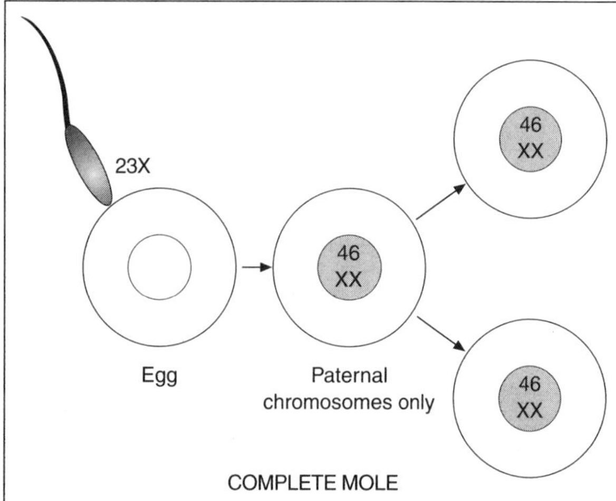

Figure 29-1 Cytogenetic makeup of complete molar pregnancy. Patterns of fertilization to account for chromosomal origin of complete (46XX) and triploid partial moles (XXY). In a complete mole, a single sperm fertilizes an egg that has lost its chromosomes. Partial moles are due to fertilization of an egg by two sperms—one 23X and one 23Y.

frequency. These may contribute to symptoms including severe nausea and vomiting (from hyperemesis gravidarum); irritability, dizziness, and photophobia (from preeclampsia); or nervousness, anorexia, and tremors (from hyperthyroidism).

Physical Examination

In a complete molar pregnancy, the pelvic examination may reveal the expulsion of **grape-like molar clusters** into the vagina or blood in the cervical os. Occasionally, the physician may find large theca lutein cysts that result from high levels of β-hCG. The abdominal examination in molar pregnancy may be remarkable for the absence of fetal heart sounds and size/date discrepancies. Similarly, the physical examination may show sequelae of pre-eclampsia or hyperthyroidism, including tachycardia, tachypnea, and hypertension.

TABLE 29-2

Symptoms Associated with Molar Pregnancy

Symptoms	Percent
Vaginal bleeding	90–97
Passage of molar vescicles	80
Discrepancy between uterine size and dates	65
Bilateral theca lutein cysts	15–30
Hyperemesis gravidarum	10–30
Pre-eclampsia before 24 weeks gestation	10–15
Hyperthyroidism	10
Trophoblastic pulmonary emboli	2

Adapted from Frederickson H, Wilkins-Haug L. OB/GYN secrets. Philadelphia: Hanley and Belfus, Inc., 1991:129.

Diagnostic Evaluation

In the presence of a molar pregnancy, quantitative serum **β-hCG levels** can be extremely high, relative to values for normal pregnancy. Confirmation of GTD is usually made using **pelvic ultrasound** that reveals a "snowstorm" pattern that is diagnostic of GTD. In the case of complete mole, no fetus is present in the uterus (Fig. 29-2).

Differential Diagnosis

The differential diagnosis for gestational trophoblastic neoplasia includes conditions that can result in an abnormally high β-hCG such as multiple gestation pregnancy, threatened spontaneous abortion, and ectopic pregnancy.

Treatment

The treatment for molar pregnancy, regardless of the duration of pregnancy, is **immediate removal of the uterine contents**. This includes suction evacuation supplemented by intravenous oxytocin to stimulate uterine contraction and minimize blood loss.

The prognosis for molar pregnancy and nonmetastatic malignant disease is excellent, with 95 to 100% cure rates. Between 15 and 25% of patients with complete molar pregnancies will develop persistent malignant disease. With chemotherapy, the cure rate for metastatic malignant disease is 95 to 100% for good-prognosis disease and 50 to 70% for poor prognosis.

Key Points

Complete molar pregnancy

1. Is diagnosed by β-hCG levels and pelvic ultrasound showing a "snowstorm" pattern;

Figure 29-2 Ultrasound scan of a hydatidiform mole (HM) with a theca-luteal cyst (TC) in the ovary.

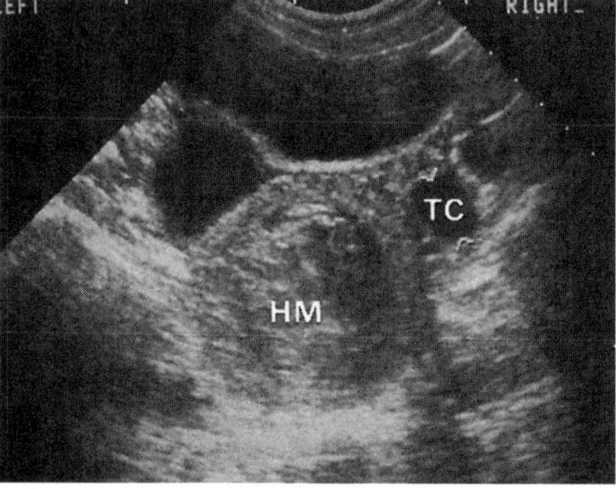

2. Comprise 90% of molar pregnancies and result from the fertilization of an empty ovum (46XX);
3. Have no associated fetus and usually present with irregular vaginal bleeding or passage of vesicles;
4. Result in persistent malignant disease in 15 to 25% of cases, which is 100% curable with chemotherapy.

▶ INCOMPLETE MOLAR PREGNANCY

Pathogenesis

An incomplete or partial mole is formed when a normal ovum is fertilized by two sperm at once (Fig. 29-3). This results in a triploid karyotype with 69 chromosomes, of which two sets are paternally derived. The most common karyotype is **69XXY** (80%). Incomplete moles often present with a **coexistent fetus** with a triploid genotype and multiple anomalies. Most fetuses associated with incomplete moles only survive several weeks *in utero* before being spontaneously aborted. Incomplete moles are almost always benign.

Clinical Manifestations

History

Patients with incomplete moles usually have similar but less severe symptoms than those with complete molar pregnancy. As a result, they may be diagnosed somewhat later. Most present with a spontaneous or missed abortion.

Physical Examination

In incomplete molar pregnancy, the physical examination is typically normal except for the absence of fetal heart sounds.

Treatment

Treatment is immediate removal of the uterine contents. Less than 4% of patients with incomplete moles will develop persistent malignant disease. Even then, the cure rate with chemotherapy is nearly 100%.

Key Points

Incomplete moles

1. Comprise 10% of molar pregnancies and result from the fertilization of an ovum by two sperm (69XXY);
2. Are comprised of molar degeneration and an abnormal fetus and usually present with spontaneous abortion;
3. Develop into malignant disease in only 4% of cases.

▶ INVASIVE MOLES

Pathogenesis

Invasive moles may represent a malignant transformation of benign disease or a recurrence of GTD. Seventy-five percent of invasive moles result from benign molar pregnancies. These moles are usually picked up when β-hCG levels are persistently elevated after uterine evacuation of a molar pregnancy. In invasive moles, the molar villi and trophoblasts penetrate locally into the myometrium, sometimes reaching through to the peritoneal cavity. Invasive moles very rarely metastasize.

Clinical Manifestations

History

Most patients with invasive moles are identified as a result of plateauing or rising β-hCG after treatment for a molar pregnancy.

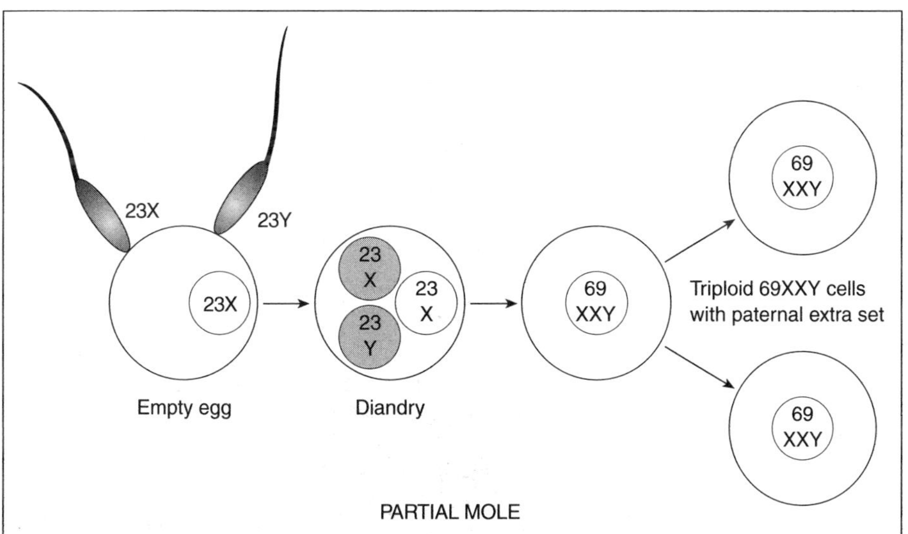

Figure 29-3 Cytogenetic makeup of incomplete molar pregnancy.

Physical Examination

The physical examination in patients with invasive mole is similar to that of molar pregnancy.

Diagnostic Evaluation

The workup for invasive moles is similar to that of benign disease including a quantitative β-hCG and pelvic ultrasound.

Treatment

GTD, even in the malignant form, is exquisitely sensitive to chemotherapy; therefore, chemotherapy is the mainstay of treatment. The treatment for **nonmetastatic** disease is single-agent chemotherapy, usually methotrexate or actinomycin-D. Either single-agent chemotherapy or a multiagent regimen (MAC: methotrexate, actinomycin-D, chlorambucil) is used for **metastatic** GTD, depending on the prognosis (Fig. 29-4).

Surgery does not generally play a role in the treatment of malignant GTD except for the removal of a focus of disease, which is refractory to chemotherapy or for hysterectomies in patients for whom childbearing is complete. Radiation is usually reserved to treat brain and liver metastases.

Key Points

Invasive moles

1. Typically result from persistent molar pregnancy and are detected by plateauing or rising β-hCGs after molar evacuation;
2. Are generally not metastatic and respond well (95 to 100% cure) to single-agent chemotherapy.

▶ CHORIOCARCINOMA

Pathogenesis

Choriocarcinoma is a malignant necrotizing tumor that can arise from trophoblastic tissue weeks to years after **any type of gestation**. Although 50% of patients who develop choriocarcinoma have a preceding molar pregnancy, 25% develop the disease after normal term pregnancies and 25% after spontaneous or induced abortions. Choriocarcinoma invades the uterine wall and blood channels with trophoblastic cells, causing destruction of uterine tissue, necrosis, and hemorrhage. This tumor is **often metastatic** and usually **spreads hematogenously** to the lungs, vagina, pelvis, brain, and liver. The staging for gestational trophoblastic neoplasia is shown in Table 29-3.

Epidemiology

Choriocarcinoma is very rare in the United States, where its incidence is only 1 in 40,000 normal pregnancies but may be as high as 1 in 114 in parts of Asia.

Clinical Manifestations

History

Patients with choriocarcinoma, unlike invasive moles, often present with symptoms of **metastatic disease**. Vaginal metastases may cause vaginal bleeding, whereas metastases to the lung may cause hemoptysis, cough, or dyspnea. Central nervous system lesions may present with headaches, dizziness, blackouts, or other symptoms common to space-occupying lesions.

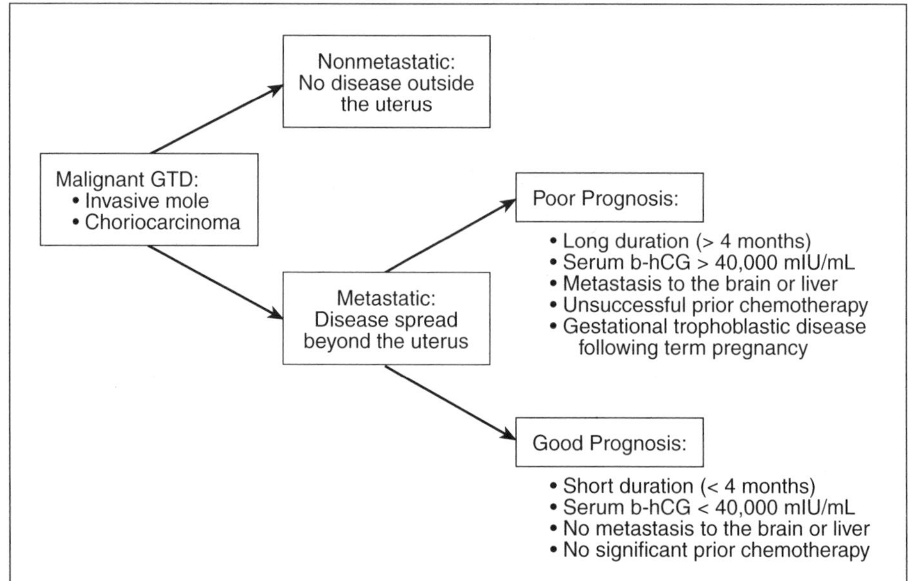

Figure 29-4 Classification of malignant gestational trophoblastic disease.

Physical Examination

Patients with choriocarcinoma often have signs of metastatic disease, including uterine enlargement, vaginal mass, and neurologic signs from central nervous system involvement.

Diagnostic Evaluation

As with invasive moles, the workup is similar to that of benign disease. Diagnostic assessment should include a thorough evaluation of metastatic disease in the lungs, liver, kidneys, spleen, and brain in addition to a quantitative β-hCG and pelvic ultrasound.

Differential Diagnosis

Choriocarcinoma is known as **the great imitator** because its signs and symptoms are similar to many disease entities. Given that choriocarcinoma can occur from **weeks to years** after any type of gestation and is relatively rare, the diagnoses is often delayed when the disease occurs outside the context of a prior molar pregnancy.

Treatment

Refer to treatment in the section on invasive moles. Briefly, because GTD is exquisitely sensitive to chemotherapy, it is the mainstay of treatment. Nonmetastatic disease uses single-agent chemotherapy, whereas metastatic GTD uses either single-agent chemotherapy or a multi-agent regimen. Surgery generally does not play a role.

Key Points

Choriocarcinoma

1. Is the rarest form of GTD and presents with signs and symptoms of metastases to the lungs, vagina, liver, brain or kidneys;
2. When metastatic, can be classified into good prognosis (95 to 100% cure rate) or poor prognosis disease (50 to 70% cure rate).

TABLE 29-3

Staging of Gestational Trophoblastic Tumors

Stage	Extent of Disease
I	Confined to the uterine corpus
II	Metastases to the pelvis or vagina
III	Metastases to the lung
IV	Distant metastases*

*Metastasis sites in order of frequency are lung, vagina, pelvis, brain, and liver

Adapted from Frederickson H, Wilkins-Haug L. OB/GYN secrets. Philadelphia: Hanley and Belfus, Inc., 1991.

Follow-Up

After evacuation of a molar pregnancy, serial β-hCG titers should be monitored using radioimmunoassay weekly and then monthly until normal for at least 1 year (longer for poor prognosis GTD). Figure 29-5 demonstrates the normal regression of β-hCG titers after molar evacuation. Because accurate monitoring depends on the ability to accurately follow β-hCG levels, it is essential to **prevent pregnancy** during the follow-up period.

Patients who are cured of the disease can have normal pregnancies after treatment with no increase in the rate of spontaneous abortion, complications, or congenital malformations. The risk of developing GTD in subsequent pregnancies is less than 5% for women with a history of GTD.

Figure 29-5 Normal regression of |gb-hCG levels after molar evacuation.

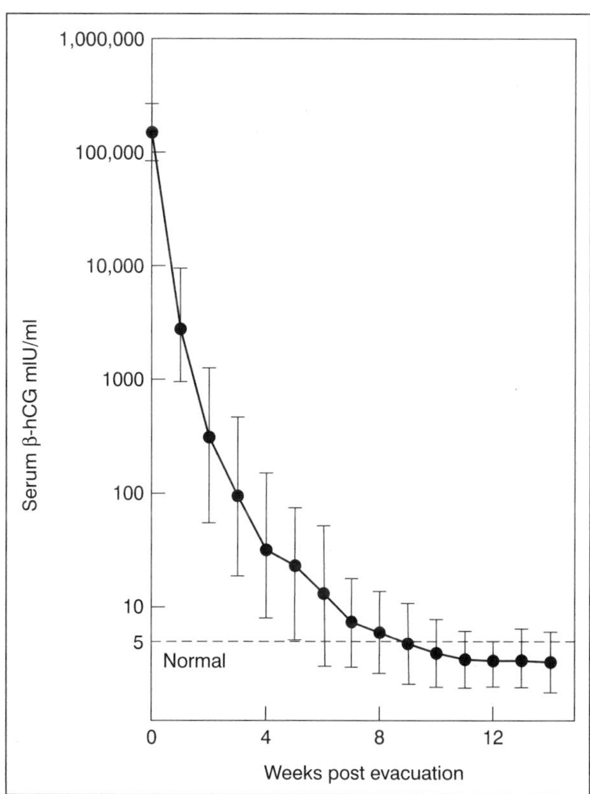

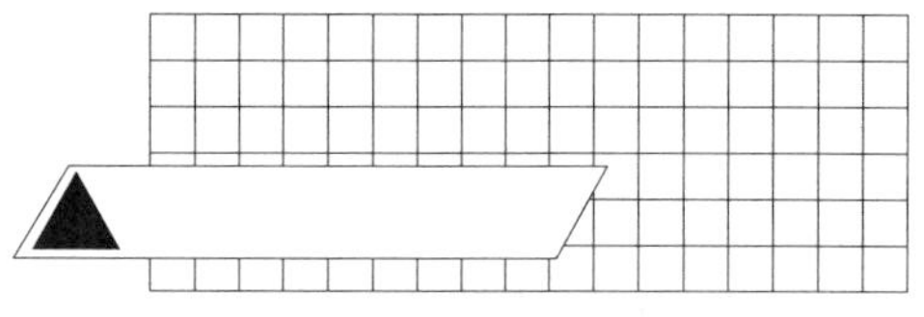

References

American College of Obstetricians and Gynecologists. Prolog: gynecologic oncology and surgery. 3rd ed. Washington DC: 1996.

Barber H. Manual of gynecologic oncology. New York: J.B. Lippincott Company, 1989.

Beckman CC, Ling F. Obstetrics and gynecology for medical students. Baltimore: Williams and Wilkins, 1992.

Benson RC, Pernoll ML. Handbook of obstetrics and gynecology. 9th ed. New York: McGraw-Hill, 1994.

Blackwell RE. Women's medicine. Boston: Blackwell Science, 1996.

Chamberlain G, Malvern J. Lecture notes on gynaecology. Oxford: Blackwell Science, 1996.

Champion RH, Burton JL, Ebling FJG, eds. Textbook of dermatology. 5th ed, Vol. II. Oxford: Blackwell Science, 1992.

Clark SL, et al. Critical care obstetrics. 2nd ed. Boston: Blackwell Science, 1991.

Clarke-Pearson DL, Dawood MY. Green's gynecology. 4th ed. Boston: Little, Brown and Co, 1990.

Cox FEG, ed. Modern parasitology: a textbook of parasitology. 2nd ed. Oxford: Blackwell Science, 1993.

Creasy RK. Management of labor and delivery. Boston: Blackwell Science, 1997.

Crissey JT, Lang H, Parish LC. Manual of medical mycology. Boston: Blackwell Science, 1995.

Cunningham FG, et al. Williams obstetrics. 19th ed. Norwalk: Appleton and Lange, 1993.

De Cherney A, Pernoll M. Current obstetric and gynecologic diagnosis and treatment. Norwalk: Appleton and Lange, 1994.

Evans MI, ed. Obstetrics and gynecology: Pretest® self assessment and review. 6th ed. New York: McGraw-Hill, 1992.

Evans MI, ed. Obstetrics and gynecology: Pretest® self assessment and review. 7th ed. New York: McGraw-Hill, 1995.

Fitzpatrick TB, et al. Color atlas and synopsis of clinical dermatology. 2nd ed. New York: McGraw-Hill, 1994.

Frederickson H, Wilkins-Haug L. OB/GYN secrets. Philadelphia: Hanley and Belfus, 1991.

Gabbe SG, Niebyl RJ, Simpson JL. Obstetrics: normal and problem pregnancies. 2nd ed. New York: Churchill Livingstone, 1991.

Hacker N, Moore JG. Essentials of obstetrics and gynecology. Philadelphia: WB Saunders, 1992.

Horowitz IR, Gomella LG. Obstetrics and gynecology on call. Norwalk: Appleton and Lange, 1993.

Hunter JAA, Savin JA, Dahl MV. Clinical dermatology. 2nd ed. Oxford: Blackwell Science, 1995.

Isselbacher KJ, et al. Harrison's principles of internal medicine. 13th ed. New York: McGraw-Hill, 1994.

Katzung B. Basic and clinical pharmacology. 4th ed. East Norwalk: Appleton and Lange, 1989.

Mead PB, Hager DW. Infection protocols for obstetrics and gynecology. Montvale: Medical Economics Publishing, 1992.

Meyer MB, Tonascia JA. Maternal smoking, pregnancy complications and perinatal mortality. Am J Obstet Gynecol 1977;128:494.

Pernoll ML. Obstetrics and gynecology. Rypins' clinical sciences review. 16th ed. Philadelphia: J.B. Lippincott Company, 1993:179–310.

Repke, JT. Intrapartum obstetrics. New York: Churchill Livingstone, 1996.

Retzky SS, Rogers RM. Clinical symposia: urinary incontinence in women. Vol. 47. Summit: Ciba Geigy, 1995.

Robbins S, Cotran R, Kumar V. Robbins pathologic basis of disease. Philadelphia: WB Saunders, 1991:1150–1170.

Sadler TW. Langman's medical embryology. 6th ed. Baltimore: Williams and Wilkins, 1990.

Shaver DC, Phelan ST, Beckmann CRB, Ling FW. Clinical manual of obstetrics. 2nd ed. New York: McGraw-Hill, 1993.

Singer A, Monaghan JM. Lower genital tract precancer: colposcopy, pathology, and treatment. Boston: Blackwell Science, 1994.

Speroff L, Darney P. A clinical guide for contraception. 2nd ed. Baltimore: Williams and Wilkins, 1996.

Speroff L, Glass RH, Kase NG. Clinical gynecologic endocrinology and infertility. 5th ed. Baltimore: Williams and Wilkins, 1994.

Tindall VR. Color atlas of clinical gynecology. Chicago: Year Book Medical Publishers, 1981.

United States Medical Licensing Examination™. 1993 Step 2 General Instructions, Content Outline, and Sample Items. Copyright © 1992 by the Federation of State Medical Boards of the United States, Inc. and the National Board of Medical Examiners®.

United States Medical Licensing Examination™. 1995 Step 3 General Instructions, Content Description, and Sample Item. Copyright © 1994 by the Federation of State Medical Boards of the United States, Inc. and the National Board of Medical Examiners®.

Weinberger SE. Principles of pulmonary medicine. Philadelphia: WB Saunders, 1992.

Index

Contraindicated

- coumadin
- ACE inhibitors
- pregnancy + Eisenmigers Synd
- pregnancy + primary pulmonary hypertension

Koconne1@
caregroup.harvard.
edu

Harvard Longwood ψ
330 Brookline Ave
Psych dept Rabb 2
Boston, MA 02215 ?

Breast CA

Tx: ocp's — Pain
Mastitis
Menses
Fibrocystic DZ

- <5% present w/ pain
- 50% caught on mammogram

Sx: Discharge - expressable clear or spontan. bloody (PPV = 15%) = most don't have CA
↓
usually benign papilloma

150-200,000 new BCA's/yr in U.S.
+ 5-10% are <30 y/o.

Sonograms are specific

2 Hits → Differentiated cell
↓
Proliferating cell w/ DNA damage (i.e. aging)
↓
cancer

Incidence just goes up with age!!

Tamoxifen → causes
Cataracts
DVT's
ischemic ♡ DZ

Raloxifine - fewer SE's than tamoxifene
↓
used for osteoporosis tx

Nabothian cyst → cervical

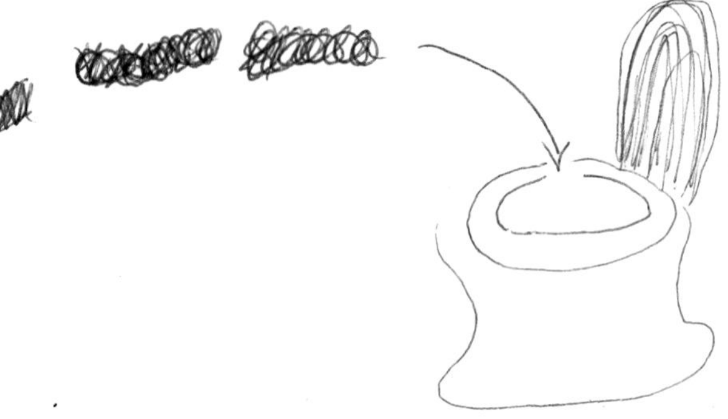